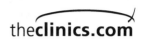
theclinics.com

CARDIOLOGY CLINICS

Emergency Cardiac Care:
From ED to CCU

GUEST EDITORS
Amal Mattu, MD
Mark D. Kelemen, MD, MSc

CONSULTING EDITOR
Michael H. Crawford, MD

February 2006 • Volume 24 • Number 1

SAUNDERS

An Imprint of Elsevier, Inc.
PHILADELPHIA   LONDON   TORONTO   MONTREAL   SYDNEY   TOKYO

W.B. SAUNDERS COMPANY
A Division of Elsevier Inc.

Elsevier Inc. • 1600 John F. Kennedy Blvd., Suite 1800 • Philadelphia, Pennsylvania 19103-2899

http://www.theclinics.com

CARDIOLOGY CLINICS   **Volume 24, Number 1**
February 2006   **ISSN 0733-8651**
Editor: Karen Sorensen   **ISBN 1-4160-3520-6**

Reprints. For copies of 100 or more, of articles in this publication, please contact the Commercial Reprints Department, Elsevier Inc., 360 Park Avenue South, New York, New York 10010-1710. Tel. (212) 633-3813 Fax: (212) 462-1935 email: reprints@elsevier.com

Cardiology Clinics (ISSN 0733-8651) is published quarterly by W.B. Saunders Company; Corporate and editorial Offices: Elsevier Inc., 1600 John F. Kennedy Blvd., Suite 1800, Philadelphia, PA 19103-2899. Accounting and circulation offices: 6277 Sea Harbor Drive, Orlando, FL 32887-4800. Periodicals postage paid at Orlando, FL 32862, and additional mailing offices. Subscription prices are $170.00 per year for US individuals, $266.00 per year for US institutions, $85.00 per year for US students and residents, $210.00 per year for Canadian individuals, $323.00 per year for Canadian institutions, $230.00 per year for international individuals, $323.00 per year for international institutions and $115.00 per year for Canadian and foreign students/residents. To receive student/resident rate, orders must be accompanied by name of affiliated institution, data of term, and the *signature* of program/residency coordinator on institution letterhead. Orders will be billed at individual rate until proof of status is received. Foreign air speed delivery is included in all *Clinics* subscription prices. All prices are subject to change without notice. POSTMASTER: Send address changes to *Cardiology Clinics*, W.B. Saunders Company, Periodicals Fulfillment, Orlando, FL 32887-4800. **Customer Service: 1-800-654-2452 (US). From outside of the US, call 1-407-345-1000.**

Cardiology Clinics is also published in Spanish by McGraw-Hill Interamericana Editores S. A., P.O. Box 5-237, 06500, Mexico D. F., Mexico; in Portuguese by Reichmann and Alfonso Editores Rio de Janeiro, Brazil; and in Greek by Dimitrios P. Lagos, 8 Pondon Street, GR115-28 Ilissia, Greece.

Cardiology Clinics is covered in *Index Medicus, Excerpta Medica, The Cumulative Index to Nursing and Allied Health Literature* (INAHL).

Printed in the United States of America.

CONSULTING EDITOR

MICHAEL H. CRAWFORD, MD, Professor of Medicine, Lucie Stern Chair in Cardiology at University of California, San Francisco; Chief of Clinical Cardiology, University of California, San Francisco Medical Center, San Francisco, California

GUEST EDITORS

AMAL MATTU, MD, Division of Emergency Medicine, Department of Surgery, University of Maryland School of Medicine, Baltimore, Maryland

MARK D. KELEMEN, MD, MSC, FACC, Associate Professor of Medicine, Director of Clinical Cardiology, Division of Cardiology, University of Maryland School of Medicine, Baltimore, Maryland

CONTRIBUTORS

MONICA AGGARWAL, MD, Division of Cardiology, University of Maryland School of Medicine, Baltimore, Maryland

THOMAS AVERSANO, MD, Professor of Medicine, Division of Cardiology, Johns Hopkins School of Medicine, Baltimore, Maryland

TOMAS H. AYALA, MD, Assistant Instructor, Division of Cardiology, University of Maryland School of Medicine, Baltimore, Maryland

ERIC T. BOIE, MD, Assistant Professor of Emergency Medicine, Mayo Clinic College of Medicine; Vice Chair, Department of Emergency Medicine, Mayo Clinic, Rochester, Minnesota

WYATT W. DECKER, MD, Chair, Department of Emergency Medicine, Mayo Clinic; Associate Professor of Emergency Medicine, Mayo Clinic College of Medicine, Rochester, Minnesota

VASKEN DILSIZIAN, MD, Professor of Medicine and Radiology, University of Maryland School of Medicine; Director of Cardiovascular Nuclear Medicine and Cardiac Positron Emission Tomography, University of Maryland Medical System, Baltimore, Maryland

ERIKA D. FELLER, MD, Assistant Professor of Medicine, University of Maryland School of Medicine, Baltimore, Maryland

STEPHEN S. GOTTLIEB, MD, Professor of Medicine and Director, Heart Failure and Transplantation, University of Maryland School of Medicine, Baltimore, Maryland

LUIS H. HARO, MD, Instructor of Emergency Medicine, Mayo Clinic College of Medicine; Consultant, Department of Emergency Medicine, Rochester Minnesota

TIMOTHY D. HENRY, MD, Director of Clinical Research, Minneapolis Heart Institute Foundation and Associate Professor of Medicine, University of Minnesota, Minneapolis, Minnesota

JUDD E. HOLLANDER, MD, Professor and Director of Clinical Research, Department of Emergency Medicine, University of Pennsylvania, Philadelphia, Pennsylvania

R.E. HOOD, MD, Assistant Professor of Medicine, Division of Cardiology, Department of Medicine, University of Maryland School of Medicine, Baltimore, Maryland

MARK D. KELEMEN, MD, MSC, FACC, Associate Professor of Medicine, Director of Clinical Cardiology, Division of Cardiology, University of Maryland School of Medicine, Baltimore, Maryland

IJAZ A. KHAN, MD, Associate Professor of Medicine, Division of Cardiology, University of Maryland School of Medicine, Baltimore, Maryland

DICK KUO, MD, Assistant Professor of Surgery, Division of Emergency Medicine, University of Maryland School of Medicine; Clinical Director, Adult Emergency Department, University of Maryland Medical System, Baltimore, Maryland

KELLY L. MILLER, MD, Assistant Instructor of Medicine, Division of Cardiology, University of Maryland School of Medicine, Baltimore, Maryland

ERIC D. PETERSON, MD, MPH, Associate Professor of Medicine and Associate Vice Chair for Quality, Duke University Medical Center; Co-Director of Cardiovascular Research and Director, Cardiovascular Outcomes Research and Quality, Duke Clinical Research Institute, Durham, North Carolina

CHARLES V. POLLACK, JR., MA, MD, FACEP, Associate Professor of Emergency Medicine and Chief, Department of Emergency Medicine, Pennsylvania Hospital, Philadelphia, Pennsylvania

RAJNISH PRASAD, MD, Assistant Professor of Medicine, Division of Cardiology, University of Maryland School of Medicine, Baltimore, Maryland

ROBERT L. ROGERS, MD, Assistant Professor of Surgery, Department of Medicine and Division of Emergency Medicine; Director of Undergraduate Medical Education for Emergency Medicine and Associate Program Director of Emergency Medicine, University of Maryland School of Medicine, Baltimore, Maryland

STEVEN P. SCHULMAN, MD, Professor of Medicine, Division of Cardiology, Johns Hopkins University School of Medicine; Director, Coronary Care Unit, the Johns Hopkins Hospital, Baltimore, Maryland

STEPHEN R. SHOROFSKY, MD, PhD, Associate Professor of Medicine and Director, Cardiac Electrophysiology Section, Division of Cardiology, Department of Medicine, University of Maryland School of Medicine, Baltimore, Maryland

AMISH C. SURA, MD, Assistant Instructor of Medicine, Division of Cardiology, University of Maryland School of Medicine, Baltimore, Maryland

LYNNET TIRABASSI, RN, BSN, Division of Cardiology, Johns Hopkins School of Medicine, Baltimore, Maryland

MARK R. VESELY, MD, Fellow of Cardiovascular Disease, Assistant Instructor of Medicine, Division of Cardiology, University of Maryland School of Medicine, Baltimore, Maryland

STANLEY WATKINS, MD, MHS, Clinical Fellow, Division of Cardiology, Johns Hopkins Hospital, Baltimore, Maryland

CHARLES S. WHITE, MD, Professor of Radiology, University of Maryland School of Medicine; Section Chief, Chest Radiology, University of Maryland Medical System, Baltimore, Maryland

R. SCOTT WRIGHT, MD, Consultant, Division of Cardiology and Cardiac Coronary Unit, Mayo Clinic; Associate Professor of Medicine, Mayo Clinic College of Medicine, Rochester, Minnesota

CONTENTS

Whether percutaneous intervention (PCI) or fibrinolytic therapy is chosen depends on a number of factors. This article reviews the data on PCI and fibrinolytics in the context of consensus guidelines, outlines adjunctive medical therapies important in the first 24 hours, and discusses a strategy for making the decisions and a hypothetical construct for evaluating new drugs and procedures in the future.

Since the plain chest radiograph was first developed, advances in technology have continued to bring new modalities for the evaluation of the heart in the emergency department. This article discusses current techniques and strategies including nuclear stress perfusion testing and stress echocardiography for risk stratification and prognosis. New-generation CT scanners and MRI techniques that are capable of producing vivid images of the coronary vessels and allow visualization of the cardiac anatomy are also presented.

This article reviews the development and utilization of risk stratification systems (RSS) in the early management of non–ST-segment elevation acute coronary syndrome (NSTE ACS). The authors discuss how guidelines and RSS help discriminate patients by risk category in order to match intensity of therapy to risk. They review the most commonly used systems as well as competing theories in risk assessment. Finally, they consider how new factors will be incorporated into risk models and propose clinical trials to compare RSS in the management of intermediate risk NSTE ACS.

This article reviews the experience of designing systems of care for primary angioplasty. These systems include the local ambulance services, a coordinated effort between community and tertiary hospitals, emergency department physicians, and cardiologists. It details the standards, training, and logistics necessary to begin this type of program. The data for prehospital management of patients who have acute myocardial infarction (AMI) is reviewed. Given the complex nature and time dependency of AMI care, the authors support ongoing quality improvement initiatives and regular interaction between the members of this unique health care team.

This article discusses the spectrum of acute coronary syndromes (ACS) but focuses primarily on patients who have non–ST-segment elevation (NSTE) ACS. After reviewing the American College of Cardiology and American Heart Association guidelines for the care of NSTE ACS patients, the article discusses current practice patterns as documented in several large registries. Gaps in patient management between that recommended in clinical practice guidelines and actual patterns of care are discussed, and areas for improvement are suggested. The article concludes with a discussion of means to overcome barriers to guideline adherence through quality improvement initiatives.

FORTHCOMING ISSUES

RECENT ISSUES

Foreword

Emergency Cardiac Care: From ED to CCU

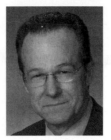

Michael H. Crawford, MD
Consulting Editor

Each year I spend considerable time on the inpatient cardiology service and on cardiology consultations. During these activities, my team interacts daily with the emergency department physicians. I am also involved administratively in putting together plans of care for various acute cardiac diseases that often arrive by way of the emergency department. I am sure that many of you share all these activities and more with your emergency department colleagues. Thus, I was delighted when Drs. Amal Mattu and Mark Kelemen of the University of Maryland agreed to edit this issue of the *Cardiology Clinics*. Representing emergency medicine and cardiology, respectively, they have assembled a group of outstanding experts from both disciplines for this issue, which is dedicated to the interface between the two fields.

Today, physician interactions concerning cardiac patients are becoming more complex, with new cardiac imaging techniques being installed in many emergency departments. Furthermore, heart failure specialists and electrophysiologists are increasingly interacting with patients in the emergency department first. This issue features articles that are dedicated to these emerging interface areas in addition to several articles on acute coronary syndromes, which represent the majority of cardiac emergency department visits. Finally, this issue will be an excellent companion to the November 2005 issue on chest pain units, which explores this aspect of emergent cardiac care.

Michael H. Crawford, MD
Division of Cardiology
Department of Medicine
University of California
San Francisco Medical Center
505 Parnassus Avenue, Box 0124
San Francisco, CA 94143-0124, USA

E-mail address:
michael.crawford@ucsfmedctr.org

0733-8651/06/$ - see front matter © 2005 Elsevier Inc. All rights reserved.
doi:10.1016/j.ccl.2005.10.002

Preface

Emergency Cardiac Care: From ED to CCU

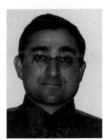 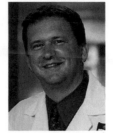

Amal Mattu, MD   Mark D. Kelemen, MD
Guest Editors

Cardiac disease is the leading cause of death in the United States. Tremendous resources in health care are devoted toward preventing and treating chronic cardiac disease. Despite this resource allocation, emergency department (ED) visits and hospital admissions for emergency cardiac conditions continue to rise. Two specialties clearly bear the greatest burden of dealing with this rising health care problem: emergency medicine and cardiology. These two specialties, though functionally and philosophically different in many ways, have discovered the importance of working together and coordinating efforts in their shared battle against the rising epidemic of cardiac disease. In this issue of the *Cardiology Clinics*, we have attempted to bridge the gap between emergency medicine and cardiology in terms of their respective approaches to treatment of various emergency cardiac conditions.

Emergency physicians are usually the first physicians to care for patients who have emergency cardiac conditions. They must initiate evidence-based therapies in a timely manner, but they must be certain to plan their initial care in conjunction with the cardiologists who continue the appropriate therapies and often provide the final definitive care. When there is poor coordination between the treatments provided by the two separate specialties, patient care suffers.

The first article in this issue provides an appropriate lead-in to the following articles on acute coronary syndrome. The authors represent both emergency medicine and cardiology and therefore are able to provide a coordinated approach to the evaluation and initial management of these patients in the ED. The subsequent article discusses some of the new concepts in atherogenesis. An understanding of the pathophysiology of atherosclerotic coronary artery disease is important if physicians are to understand the newer treatment of patients with acute coronary syndrome (ACS). This article and the following articles then discuss the evidence-based work-up and therapies for patients who have ACS. With the understanding that optimal management of patients who have ACS requires a multidisciplinary health care team that includes prehospital providers, ED providers, and in-hospital providers, this issue also features an article that focuses on methods of improving community systems of care to optimize treatment of patients with ACS.

The use of cocaine has increased in recent years, both in inner-city and suburban areas. Consequently, ED visits for cocaine-related chest pain are on the rise. The recent literature has demonstrated that rapid rule-out protocols are safe and effective for these patients. This issue features an article that discusses some of the pathophysiology of cocaine-related chest pain and ACAD. The authors also describe protocols for the evaluation and management of these patients.

0733-8651/06/$ - see front matter © 2005 Elsevier Inc. All rights reserved.
doi:10.1016/j.ccl.2005.10.001

cardiology.theclinics.com

Congestive heart failure (CHF) is common in the United States, and the prevalence of CHF is expected to rise as the population ages. ED visits for decompensated CHF are on the rise as well. The use of traditional medications that had been used for many years is now being questioned, and some of the newer therapies are equally controversial. A chapter addresses these controversies and provides suggestions for reasonable emergency management of patients who have decompensated CHF.

The final two articles address the emergency management of cardiac arrhythmias and severe hypertension, respectively. Many advances in pharmacology have resulted in improvements in our ability to treat acute arrhythmias and hypertension. The authors of these two articles address some of the new medications available for treatment, and they suggest optimal management strategies.

In overseeing the development of this issue of *Cardiology Clinics*, we have tried to maintain both an emergency medicine as well as a cardiology perspective on the content of the articles. We believe that physicians from both specialties will benefit from the topics and the content. Traditionally there has been a gap between the specialties of emergency medicine and cardiology with regard to their respective approaches to caring for patients who have emergency cardiac conditions.

However, there is no doubt that both specialties must overcome that gap if they are to optimize the management of these patients. We hope that this issue helps to bridge the gap.

We would like to thank the dedicated authors of this issue of the *Cardiology Clinics*, all of whom contributed significant time researching and writing the articles. We would also like to thank Karen Sorensen and Elsevier for their support of this issue. Finally, we thank our families for their patience, support, and encouragement throughout this process.

Amal Mattu, MD
Division of Emergency Medicine
Department of Surgery
University of Maryland School of Medicine
110 S. Paca Street, Sixth Floor, Suite 200
Baltimore, MD 21201, USA

E-mail address: amattu@smail.umaryland.edu

Mark D. Kelemen, MD
Division of Cardiology
University of Maryland School of Medicine
22 South Greene Street
Baltimore, MD 21202, USA

E-mail address:
mkelemen@medicine.umaryland.edu

CARDIOLOGY
CLINICS

ELSEVIER
SAUNDERS

Cardiol Clin 24 (2006) 1–17

Initial Approach to the Patient who has Chest Pain

Luis H. Haro, MD[a,b,*], Wyatt W. Decker, MD[a,b],
Eric T. Boie, MD[a,b], R. Scott Wright, MD[a,c]

[a]Mayo Clinic College of Medicine, 200 First Street SW, Rochester, MN 55905, USA
[b]Department of Emergency Medicine, Mayo Clinic, 200 First Street SW, Rochester, MN 55905, USA
[c]Division of Cardiology and Cardiac Coronary Unit, Mayo Clinic, 200 First Street SW, Rochester, MN 55905, USA

Scope of the problem

According to Center for Disease Control 2001–2002 National Hospital Ambulatory Medical Care Survey, an estimated 107 to 110 million visits were made to hospital emergency departments. Of these, approximately 3.5 to 5.4 million visits (3.4% to 5.3%) were patients who presented with chest pain as their chief complaint [1]. In 2001, first-listed and secondary hospital discharge data from the National Registry of Myocardial Infarction-4 (NRMI-4) indicate there were 1,680,000 unique discharges for acute coronary syndrome (ACS) [2].

In evaluating acute chest pain, the immediate goal is to determine the accurate diagnosis and to initiate the appropriate life-saving therapies as quickly as possible. It is particularly important to identify as quickly as possible those patients presenting with ST-segment elevation myocardial infarction (STEMI) so that the appropriate reperfusion therapies can be initiated with as little delay as possible. Recent work estimates that at least 500,000 patients each year qualify for acute reperfusion therapy for STEMI [3].

The particular challenge facing today's practitioners of emergency medicine is to evaluate every patient who presents with acute chest pain for a variety of life-threatening causes of chest pain, such as ACS, acute aortic dissection (AD), pulmonary embolism (PE), pericardial disease with

tamponade physiology, penetrating ulcer, and tension pneumothorax (Box 1). Once these entities are excluded, other benign causes of chest pain are considered. Most of the cases presenting with acute chest pain are of benign origin.

This article focuses on assessment; diagnosis, and management within the first 2 to 3 hours of emergency department presentation of patients who have a chief complain of chest pain and whose clinical status or diagnosis merits admission to the coronary care unit or medical ICU.

Prehospital evaluation and interventions

A patient complaining of chest pain who is at risk for ACS should be transported from home or the outpatient clinic to the emergency department by an ambulance with advanced life-support (ALS) capabilities. Only ALS ambulance personnel can obtain intravenous access, provide sublingual nitroglycerin and morphine, and provide advanced cardiac life support if the patient's condition deteriorates in route.

Advanced emergency medical services (EMS) can also perform and transmit prehospital ECGs (PH-ECGs), stabilize a compromised airway including endotracheal intubation and initiation of mechanical ventilation, and initiate pharmacologic support in situations of hemodynamic compromise before arrival at the emergency department.

Many patients who have acute myocardial infarction (AMI) suffer cardiac arrest in the first few hours of the event. Many of these patients die at home suddenly. The use of an ALS-based EMS offers the best option for early, rapid management of cardiac arrhythmias and sudden cardiac death. Lives are saved by having excellent prehospital

* Corresponding author. Department of Emergency Medicine, Mayo Clinic, 200 First Street SW, Rochester, MN 55905.

E-mail address: haro.luis@mayo.edu (L.H. Haro).

Box 1. Differential diagnosis of chest pain

Life-threatening causes
Acute coronary syndrome
Aortic dissection
Pulmonary embolus
Tension pneumothorax

Other cardiovascular and nonischemic
  causes
Pericarditis
Atypical angina
Hypertrophic cardiomyopathy
Vasospastic angina

Other noncardiac causes
Boerhaave's syndrome (esophageal
  rupture with mediastinitis)
Gastroesophageal reflux and spasm
Chest-wall pain
Pleurisy
Peptic ulcer disease
Panic attack
Biliary or pancreatic pain
Cervical disc or neuropathic pain
Somatization and psychogenic pain
  disorder

---

care for patients who are in ventricular fibrillation arrest, for whom survival rates to hospital discharge with acceptable neurologic function can reach 40% [4].

Unfortunately, ambulance services are not always requested. Despite many national education campaigns, patients continue to bypass the EMS systems and arrive by other means. In NRMI-2, 53% of patients who had STEMI arrived by private means [5]. In other studies, the average percentage of patients who had a confirmed coronary event and used EMS was 23%, with a range of 10% to 48%. It is a matter of concern that 16% drove themselves to the emergency department [6], especially considering that approximately 1 in every 300 patients transported to the emergency department by private vehicle goes into cardiac arrest in route [7]. When they do call an ambulance, the average patient who has STEMI does not seek medical care for approximately 2 hours after symptom onset, and this pattern seems to be unchanged during the last decade [8–10]. Average and median delays in

obtaining treatment for patients who had STEMI were 4.7 and 2.3 hours, respectively, from the 14-country Global Registry of Acute Coronary Events project [11].

The reasons given by patients in the United States for delay in seeking care have been studied in the REACT project. The investigators conducted focus groups ($N = 34,207$ participants) in major regions of the United States. Target groups included adults who had had previous heart attacks, those at higher risk for heart attack, and bystanders to heart attacks. Reasons given by the target groups for delaying seeking help were (1) they expected heart attack symptoms to be more dramatic; (2) they unrealistically judged their personal risk as low; (3) they understood little about the benefits of rapid interventions; (4) they were unaware of the benefits of using EMS instead of alternative transport; and (5) they seemed to need the "permission" or advice of health care providers or family to act [9,12,13].

Prehospital ECGs

PH-ECGs are an underused component in modern ACS care. In most places in the United States they can be obtained easily by advanced EMS personnel and transmitted en route to an emergency department control center. If transmission is a problem, delays in the emergency department can be avoided, because the computer readout is highly accurate and can be called in to the receiving emergency department. Doing so allows emergency department personnel to alert the coronary care unit and be ready for fibrinolysis or primary percutaneous intervention (PPCI). The use of PH-ECGs reduces door-to-needle time for in-hospital fibrinolysis by a mean of 10 minutes; NRMI-2 found the use of PH-ECGs reduced the door-to-balloon- time for primary PCI by a mean of 23 minutes [5].

Prehospital triage

The use of PH-ECGs can also help EMS triage more efficiently. In general, patients who have STEMI should be transported to the nearest facility that best handles the situation. For example, a patient who has an uncomplicated STEMI can be transported to the nearest facility that offers acute reperfusion therapy. The patient who has STEMI and who is also in cardiogenic shock should be transported preferentially to a facility capable of performing PPCI or coronary artery bypass graft surgery rather than being transported to a facility that has only intravenous fibrinolysis available, if the transport times are not significantly different. The Should We Emergently Revascularize Occluded Arteries in Cardiogenic Shock (SHOCK) trial demonstrated that emergency revascularization improved 1-year survival, achieving an absolute 12.8% reduction in 6-month mortality in patients treated with early revascularization ($P = .027$) [14]. Because much of the mortality in patients in cardiogenic shock occurs early in the time course, it is prudent to transport patients rapidly to the nearest center of excellence that is best equipped to provide the optimal cardiovascular care.

Initiation of prehospital fibrinolysis

Recent work has suggested that time to reperfusion remains one of the most important determinants of the degree of salvaged myocardium [15,16]. Fig. 1 suggests that the earlier reperfusion is initiated, the more myocardium one can salvage. Fig. 1 also reveals that a strategy that significantly delays primary reperfusion therapy may result in little myocardial salvage. Such data have inspired clinical trails to perform prehospital fibrinolysis (PHF). A meta-analysis of PHF trials showed time to treatment was reduced by a mean of 58 minutes, with a range of 33 minutes (Seattle, WA) to 130 minutes (rural Scotland). The pooled data demonstrated a 17% relative risk (RR) reduction in early mortality [17]. A more real-world contemporary analysis of PHF versus other

reperfusion therapies has been provided by the French nationwide Unité de Soins Intensifs Coronaires 2000 registry [18]. In November 2000 in France use of PHF was used for 9% of the patients who had STEMI (range, 7%–26%; N = 180). This therapy seemed to offer the best survival benefit (Fig. 2). One-year survival was 94% for patients treated with PHF, 89% for patients treated with in-hospital fibrinolysis or PPCI, and 79% for patients who did not receive reperfusion therapy.

The American College of Cardiology (ACC) and the American Heart Association (AHA) recommend establishment of a PHF protocol in systems where the prehospital transport times are more than 20 minutes and ALS-EMS units have high volume (>25,000) runs per year [3]. It also recommended that the PHF team include full-time paramedics, have available PH-ECG technology with physician support, and be overseen by a medical director committed to developing and maintaining a quality PHF program. Unfortunately, no single study in the United States has demonstrated a reduction in short-term mortality risks compared with hospital-based fibrinolysis. (An in-depth discussion of options for reperfusion is given elsewhere in this issue.)

Emergency department evaluation

Once a patient arrives at the emergency department, the initial nursing triage of patients who have chest pain and are at risk for ACS must be to a telemetry bed staffed with nurses and physicians capable of performing an immediate assessment and delivering advanced cardiac life support.

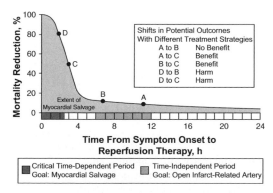

Fig. 1. Hypothetical construct of the relationship among the duration of symptoms of acute myocardial infarction before reperfusion therapy, mortality reduction and extent of myocardial salvage. (*From* Gersh JB, Stone WG, White DH, et al. Pharmacological facilitation of primary percutaneous coronary intervention for acute myocardial infarction. JAMA 2005;293(8):980; with permission.)

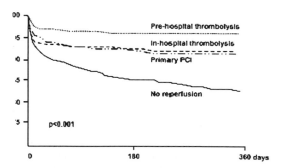

Fig. 2. Age-adjusted Kaplan-Meier 1-year survival according to reperfusion strategy. PCI, percutaneous primary intervention. (*From* Danchin N, Blanchard D, Steg GP, et al. Impact of prehospital thrombolysis for acute myocardial infarction on 1-yr outcome. Circulation 2004;110:1913; with permission.)

Placement on a monitor, intravenous access, oxygen administration, and administration of aspirin (ASA) or clopidogrel (if the patient is allergic to ASA) should be done within 5 minutes of patient arrival. These actions should be driven by nursing care to minimize the time to initiation of therapy. In the critically ill patient whose vitals signs are compromised (ie, cardiac arrest, tachyarrhythmias, severe bradycardia, shock, or hypotension), the advanced cardiac life support guidelines developed by the AHA should be followed. (Detailed management of particular arrhythmias is discussed elsewhere in this issue.)

If the patient is stable, and if no PH-ECG is available, an ECG should be obtained within 10 minutes of arrival at the emergency department, according to the ACC/AHA guidelines [3]. No study to date has shown that this can be done consistently, however. Barriers to optimizing early care for patients who have chest pain are relatively trivial but are common in busy emergency departments. Such barriers include large or demanding clinical volumes and time spent undressing the patient (especially the elderly), in monitor placement, in obtaining intravenous access, and in administering ASA and oxygen. These are important and necessary tasks, but they should not delay the acquisition of an ECG. The authors encourage all emergency department personnel to create a systems-based approach that intentionally works to minimize door-to-ECG-acquisition time in a way that facilitates clinical decision making and improves patient outcomes. To evaluate better the patient presenting with chest pain, they advocate using a standard 12-lead ECG and additional ECG techniques including right-sided leads (V_3R through V_6R), posterior leads (V_7, V_8, and V_9), and continuous ST-segment monitoring in selected patients who have ongoing chest pain and high pretest probability of ACS. Approximately 20% of patients who present to the emergency department with chest pain have a completely normal 12-lead ECG. The use of these additional techniques helps uncover a significant number of patients who have AMI but whose 12-lead ECG is not diagnostic. The rate of AMI in patients who have chest pain and a totally normal ECG remains around 1% to 4% [19].

Patient history and examination

The initial history and physical examination optimally should be performed within 10 minutes of patient arrival. The initial encounter should be focused and is done to identify best those who have life-threatening cardiac and noncardiac situations.

The pain characteristics in ACS are frequently substernal and are characterized as crushing, aching, vise-like, or pressure. The pain commonly radiates to the neck, jaw, and left arm. Associated symptoms include dyspnea, nausea, vomiting, diaphoresis, and presyncope. Pain often begins abruptly, lasting 15 minutes or longer and taking several minutes to reach maximal intensity. The pain is worse with activity and improves with rest. Although sharp, stabbing, or fleeting pain is regarded as atypical for ischemic pain, such pain is seen in 5% of patients who have AMI [20]. Elderly patients who have ACS can present with a range of complaints including generalized weakness, altered mental status, syncope, atypical chest pain, and dyspnea. Dyspnea is the single most common presenting symptom of angina in patients who are more than 85 years old [21]. Women presenting with ACS tend to be older on average than their male counterparts, to have more comorbid disease (eg, diabetes and hypertension), and to have a longer delay from symptom onset to presentation in the emergency department [22].

Assessment of cardiac risk factors is traditionally considered a routine element of the patient history, but its value in the emergency department has been disputed. Patient age, sex, body habitus, family history of coronary artery disease, and comorbid illness including diabetes mellitus, hypertension, hypercholesterolemia, and tobacco abuse are all classic coronary risk factors. Aside from age, sex, and family history of premature coronary artery disease, the actual role of risk factors in predicting ACS or AMI in patients presenting to the emergency department with chest pain seems minimal [23]. Risk factors are based on population studies and thus are more predictive of development of coronary artery disease over a lifetime, not of whether a patient experiencing chest pain in the emergency department is likely to have ACS [21]. One should not dwell on this component of the history.

The initial physical examination should focus on the cardiovascular system. The clinician should evaluate the jugular venous pressure, looking for elevation, the presence of a Kussmaul's sign, and the presence of hepato-jugular reflux. The lung fields should be examined for signs of congestion and wheezing. The heart and peripheral vasculature should be examined for abnormalities. The abdomen should also be examined for signs of hepatic congestion and abdominal aortic pathology.

Cardiac biomarker and laboratory assessment

The use of cardiac biomarkers is well established in patients who have ACS. These biomarkers provide the most accurate diagnosis of acute myocardial injury and are considered the reference standard for the diagnosis of AMI [3,24,25]. In addition to diagnostic accuracy, the troponins provide prognostic data [26].

Additional cardiac biomarkers that provide prognostic data in STEMI and non-STEMI patients include B-type natriuretic peptide (BNP) and C-reactive protein [27] Patients who had elevations of several of these biomarkers faced the greatest risks. In the Orbofiban in Patients with Unstable Coronary Syndromes Trial 16 study, baseline measurements of troponin I, C-reactive protein, and BNP were performed in 450 patients. Elevations in troponin I, C-reactive protein, and BNP were independent predictors of the composite of death, myocardial infarction (MI), or congestive heart failure. When patients were categorized on the basis of the number of elevated biomarkers at presentation, there was a near doubling of the mortality risk for each additional biomarker that was elevated ($P = .01$) [28].

Recent work suggests a prognostic role for soluble CD-40 ligand and myeloperoxidase in patients who have AMI, but additional work is needed to confirm the long-term prognostic role of these newer markers and what value they add when combined with troponin, BNP, and C-reactive protein in patients who have AMI.

The authors recommend additional laboratory testing in patients presenting with chest pain. Glucose, creatinine, and electrolyte levels and a complete blood cell count should be obtained. In patients in whom acute pulmonary embolism is suspected, a D-dimer should be obtained. All these laboratory measures should be obtained as soon as possible.

Reperfusion strategies in ST-segment elevation myocardial infarction

A detailed discussion of reperfusion strategies in STEMI is given elsewhere in this issue. Following is a brief discussion of initial considerations.

When faced with a patient whose ECG demonstrates STEMI or new left bundle branch block, it is important to have pre-established multidisciplinary guidelines in place to indicate the best and

the most expeditious reperfusion management. The authors recommend the use of intravenous fibrinolytic therapy (IFT) in hospitals without on-site and experienced catheterization laboratories. The use of IFT should be restricted to patients who present within 6 hours of symptom onset and have clear-cut ST segment elevation or new left bundle branch block. IFT should not be used in asymptomatic patients whose symptoms began more than 24 hours previously [3]. This therapy is most useful in the first 3 hours after symptom onset and restores coronary flow completely in about half the patients treated with it. The success rate, defined as Thrombolysis in Myocardial Infarction (TIMI)-3 flow at 90 minutes after the start of treatment, varies between 32% and 55%. The great risk of IFT is hemorrhage, including a 0.5% to 1.2% risk of intracranial hemorrhage and a 3% to 6% risk of other major bleeding complications (gastrointestinal bleeding, retroperitoneal bleeding, a $\geq$ 4-g drop in hemoglobin) [29]. PPCI can be performed in nearly all patients who have STEMI and is more successful than IFT at restoring TIMI-3 flow [30,31]. PPCI has a lower risk of intracranial hemorrhage and reinfarction compared with IFT [3,18]. PPCI must be done promptly. Several groups have reported increased mortality with increased door-to-balloon time [32,33,34]. De Luca and colleagues [35,36], in a study population of 1791 patients who had STEMI treated with emergent PCI, demonstrated that for every 30-minute delay in reperfusion therapy with PPCI, there was an increased 1-year mortality of 7.5%. ACC/AHA guidelines stipulate, that after adjusting for baseline characteristics, time from symptom onset to balloon inflation is significantly correlated with 1-year mortality (RR, 1.08 for each 30-minute delay; $P = .04$). The ACC recommends a door-to-balloon time of 60 to 120 minutes [3]. This goal can be achieved only if specific intradepartmental time goals are reached for the critical emergency department actions:

1. The diagnosis: door-to-ECG (preferably less than 10 minutes)
2. The decision to treat: door-to-catheterization team activation (preferably within 15–25 minutes and preferably performed by the emergency physician on call to minimize delays in consultation)
3. The transition in care: door-to-emergency department departure (preferably within 45–60 minutes)

This flow allows a 30-minute response time for the catheterization team members to respond after hours. Most invasive cardiologists are able to perform the first balloon inflation within 45 minutes after the patient's arrival at the catheterization laboratory. This flow would allow a door-to-balloon time of 90 to 120 minutes. Although it is impossible to achieve this flow for 100% of patients, maintaining these goals and making efforts to achieve such timelines are essential steps in achieving consistency in care and making health care more reliable. Future quality-assurance efforts in emergency medicine and cardiology will be to study, publish, and advise on best practice models that can serve as blueprints to achieve such goals.

High-risk ST-segment elevation myocardial infarction

In certain situations, slightly delayed PPCI is preferable to immediate IFT. Patients who present in cardiogenic shock have a high mortality risk, and the data from the SHOCK trial suggested that immediate revascularization is superior to delayed revascularization [14]. In practice, for such patients it is preferable to initiate reperfusion therapy with PPCI, even delayed PPCI, rather than immediate IFT if one can activate a team for PPCI reasonably quickly. Additionally, observational data from the NRMI registry have suggested that patients who have more advanced CHF (Killip class $\geq$ II) have better outcomes with PPCI than with IFT [5].

Risk of bleeding

A rare but important clinical conundrum is the patient who does not have a high risk of STEMI and who has a perceived high risk for bleeding from IFT. What should one do? Delay treatment with IFT and transfer the patient to a facility with PPCI, accept the risk and administer IFT anyway, or withhold all reperfusion therapies? One potential decision is to withhold IFT in any patient who has a greater than 4% risk for life-threatening bleeding and to transfer the patient to another facility for PPCI. To assess risk of bleeding, the ACC/AHA has defined contraindications and cautions for fibrinolysis use [3]. Risk scores (based on points for bleeding risks) are better predictors, and among these the best are those derived from observational studies [37]. In centers where immediate PPCI is not available, the use of such risk scores is highly recommended.

Delayed primary percutaneous coronary revascularization

In the United States the balance of risk–benefit between the expedited transfer of patients for PPCI and more immediate treatment with IFT remains an uncertain science. The decision regarding transfer must be based on multiple factors, and transfer should be made only when there is a clear-cut benefit for the patient. Although there is little consensus in the United States regarding a role for delayed PPCI in patients presenting to community hospitals without PPCI capability, the data from Danish Acute Myocardial Infarction-2 trial are provocative. The investigators demonstrated that patients transferred for PPCI within 2 hours of presentation had a better composite outcome (death, stoke, and recurrent nonfatal MI) than if treated with fibrinolysis at the local hospital [33,35,38]. No consensus has emerged in the United States regarding this issue, and ongoing randomized clinical trials are testing this strategy along with a strategy of facilitated PPCI using upstream administration of IFT before PPCI.

From the current literature, it is not possible to state that a particular reperfusion strategy is applicable to all STEMI, in all clinical settings, and in all hours of the day. It is most important to choose the appropriate reperfusion strategy based on the patient's clinical presentation and symptom onset and to provide the therapy in a timely fashion.

Early therapy for acute cardiac syndromes
Oxygen

Supplemental oxygen administration has become routine for all patients presenting with chest pain. Experimental results indicate that breathing oxygen might limit ischemic myocardial injury, and there is evidence that it reduces ST-segment elevation. Therefore, the use of oxygen is recommended for all AMI patients during in the first 6 hours and longer if the AMI is complicated by congestive heart failure, PE, or other significant underlying disease causing hypoxemia.

Aspirin

Aspirin (162–325 mg) should be chewed immediately at arrival if no ASA allergy exists. ASA produces a rapid antithrombotic effect by near-total inhibition of thromboxane A_2. The second International Study of Infarct Survival Collaborative (ISIS-2) demonstrated an absolute risk difference in 35-day mortality of 2.4% (RR,

23%) [39]. When combined with IFT, the absolute difference in mortality was 5.2% (RR, 25%) [40]. In patients who are allergic to ASA, clopidogrel should be substituted.

Unfractionated heparin

The authors recommend the routine use of unfractionated heparin (UFH) in all patients who have AMI, and it is essential for those undergoing IFT. UFH administration should precede IFT in all circumstances. The authors recommend weight-adjusted UFH administration including a bolus of 60 U/kg (maximum of 4000 U) followed by a 12-U/kg/hour infusion (maximum of 1000 U/hour) adjusted to a partial thromboplastin time at 1.5 to 2.0 times control. If a nonselective fibrinolytic (streptokinase, urokinase, or anistreplase) is used, UFH can be given only to patients who have a high risk of systemic emboli, such as large or anterior MI, atrial fibrillation, or known left ventricular thrombus. For patients who will receive PPCI, the authors recommend a weight-adjusted bolus dose of UFH of 50 to 70 U/kg accompanied by a 12-U/kg/hour infusion (maximum of 1000 U/hour).

Low molecular weight heparin

Low molecular weight heparin is an acceptable alterative to UFH for patients younger than 75 years, provided that serum creatinine is not greater than 2.5 mg/dL in men or 2.0 mg/dL in women.

The authors recommend the use of enoxaparin as a 30-mg intravenous bolus followed by 1.0 mg/kg injected subcutaneously every 12 hours for 48 to 72 hours. In the United States, the Food and Drug Administration has not yet approved enoxaparin for treatment of IFT, but ongoing studies are testing the efficacy of this combination.

Nitroglycerin

Patients who have ongoing chest discomfort should receive sublingual nitroglycerin (0.4 mg) every 5 minutes for a total of three doses, after which the need for intravenous infusion is assessed. Nitrates reduce preload and afterload through peripheral arterial and venous dilatation, relax the epicardial coronary arteries to improve coronary flow, and dilate collateral vessels, potentially creating a favorable subendocardial-to-epicardial flow ratio. Nitrates are harmful in patients who have hypotension, bradycardia, or a suspected right ventricular infarction and in those who have taken a phosphodiesterase inhibitor-5 for erectile dysfunction within the last 24 hours.

Morphine sulfate

Pain increases sympathetic activity, and surges in catecholamine levels have been implicated as having a role in plaque fissuring and thrombus propagation in AMI, as well as reducing the threshold for ventricular fibrillation. Morphine is useful in controlling the pain of AMI but should be used judiciously. When necessary, morphine sulfate should be given in 2 to 4 mg doses intravenously with increments 2 to 8 mg at 5- to 15-minute intervals. Recent data from Can Rapid Risk Stratification Of Unstable Angina Patients Suppress Adverse Outcomes With Early Implementation Of The ACC/AHA Guidelines study [41] suggest that the use of morphine, alone or in combination with nitroglycerin for patients presenting with non-STEMI, is associated with adverse outcomes. The rate of AMI increased from 3.0% in the group of patients not receiving morphine (n = 40,036) to 3.8% in the group of patients receiving morphine (n = 17,003). Death increased from 4.7% to 5.5%, respectively, and the composite endpoint of death and AMI increased from 7.1% to 8.5%, respectively. There might be a selection bias, because the morphine group had higher incidence of ST-segment depression, transient ST-segment elevation, and positive cardiac markers and was more likely to receive an ECG within 10 minutes of arrival and to be cared for by a cardiologist. The authors address this potential by providing a risk adjustment and a propensity score matched-pair analysis for 33,972 of the patients. They conclude that the use of morphine is associated with a higher mortality and raise concerns regarding the safety of using morphine for this selected population. They hypothesize that common side effects such as hypotension, bradycardia, and respiratory depression result in decreased myocardial oxygen delivery, increased arterial carbon dioxide, and perhaps even decreased cerebral perfusion. Unfortunately, these parameters were not evaluated in this observational study. The authors' observation and conclusions are interesting and deserve future study. To date the ACC/AHA recommendations support the use of morphine as a class I indication (conditions for which there is evidence or general agreement that a given procedure or treatment is beneficial, useful, and effective), level of evidence C (only consensus opinion of experts, case studies, or standard of care exists). It is possible that this classification will change to a class IIB (usefulness/efficacy less well established by evidence/opinion).

Beta-blockers

Intravenous or oral beta-blockers should be given promptly to patients who have AMI and who do not have a contraindication. Immediate beta-blocker therapy seems to reduce the magnitude of infarction and the incidence of associated complications in patients not receiving fibrinolysis, to reduce the rate of reinfarction in those receiving fibrinolysis, and to reduce the frequency of life-threatening arrhythmias. During the first few hours of STEMI, beta-blockers diminish myocardial oxygen demand by reducing heart rate, systemic arterial pressure, and myocardial contractility. In addition, prolongation of diastole may augment perfusion to ischemic myocardium, particularly the subendocardium. In the ISIS-1 trial, immediate oral atenolol, 5 to 10 mg, followed by atenolol, 100 mg daily, reduced 7-day mortality from 4.3% to 3.7% ($P < .02$; 6 lives saved per 1000 treated). In the Metoprolol in Acute Myocardial Infarction trial [42], metoprolol, 15 mg administered intravenously in three divided doses followed by 50 mg orally every 6 hours for 48 hours and then 100 mg daily, reduced 15-day mortality from 4.9% to 4.3% as compared with placebo. The benefits of routine early intravenous use of beta-blockers in the fibrinolytic era have been challenged by two later randomized trials and by a post hoc analysis of the use of atenolol in the Global Utilization of Streptokinase and TPA (alteplase) for Occluded Coronary Arteries (GUSTO-1) trial [43,45].

Beta-blocker therapy is contraindicated in patients who have STEMI and moderate left ventricular failure until compensated and in patients who have bradycardia, hypotension, shock, a PR interval greater than 0.24 second, second- or third-degree atrioventricular block, active asthma, or reactive airway disease. Beta-blockers are also contraindicated in cocaine-induced chest pain because of the risk of inducing coronary spasm.

Glycoprotein IIb/IIIa inhibitors

Antagonism of glycoprotein (Gp) IIb/IIIa receptor blocks the final common pathway of platelet aggregation. Three such agents are available in the United States: abciximab, tirofiban, and eptifibatide. The use of these agents with IFT is not proven despite two large trials (GUSTO-V and Assessment of the Safety and Efficacy of a New Thrombolytic-3), which tested the efficacy of combined therapy. It is reasonable to start an intravenous Gp IIB/IIIA antagonist before initiation of PPCI in selected patients. In STEMI, the evidence favors abciximab for patients receiving immediate PPCI, but there are no direct comparisons of abciximab and eptifibatide. Decisions regarding upstream use of a Gp IIb/IIIa agent should be made in consultation with the consulting interventional cardiologist.

The use of Gp IIb/IIIa inhibitors in unstable angina and non-STEMI was best evaluated by Boersma and colleagues [45] who published a comprehensive meta-analysis that included six investigations (PARAGON A, Platelet Receptor Inhibition in Ischemic Syndrome Management, Platelet Receptor Inhibition in Ischemic Syndrome Management in Patients Limited By Unstable Signs And Symptoms, GUSTO IV-ACS, Platelet IIb/IIIa Antagonist for the Reduction of Acute Coronary Syndrome Events in a Global Organization Network B (PARAGON B), and Platelet Glycoprotein IIb/IIIa in Unstable Angina: Receptor Suppression Using Integrilin Therapy (PURSUIT) The primary endpoint was death or nonfatal MI. The meta-analysis included 31,402 patients. Patients who received the Gp inhibitor had a 1.2% risk reduction in the odds of death or MI after randomization (5.7% versus 6.9%; $P = .0003$). Recently, the Treat Angina with Aggrastat and Determine Cost of Therapy with an Invasive or Conservative Strategy-TIMI 18 trial combined early PCI with a Gp IIb/IIIa antagonist and demonstrated a benefit from the use of the combination [46]. The authors believe that initiation of these agents in the emergency department is reasonable and may facilitate successful early PCI. (A detailed discussion of early management of non-ST-segment elevation ACS appears later in this issue).

Undifferentiated chest pain: the threats to life

If the ECG obtained has no significant ST-segment abnormalities, the evaluation of acute chest pain continues with an in-depth clinical history taking that focuses on the characteristics of pain, the time of onset, and the duration of symptoms, associated symptoms, risk assessment for ACS, PE, AD, and pericardial disease with tamponade physiology, and an examination that emphasizes vital signs and cardiovascular, pulmonary, and neurologic status. Most physicians do a mental exercise; others use an algorithmic approach; but the focus of the evaluation *is* not on determining the most likely cause of chest pain. Instead, the question is: What life threatening entity could cause this patients chest pain (even if the possibility is less than 5%), and how will I make sure that I exclude it? As with missed AMI, the medical community, patients, and certainly the judicial system have no tolerance for missed life-threatening entities. The discussion that follows is based on the two most important threats to life, AD and PE.

Acute aortic dissection

Epidemiology

AD is the most common and most lethal aortic emergency [45,47,48]. The true incidence has been difficult to determine, because many incorrectly diagnosed cases escape notice. The occurrence of AD was reported to be between 5 and 20 per million population [49]. The incidence of hospital admission for AD ranged between 1 in 5335 to 1 in 16,550 [50]. Among the life-threatening causes of chest pain, AD has the highest mortality—an estimated 1% to 2% per hour for the first 48 hours [44]. Unfortunately, when initially evaluating patients who have AD, physicians correctly suspect the diagnosis in as few as 15% to 43% of cases [51–53]. Diagnostic delays of more than 24 hours after hospitalization are common and occur in up to 39% of the cases (31% for proximal AD and 53% for distal AD) [54]. Finally, when the diagnosis is made, it is often an incidental discovery made during an advanced imaging procedures requested to assess for other diagnoses. Several factors drive this poor performance. The most frustrating combination for a physician to face when evaluating a patient is a chief complaint (ie, chest pain) that has no typical presentation and is life threatening. Unfortunately, that combination is the rule in AD: classic findings such as ripping interscapular back pain, diastolic murmur, and a wide mediastinum are present less than one third of the cases [51,53,55].

During the last decade a substantial number of studies have evaluated the predictive value of several historical clues and physical examination findings in AD. Particularly useful is Klompas' [53] comprehensive review of the literature and the International Registry of Aortic Dissection (the IRAD database) whose inception and structure is based on 18 large referral centers in six countries [55]. Following are some of the most recent advances in understanding the clinical presentation of AD, based on these and other studies.

Clinical manifestations of aortic dissection

Traditionally, AD occurs in patients in the later decades of life: 95% of these patients are older than 40 years, and the mean age at presentation is 65 years [51,53,55]. Risk factors for AD include hypertension, male sex, non-white race, connective tissue disease (ie, Ehlers-Danlos syndrome or Marfan's syndrome), bicuspid aortic valve, coarctation of the aorta, and drug use including methamphetamine and cocaine. Januzzi and colleagues [56] evaluated patients younger than 40 years who had AD. Of 1078 patients in IRAD who had AD, 69 (6.4%) were younger than 40 years old. In these 69 patients, traditional risk factors such as hypertension and atherosclerosis were significantly lower than in the overall population of patients who had AD. The incidence of Marfan's syndrome, bicuspid aortic valve, and prior aortic valve surgery was significantly higher in these patients ($P < .0001$).

Clinical manifestations of AD are often dominated by the pathoanatomic characteristics of a malperfusion syndrome from a dissection-related side branch obstruction [57]. Severe pain is the most common presenting symptom; 74% to 84% of the patients recall an abrupt onset [51,53,55]. This symptom alone should trigger suspicion of an AD. Anterior chest pain is more frequent in patients who have AD involving the aortic arch, whereas patients who have AD distal to the left subclavian more often experience back pain and abdominal pain (29% of all patients who have AD; 42% of the patients who have distal AD) [55]. Contrary to common belief, pain is described as sharp more often than tearing or ripping. Pain that migrates throughout the chest is present in only 28% of the patients, with no difference between type A or type B.

Less frequent presentations of AD are stroke (carotid occlusion), heart failure (aortic valve insufficiency), syncope (tamponade, central nervous system ischemia), buttock and leg pain with or without lower extremity weakness (femoral artery occlusion), back and flank pain (renal artery occlusion), abdominal pain (mesenteric ischemia or celiac trunk involvement), and of course the infamous painless AD.

Of particular importance is the presence of syncope as a symptom of AD. In 2001, IRAD had identified 728 patients who had AD. Syncope was found in 96 patients (13%), including 24 (3%)

who described it in isolation without any symptoms of chest or back pain [56]. Syncope is more frequent in proximal AD than in distal AD (19% versus 3%; $P > .001$). Those who had syncope were more likely to have cardiac tamponade (28% versus 8%; $P > .001$), stroke (18% versus 4%; $P > .001$), and other neurologic deficits such as decreased level of consciousness, coma, and spinal cord ischemia (25% versus 14%; $P > .005$). In 46% of patients, a cause was not found.

Other symptoms that require particular attention are transient ischemic attack and other focal neurologic complaints. These findings are documented in 4.7% to 17% of the cases [51,53,55]. A complaint of focal deficits paired with chest pain has one of the highest likelihood ratios of being AD (positive likelihood ratio, 6.6–33) [53].

Findings on physical examination

Physical examination findings associated with AD are typically present in less than half the cases [53]. Among the most useful signs able to predict AD is a pulse deficit. A pulse deficit between the carotid, radial, or femoral arteries is relatively infrequent (25%–30%) but when present is strongly suggestive of AD in the setting of chest or back pain (positive likelihood ratio, 5.7; 95% CI, 1.4–23.0) [53]. This finding can predict in-hospital complications and mortality. Bossone and colleagues [58] noted that in-hospital mortality is higher when pulses absent (41% versus 25%). The more absent pulses the higher mortality. Blood pressure on presentation does not seem to be helpful in predicting who might have AD. Although approximately half the patients present with elevated blood pressure, an equal proportion are either hypertensive or normotensive [52,53,55]. A history of chronic hypertension as a risk factor is helpful, however, because it is the most frequent risk factor. Other physical findings are murmur of aortic insufficiency (detected in one third of the cases) and muffled heart tones and jugular venous distention that point toward cardiac tamponade.

Biomarkers in the workup of aortic dissection

The lack of symptoms or signs that have a good negative predictive value has forced investigators to look at serologic means to diagnose AD. This concept is particularly attractive because a serum test with a good negative predictive value would obviate the need for imaging. In the last decade several efforts have been made toward achieving this goal. Investigators have looked at soluble elastic compounds, D-dimer, and smooth muscle myosin heavy chain (SMMHC).

SMMHC is a major component of smooth muscle. Katoh and Suzuki [59] first described the use of SMMHC in AD in Japan in 1995. SMMHC was tested in serum of healthy subjects with levels of 0.9 ± 0.9 ng/mL and in four patients who had AD confirmed by surgery, all four of whom demonstrated elevated levels at presentation (> 7 ng/mL) that dropped to normal values after 24 hours. The immunoassay showed a sensitivity of 90% in the first 12 hours after onset of symptoms with a specificity of 97%. Most recently, Suzuki and colleagues [60] documented 25 patients enrolled in the IRAD whose measured SMMHC showed elevated levels of 19.6 ± 56.6 ng/mL (normal < 2.5 ng/mL) with a presentation time of 6.1 hours $\pm$ 4.5 hours. This study showed superior diagnostic performance in the early hours after onset ($> 90\%$ sensitivity in the first 3 hours after onset). The sensitivity decreased to 44% after 3 hours, however, and decreased most significantly after 6 hours [60].

Elastin is one of the major components of the arterial wall. An ELISA to measure soluble elastin fragments, a product of human aortic elastin, was developed by Shinohara and colleagues [61]. They reported that 16 of 25 patients who had AD had elevated soluble elastin fragments; unfortunately, all patients who did not have a patent false lumen had normal levels. Although the authors conclude that the test might be helpful in the diagnosis and screening of AD, one patient who had AMI had elevated levels, the study was retrospective, and the negative predictive value was poor and therefore not useful to exclude AD.

D-dimer is frequently used to exclude thromboembolic disease in low-risk patients. It is a cross-linked fiber degradation product formed by plasmin, which serves as a marker of clot lysis. Weber and colleagues [62] prospectively tested D-dimer levels in 10 patients suspected of having AD. In addition, they retrospectively reviewed 14 patients who had proven AD; 35 patients served as a control group. D-dimer was elevated in all patients who had AD. No patients who did not have AD had elevated D-dimer. The authors concluded that the presence of AD is unlikely in the setting of a negative D-dimer [62]. This conclusion is thought provoking and currently is being evaluated in a multicenter study along with soluble elastin fragments and SMMHC (L.H. Haro, personal communication, 2004).

ECG findings suggesting ST-segment elevation myocardial infarction

Emergency physicians and cardiologists are frequently challenged by a patient who presents with chest pain that radiates to the back and an ECG with ST-segment elevation suggestive of an AMI. In these cases, therapy is frequently delayed, because patients often go to CT or transfer without fibrinolytic therapy to rule out dissection. The frequency of ST-segment elevation and Q waves suggestive of an AMI in AD are well documented in the literature. In the initial IRAD publication, the finding was documented in 4.6% of type A and in 0.7% of type B [55]. In Komplas' review [53], new MI on ECG was present in 7% of the cases (95% CI, 4–14). Coronary artery involvement (CAI) in AD and ST abnormalities in the ECG do not go hand-in-hand, however. Bossone and colleagues [63] evaluated the clinical characteristics and outcomes of 475 patients who had AD, of whom 64 (13.5%) had CAI. When they reviewed the ECGs, patients who had CAI were more likely to show new Q wave or ST-segment elevation (16.7% versus 4.3%; *P* = .0001). Thus, these ECG findings were present in only one of six patients who had CAI. Therefore, ST-segment elevation in AD seems to be uncommon, and the ECG often is not diagnostic even when AD with CAI is present. The low frequency of AD with ST-segment elevation compared with actual STEMI would argue for selected and infrequent need for imaging. (The US Census Bureau projected a 296,042,501 population for May 2005. The best estimate of the occurrence of AD is between 5 and 20 per million population, or approximately 1400 to 6000 new dissections per year, 62% of which would be type A. Five percent to 7% of those type A dissections would have ST-segment abnormalities suggestive of a STEMI, representing less than 300 cases in the United States each year. Approximately 500,000 patients in the United States have STEMI each year.)

In general, when a patient presents with chest pain and ST-segment elevation in the ECG, one should assume STEMI and treat accordingly. The authors believe that reperfusion therapy with PPCI is the safest way to proceed. If no culprit artery is found, arteriography or intraoperative transesophageal echocardiography (TEE) can be performed. If PPCI is not available, and symptom onset occurred more than 3 hours previously, the benefit of fibrinolysis is low. Obtaining a CT emergently or transferring the patient for PPCI is the best option. Heparin can be withheld. In a patient who demonstrates ST-segment elevation in the ECG, an anterior distribution, and more than 3 hours of pain with no findings highly suggestive of AD (severe abrupt pain, focal deficit, pulse deficit), and a completely normal chest radiograph, the likelihood of AD is low (likelihood ratio, 0.07%; 95% CI, 0.03–0.17) [18], and the morbidity and mortality of STEMI are high. The authors recommend fibrinolysis while awaiting transfer or further imaging such as CT or TEE.

Imaging

The choice of imaging modality is usually based on availability and the patient's stability. CT and TEE are frequent choices [55]. CT is the most readily available, widely used, noninvasive technique for the diagnosis of AD. The sensitivity and specificity of CT approaches 100% for the diagnosis of AD [64]. Aortography was the traditional method for making the diagnosis of AD, with an accuracy of 95% to 99% [65]. Aortography, however, is highly invasive, requires the patient be out of the emergency department for an extended period of time, and exposes the patient to a significant contrast load [47]. TEE is being used with increasing frequency and has been shown to be safe, even in critically ill patients [58,66,67]. The sensitivity of TEE for detecting both proximal and distal dissections is 100% [59]. The main limitations to the use of the TEE is a lack of widespread, 24-hour availability. Finally, MRI is the newest imaging method for the diagnosis of AD. It is highly sensitive and specific and does not require exposing the patient to contrast material. It is not ideal in ventilated or monitored patients and is not widely available.

Treatment of aortic dissection

Treatment of AD is aimed at eliminating the forces that favor progression of the dissection. Prompt production of blood pressures can be accomplished through use of sodium nitroprusside with a rate adjusted to achieve a systolic blood pressure between 100 and 120 mm Hg [44,47,57]. Concomitant use of a beta-blocker to avoid reflex tachycardia secondary to the nitroprusside use is desirable to decrease further the shear forces that promote propagation. A target heart rate of 60 to 80 beats per minute is desirable [44,57].

Patients who have acute dissection involving the ascending aorta should receive rapid surgical consultation. An exception might be isolated arch dissection; most physicians consider this a surgical entity. Richartz and colleagues [68] published the international experience with isolated arch dissections. Of 989 patients, 92 (9%) had isolated arch dissection. Of these, 39 (42%) were treated surgically, and 53 (58%) were treated medically. Thirty-day mortality was 17% (23% with surgery and 13% with medical management) and therefore was much lower than typical for type A dissections (35% with surgery and 65% with medical management). Complications were the same. The conclusion was that isolated arch dissections are best managed conservatively. Distal ADs are in general traditionally treated medically. Surgery is indicated in distal dissections when there is evidence of lower extremity or visceral ischemia, renal failure, or paraplegia [47].

Percutaneous management of aortic dissection

Complicated type B dissections have been subject to novel percutaneous therapies such as percutaneous fenestration (restoring flow to the true lumen by creating a tear in the dissection flap between the true and false lumen) and percutaneous stent–graft placement. With these techniques compromised flow can be restored in 90% of the cases (range, 70%–100%). If a patient survives the intervention, postoperative average 30-day mortality is 10% (range, 0%–25%), and additional surgical intervention is rarely needed [69].

Pulmonary embolism

Missed PE is a major source of malpractice litigation in emergency medicine [70]. It is estimated that the diagnosis of PE is missed 400,000 times annually, leading to 100,000 preventable deaths [71]. Other studies have estimated that only 30% of PE is diagnosed ante mortem [72]. The mortality rate for untreated PE is 18.4%—seven times greater than that of appropriately treated PE [73]. Certainly, failure to be diagnosed is the greatest threat to the patient who has PE [74]. The challenges faced in the diagnosis of PE are similar to those discussed for ACS and AD.

In general, the presentation of PE is nonspecific. Young patients who have excellent cardiac reserve tend to have mild, transient, or no symptoms at all [74]. Patients may complain of chest pain which is typically sudden in onset and pleuritic in nature. Dyspnea, palpitations, presyncope, or syncope may also be presenting complaints. Accurate diagnosis is clouded when clinical presentations coexist with underlying obstructive lung disease, pneumonia, or underlying congestive heart failure. In such cases, PE can present with the symptoms of any of these entities [75].

The clinical likelihood of a patient's having PE has long been estimated by implicit means. Physician judgment is based on the patient's clinical presentation, history and physical evaluation, and risk factor assessment. Studies, however, have shown poor agreement among physicians in estimating pretest probability of disease [76]. Physician experience affects pretest probability assessment, with less experienced clinicians demonstrating less ability to assign pretest probability accurately [77]. Implicit assessment results in a large group of patients being placed in the moderate-risk category. Thus, clinical judgment has yielded disappointing results in accurately determining the pretest probability of disease.

Therefore, clinical scoring systems have been developed. Wells and colleagues [78] and Anderson and others [79] have created a seven-feature bedside assessment tool to categorize patients as having low, moderate, or high pretest probability of PE. Even with Wells' criteria, studies have shown poor agreement among physicians on the assignment of pretest probability and poor accuracy for the same [80]. Until a reliable, validated clinical scoring system can be developed, the assignment of pretest probability of PE will remain a challenge.

History and physical examination

As in the entities previously described, history taking in a patient presenting with chest pain suspicious for PE should focus on features of the pain and associated symptoms. Particularly important in patients suspected of having PE is risk factor assessment. Box 2 lists the many of risk factors that need to be considered in a patient who has possible PE [74]. The physical examination in a patient suspected of having PE should focus on vital signs and pulmonary findings. Tachycardia and tachypnea are classically described, but the former is often absent in younger patients, and the later is absent in up to 13% of patients who have documented PE [74]. The physical examination may show pleural rub, rales, or findings consistent with pulmonary consolidation. In summary, no physical finding is sensitive or specific for the diagnosis of PE. Physical examination offers no clues to the diagnosis in 28% to 58% of cases [74].

Box 2. Risk factors for pulmonary embolism

Inherited disorders (thrombophilias)
Elevated individual clotting factor levels
(VIII, IX, XI)
Factor V_{Leiden} mutation
Hyperhomocystinemia
Protein C, protein S, or antithrombin III
deficiency
Prothrombin G20210A mutation

Acquired—persistent
Age
Antiphospholipid antibodies (lupus
anticoagulant, anticardiolipin
antibody)
History of pulmonary embolism/deep
venous thrombosis
History of superficial thrombophlebitis
Hyperviscosity syndrome (polycythemia
vera, malignant melanoma)
Immobilization (bedridden, paresis, or
paralysis)
Malignancy
Medical conditions

Congestive heart failure
Obesity
Nephrotic syndrome

Tobacco abuse
Acute myocardial infarction
Varicose veins

Acquired—transient
Central venous catheter/pacemaker
placement
Hormone replacement therapy
Immobilization—isolated extremity
Long distance travel/air travel
Oral contraceptive pills
Pregnancy and puerperium
Surgery
Trauma

From Sadosty AT, Boie ET, Stead LG. Pulmonary embolism. Emerg Med Clin North Am 2003;21(2):363–84; with permission.

D-dimer assays

The advent of quantitative ELISA has improved the sensitivity of D-dimer assays tremendously [81]. D-dimer assays as a whole have poor specificity, with numerous conditions resulting in false-positive results. They are most useful when combined with other noninvasive imaging or clinical probability assessment scoring systems. In this way, a negative D-dimer can be incorporated into diagnostic algorithms to withhold anticoagulation safely in patients who have a low pretest probability for PE [81]. Recent studies report the negative likelihood ratios for a negative result on a quantitative rapid ELISA D-dimer make them as predictive as a normal V/Q scan or negative duplex ultrasound [82].

Eleven prospective clinical studies have evaluated the role of D-dimer in excluding venous thromboembolic disease. In patients who have a high clinical pretest probability of PE but a negative D-dimer, there is not enough evidence to support stopping an investigation for PE [73]. In contrast, it has become increasingly accepted that the diagnosis of PE is effectively ruled out in patients who have a low clinical pretest probability of disease and a negative quantitative rapid ELISA D-dimer [82]. Controversy still exists over the extent of workup necessary in patients who have a moderate pretest clinical probability and a negative D-dimer assay.

One significant limitation affecting widespread use of D-dimer is the numerous commercially available assays that are not interchangeable, differing significantly in sensitivity and negative likelihood ratios [81]. Latex glutination assays and whole-blood qualitative assays do not demonstrate the same negative predictive value as quantitative ELISA assays and should not be incorporated in diagnostic algorithms similarly.

V/Q scanning

The Prospective Investigation of Pulmonary Embolism Diagnosis investigators employed V/Q scanning as the primary advanced imaging diagnostic modality for patients suspected of having PE [83]. Ventilation/perfusion scans are most helpful when they are read as either normal or high probability. Results of V/Q scans, however, fail to provide definitive indications for withholding or administering anticoagulation in up to 70% of patients on whom the test is performed [74].

CT scanning

CT is widely available, noninvasive, increasingly sensitive, and has the advantage of revealing alternative diagnoses when PE is not found [84]. CT can miss subsegmental PE. Some authors have argued that this finding is insignificant and that outcome studies of rate of subsequent or recurrent PE and death would be more a appropriate reference standard than comparisons to the standard of angiographic subsegmental PE detection rates [85]. Eleven such studies exist, both prospective and retrospective, which demonstrate patient outcome is not adversely affected when anticoagulation is withheld based on a negative spiral CT [86].

Diagnostic evaluation summary

A review by Fedullo and Tapson [87] provides rational guidance to the approach to the patient suspected of having PE, using a combination of pretest probability assessment, D-dimer assays, and advanced imaging modalities to rule in or rule out effectively the diagnosis of PE.

Patients who have a low pretest probability of PE account for 25% to 65% of all patients evaluated for PE, with subsequent diagnosis of PE in 5% to 10% of cases [78,88–90]. For these patients at low clinical probability, a negative quantitative ELISA D-dimer effectively rules out the diagnosis of PE.

Patients who have a high pretest probability for PE comprise 10% to 30% of all patients evaluated for PE, with subsequent diagnosis of PE in 70% to 90% [78,88–90]. D-dimer has no significant role in this patient population, because a negative result does not rule out the presence of PE. Spiral CT should be performed in these patients. If CT is negative, duplex ultrasound or CT venography of the lower extremities may be indicated. If lower extremity studies are also negative in this high-risk patient population, pulmonary angiogram is indicated to rule out the presence of PE.

Intermediate-risk patients comprise 25% to 65% of all patients examined for PE, with subsequent diagnosis of PE in 25% to 45% [78,88–90].

References

[1] McCaig LF, Burt CW. National hospital ambulatory medical care survey: 2002 emergency department summary. Adv Data 2004;(340):1–34.
[2] American Heart Association. Heart disease and stroke statistics—2004 update. Available at: http://www.americanheart.org/presenter.jhtml?identifier=3000090. Accessed November 15, 2003.
[3] Antman EM, Anbe DT, Armstrong PW, et al. ACC/AHA guidelines for the management of patients with ST-elevation myocardial infarction; a report of the American College of Cardiology/American Heart Association Task Force on Practice Guidelines (Committee to Revise the 1999 Guidelines for the Management of Patients with Acute Myocardial Infarction). J Am Coll Cardiol 2004;44(3):671–719.
[4] Bunch TJ, White RD, Gersh BJ, et al. Outcomes and in-hospital treatment of out-of-hospital cardiac arrest patients resuscitated from ventricular fibrillation by early defibrillation. Mayo Clin Proc 2004; 79(5):613–9.
[5] Canto JG, Zalenski RJ, Ornato JP, et al, for the National Registry of Myocardial Infarction 2 Investigators. Use of emergency medical services in acute myocardial infarction and subsequent quality of care: observations from the National Registry of Myocardial Infarction 2. Circulation 2002;106:3018–23.
[6] Brown AL, Mann NC, Daya M, et al. Demographic, belief, and situational factors influencing the decision to utilize emergency medical services among chest pain patients: Rapid Early Action for Coronary Treatment (REACT) study. Circulation 2000; 102:173–8.
[7] Becker L, Larsen MP, Eisenberg MS. Incidence of cardiac arrest during self-transport for chest pain. Ann Emerg Med 1996;28:612–6.
[8] Rogers WJ, Canto JG, Lambrew CT, et al. Temporal trends in the treatment of over 1.5 million patients with myocardial infarction in the US from 1990 through 1999: the National Registry of Myocardial Infarction 1, 2 and 3. J Am Coll Cardiol 2000;36:2056–63.
[9] Goff DC, Feldman HA, McGovern PG, et al, for the Rapid Early Action for Coronary Treatment (RE-ACT) Study Group. Prehospital delay in patients hospitalized with heart attack symptoms in the United States: the REACT trial. Am Heart J 1999; 138:1046–57.
[10] Welsh RC, Ornato J, Armstrong PW. Prehospital management of acute ST-elevation myocardial infarction: a time for reappraisal in North America. Am Heart J 2003;145:1–8.
[11] Steg PG, Goldberg RJ. Baseline characteristics, management practices and in-hospital outcomes of patients hospitalized with acute coronary syndromes in the Global Registry of Acute Coronary Events (GRACE). Am J Cardiol 2002;90(4):358–63.
[12] Finnegan JR Jr, Hendrika Meischke H, Zapka JG, et al. Patient delay in seeking care for heart attack symptoms: findings from focus groups conducted in five US regions. Prev Med 2000;31:205–13.
[13] Goff DC Jr, Mitchell P, Finnegan J, et al, for the RE-ACT Study Group. Knowledge of heart attack symptoms in 20 US communities. Results from the Rapid Early Action for Coronary Treatment Community Trial. Prev Med 2004;38(1):85–93.
[14] Hochman JS, Sleeper LA, White HD, et al, for the Should We Emergently Revascularize Occluded Coronaries for Cardiogenic Shock (SHOCK)

Investigators. One-year survival following early revascularization for cardiogenic shock. JAMA 2001; 285:190–2.

[15] Gersh JB, Stone WG, White DH, et al. Pharmacological facilitation of primary percutaneous coronary intervention for acute myocardial infarction. JAMA 2005;293(8):979–86.

[16] Reimer KA, Lowe JE, Rasmussen MM, et al. The wavefront phenomenon of ischemic cell death: 1. Myocardial infarct size vs duration of coronary occlusion in dogs. Circulation 1977;56:786–94.

[17] The European Myocardial Infarction Project Group. Prehospital thrombolytic therapy in patients with suspected acute myocardial infarction. N Engl J Med 1993;329:383–9.

[18] Danchin N, Blanchard D, Steg GP, et al. Impact of prehospital thrombolysis for acute myocardial infarction on 1-yr outcome. Circulation 2004;110: 1909–15.

[19] Brady WJ, Roberts D, Morris F. The nondiagnostic ECG in the chest pain patient: normal and nonspecific initial ECG presentations of acute MI. Am J Emerg Med 1999;17(4):394–7.

[20] Lim SH, Sayre MR, Gibler WB. 2-D echocardiography prediction of adverse events in ED patients with chest pain. Am J Emerg Med 2003;21(2):106–10.

[21] Jones ID, Slovis CM. Emergency department evaluation of the chest pain patient. Emerg Med Clin North Am 2001;19(2):269–82.

[22] Boccardi L, Verde M. Gender differences in the clinical presentation to the emergency department for chest pain. Ital Heart J 2003;4(6):371–3.

[23] Kontos MC. Evaluation of the emergency department chest pain patient. Cardiol Rev 2001;9(5): 266–75.

[24] Alpert JS, Thygesen K, Antman E, et al. Myocardial infarction redefined: a consensus document of the Joint European Society of Cardiology/American College of Cardiology Committee for the redefinition of myocardial infarction. J Am Coll Cardiol 2000;36:959–69.

[25] Wu AH, Apple FS, Gibler WB, et al. National Academy of Clinical Biochemistry Standards of Laboratory Practice: recommendations for the use of cardiac markers in coronary artery diseases. Clin Chem 1999;45:1104–21.

[26] Antman EM, Tanasijevic MJ, Thompson B, et al. Cardiac specific troponin I levels to predict the risk of mortality in patients with acute coronary syndromes. N Engl J Med 1996;335:1342–9.

[27] Lindahl B, Toss H, Siegbahn A, et al, for the FRISC Study Group. Markers of myocardial damage and inflammation in relation to long-term mortality in unstable coronary artery disease. N Engl J Med 2000;16(343):1139–47.

[28] Sabatine MS, Morrow DA, de Lemos JA, et al. Multimarker approach to risk stratification in non-ST elevation acute coronary syndromes simultaneous assessment of troponin I, C-reactive protein, and B-type natriuretic peptide. Circulation 2002;105: 1760.

[29] Weaver WD, Simes RJ, Betriu A, et al. The most effective therapy for MI reperfusion in primary percutaneous coronary revascularization (PPCI). It is superior to IFT (comparison of primary coronary angioplasty and intravenous thrombolytic therapy for acute myocardial infarction: a quantitative review). JAMA 17;278(23):2093–8.

[30] Brodie BR, Stuckey TD, Wall TC, et al. Importance of time to reperfusion for 30-day and late survival and recovery of left ventricular function after primary angioplasty for acute myocardial infarction. J Am Coll Cardiol 1998;32:1312–9.

[31] Brodie BR, Stone GW, Morice MC, et al, for the Stent Primary Angioplasty in Myocardial Infarction Study Group. Importance of time to reperfusion on outcomes with primary coronary angioplasty for acute myocardial infarction (results from the Stent Primary Angioplasty in Myocardial Infarction Trial). Am J Cardiol 2001;88:1085–90.

[32] Berger PB, Ellis SG, Holmes DR, et al. Relationship between delay in performing direct coronary angioplasty and early clinical outcome in patients with acute myocardial infarction: results from the Global Use of Strategies to Open Occluded Arteries in Acute Coronary Syndromes (GUSTO-IIb) trial. Circulation 1999;100:14–20.

[33] Cannon CP, Gibson CM, Lambrew CT, et al. Relationship of symptom-onset-to-balloon time and door-to-balloon time with mortality in patients undergoing angioplasty for acute myocardial infarction. JAMA 2000;283:2941–7.

[34] Widimsky P, Groch L, Zelizko M, et al, on behalf of the PRAGUE Study Group Investigators. Multicentre randomized trial comparing transport to primary angioplasty vs immediate thrombolysis vs combined strategy for patients with acute myocardial infarction presenting to a community hospital without a catheterization laboratory The PRAGUE Study. Eur Heart J 2000;21:823–31.

[35] De Luca G, Suryapranata H, Ottervanger JP, et al. Time delay to treatment and mortality in primary angioplasty for acute myocardial infarction: every minute of delay counts. Circulation 2004;109:1223–5.

[36] Williams DO. Treatment delayed is treatment denied. Circulation 2004;109:1806–8.

[37] Brass LM, Lichtman JH, Wang Y, et al. Intracranial hemorrhage associated with thrombolytic therapy for elderly patients with acute myocardial infarction: results from the Cooperative Cardiovascular Project. Stroke 2000;31:1802–11.

[38] Andersen HR, Nielsen TT, Rasmussen K, et al, for the DANAMI- 2 Investigators. A comparison of coronary angioplasty with fibrinolytic therapy in acute myocardial infarction. N Engl J Med 2003; 349:733–42.

[39] Second International Study of Infarct Survival Collaborative Group (ISIS-2). Randomised trial of

intravenous streptokinase, oral aspirin, both, or neither among 17,187 cases of suspected acute myocardial infarction: ISIS-2. Lancet 1988;2:349–60.

[40] Roux S, Christeller S, Lüdin E. Effects of aspirin on coronary reocclusion and recurrent ischemia after thrombolysis: a metaanalysis. J Am Coll Cardiol 1992;19:671–7.

[41] Meine TJ, Roe MT, Chen AY, et al, for the CRUSADE Investigators. Association of intravenous morphine use and outcomes in acute coronary syndromes: results from the CRUSADE Quality Improvement Initiative. Am Heart J 2005; 149.

[42] The MIAMI Trial Research Group. Metoprolol in acute myocardial infarction: patient population. Am J Cardiol 1985;56:10G–4G.

[43] Pfisterer M, Cox JL, Granger CB, et al. Atenolol use and clinical outcomes after thrombolysis for acute myocardial infarction: the GUSTO-I experience. Global Utilization of Streptokinase and TPA (alteplase) for Occluded Coronary Arteries. J Am Coll Cardiol 1998;32:634–40.

[44] Hals G. Acute thoracic aortic dissection: Current evaluation and management. Emerg Med Rep 2000;21:1.

[45] Boersma E, Harrington RA, Moliterno DJ, et al. Platelet glycoprotein IIb/IIIa inhibitors in acute coronary syndromes: a meta-analysis of all major clinical randomized trials. Lancet 2002;359:189–98.

[46] Cannon PC, Weintraub WS, Demopoulos LA, et al. Comparison of early invasive and conservative strategies in patients with unstable coronary syndromes treated with the glycoprotein IIb/IIIa inhibitor tirofiban. N Engl J Med 2000;25(344):1879–87.

[47] Salkin MS. Thoracic aortic dissection: avoiding failure to diagnose. ED Legal Letter 1997;8(11):107–18.

[48] Thoracic and abdominal aortic aneurysms. In: Tintinalli JE, Krome RL, et al, editors. Emergency medicine—a comprehensive study guide. 3rd edition. New York: McGraw Hill; 1992. p. 1384.

[49] Pate JW, Richardson RL, Eastridge CE. Acute aortic dissection. Am J Surg 1976;42:395–404.

[50] Hirst AE, Johns VJ, Kime SW, et al. Dissecting aneurysm of the aorta. A review of 505 cases. Medicine 1958;37:217–22.

[51] Spitell PC, Spitell JA, Joyce JW, et al. Clinical features and differential diagnosis of aortic dissection: experience with 236 cases (1980–1990). Mayo Clin Proc 1993;68:642–51.

[52] Meszaros I, Morocz J, Szlavi J, et al. Epidemiology and clinicopathology of aortic dissection: a population-based longitudinal study over 27 years. Chest 2000;117:1271–8.

[53] Klompas M. Does this patient have an acute thoracic aortic dissection? JAMA 2002;287(17):2262–72.

[54] Viljanen T. Diagnostic difficulties in aortic dissection: retrospective study of 89 surgically treated patients. Ann Chir Gynaecol 1986;75:328–32.

[55] Hagan PG, Nienaber CA, Isselbacher EM, et al. The international registry of acute aortic dissection (IRAD): new insights into an old disease. JAMA 2000;283:897–903.

[56] Januzzi JL, Isselbacher EM, Fatorri R, et al. Characterizing the young patient with aortic dissection: results from the international registry of aortic dissection (IRAD) [abstract 1081–154]. J Am Coll Cardiol 2003;41:253A.

[57] Nienamber CA, Eagle KA. Aortic dissection: new frontiers in diagnosis and management. Circulation 2003;108:628–35.

[58] Bossone E, Vincenzo R, Nienamber CA, et al. Usefulness of pulse deficit to predict in-hospital complications and mortality in patients with type A aortic dissection. Am J Cardiol 2002;89:851–5.

[59] Katoh H, Suzuki T. A novel immunoassay of smooth muscle myosin heavy chain in serum. J Immanuol Methods 1995;185:57–63.

[60] Suzuki T, Trimarchi S, Smith D, et al. Early diagnosis of acute aortic dissection: identification of clinical variables associated with early diagnosis and determination of the usefulness of biochemical diagnosis as shown by the international registry of acute aortic dissection (IRAD) database. Circulation 2004; 110(17):370.

[61] Shinohara T, Suzuki K, Okada M, et al. Soluble elastin fragments in serum are elevated in acute aortic dissection. Thromb Vasc Biol 2003;23:1839–44.

[62] Weber T, Hogler S, Auer J, et al. D-dimer in acute aortic dissection. Chest 2003;123(5):1375–8.

[63] Bossone E, Mehta RH, Trimarchi S, et al. Coronary involvement in patients with acute type A aortic dissection. J Am Coll Cardiol 2003;235A:1034–41.

[64] Yoshida S, Akiba H, Tamakawa M, et al. Thoracic involvement of type A aortic dissection and intramural hematoma: diagnostic accuracy—comparison of emergency helical CT and surgical findings. Radiology 2003;228(2):430–5.

[65] Eagle KA, Quertermous T, Kritzer GA, et al. Spectrum of conditions initially suggesting acute aortic dissection but with negative aortograms. Am J Cardiol 1986;57(4):322–6.

[66] Kouchoukos NT, Dougenis DD. Surgery of the thoracic aorta. N Engl J Med 1997;336:1876–86.

[67] Nienaber CA, Spielmann RP, von Kodolitsch Y, et al. Diagnosis of thoracic aortic dissection. Magnetic resonance imaging versus transesophageal echocardiography. Circulation 1992;85(2):434–47.

[68] Richartz B, Schiller F, Bossone E, et al. Aortic arch dissection as a distinct entity: lessons learned from IRAD. Circulation 2002;106:473.

[69] Nienaber CA, Eagle KA. Aortic dissection: new frontiers in the diagnosis and management. Part II: therapeutic management and follow-up. Circulation 2003;108:772–8.

[70] Laack TA, Goyal DG. Pulmonary embolism: an unsuspected killer. Emerg Med Clin North Am 2004; 22(4):961–83.

[71] Feied C. Pulmonary embolism. In: Rosen P, Barkin R, Daniel DF, editors. Emergency medicine:

concepts and clinical practice. St. Louis (MO): Mosby-Year Book; 1998. p. 1770–2.

[72] Morgenthaler TI, Ryu JH. Clinical characteristics of fatal pulmonary embolism in a referral hospital. Mayo Clin Proc 1995;70:417–24.

[73] Carson JL, Kelley MA, Duff A, et al. The clinical course of pulmonary embolism. N Engl J Med 1992;326(19):1240–5.

[74] Sadosty AT, Boie ET, Stead LG. Pulmonary embolism. Emerg Med Clin North Am 2003;21(2):363–84.

[75] Goldhaber SZ. Pulmonary embolism. Lancet 2004; 363(7417):1295–305.

[76] Jackson RE, Rudoni RR, Pascual R. Emergency physician (EP) assessment of the pre-test probability of pulmonary embolism (PE). Acad Emerg Med 1999;6:437.

[77] Kline JA, Wells PS. Methodology for a rapid protocol to rule out pulmonary embolism in the emergency department. Ann Emerg Med 2003;42(2):266–75.

[78] Wells PS, Ginsberg JS, Anderson DR, et al. Use of a clinical model for safe management of patients with suspected pulmonary embolism. Ann Intern Med 1998;129(12):997–1005.

[79] Anderson DR, Wells PS, Stiell I, et al. Thrombosis in the emergency department: use of a clinical diagnosis model to safely avoid the need for urgent radiological investigation. Arch Intern Med 1999;159(5):477–82.

[80] Sanson BJ, Lijmer JG, MacGillavry MR, et al. Comparison of a clinical probability estimate and two clinical models in patients with suspected pulmonary embolism. ANTELOPE-Study Group. Thromb Haemost 2000;83(2):199–203.

[81] Frost SD, Brotman DJ, Michota FA. Rational use of D-dimer measurement to exclude acute venous thromboembolic disease. Mayo Clin Proc 2003; 78(11):1385–91.

[82] Stein PD, Hull RD, Patel KC, et al. D-dimer for the exclusion of acute venous thrombosis and pulmonary embolism: a systematic review. Ann Intern Med 2004;140(8):589–602.

[83] PIOPED Investigators. Value of the ventilation/perfusion scan in acute pulmonary embolism. Results of the Prospective Investigation of Pulmonary Embolism Diagnosis (PIOPED). JAMA 1990;263(20): 2753–9.

[84] Perrier A, Howarth N, Didier D, et al. Performance of helical computed tomography in unselected outpatients with suspected pulmonary embolism. Ann Intern Med 2001;135(2):88–97.

[85] Wolfe TR, Hartsell SC. Pulmonary embolism: making sense of the diagnostic evaluation. Ann Emerg Med 2001;37(5):504–14.

[86] Schoepf UJ, Goldhaber SZ, Costello P. Spiral computed tomography for acute pulmonary embolism. Circulation 2004;109(18):2160–7.

[87] Fedullo PF, Tapson VF. Clinical practice. The evaluation of suspected pulmonary embolism. N Engl J Med 2003;349(13):1247–56.

[88] Khorasani R, Gudas TF, Nikpoor N, et al. Treatment of patients with suspected pulmonary embolism and intermediate probability lung scans: is diagnostic imaging underused? AJR 1997;169(5): 1355–7.

[89] Miniati M, Pistolesi M, Marini C, et al. Value of perfusion lung scan in the diagnosis of pulmonary embolism: results of the Prospective Investigative Study of Acute Pulmonary Embolism Diagnosis (PISA-PED). Am J Respir Crit Care Med 1996; 154(5):1387–93.

[90] Miniati M, Monti S, Bottai M. A structed clinical model for predicting the probability of pulmonary embolism. Am J Med 2003;114(3):173–9.

ELSEVIER
SAUNDERS

Cardiol Clin 24 (2006) 19–35

CARDIOLOGY
CLINICS

Pathogenesis and Early Management of Non–ST-segment Elevation Acute Coronary Syndromes

Tomas H. Ayala, MD[a],*, Steven P. Schulman, MD[b,c]

[a]*Division of Cardiology, University of Maryland School of Medicine, 22 South Greene Street, Baltimore, MD 21201, USA*
[b]*Johns Hopkins University School of Medicine, 600 North Wolfe Street, Baltimore, MD 21287, USA*
[c]*Coronary Care Unit, the Johns Hopkins Hospital, 600 North Wolfe Street, Baltimore, MD 21287, USA*

In 2001, there were more than 5.6 million visits to United States emergency departments because of chest pain or related symptoms [1]. Of these, nearly 1.4 million patients were admitted with acute coronary syndromes (ACS) [2]. The term "ACS" has evolved into a useful descriptor of a collection of symptoms associated with acute myocardial ischemia caused by sudden restriction of coronary blood flow. It is used to describe collectively acute myocardial infarction (AMI), both with and without ST-segment elevation, and unstable angina. By definition, then, it is a deliberately broad term that encompasses a range of related clinical conditions with varying degrees of host response, injury, prognosis, and, therefore, treatment.

In its very lack of specificity, the term "ACS" reflects the difficulty often encountered in differentiating between myocardial infarction (MI) (especially without ST segment elevation) and unstable angina at the time of presentation. As reflected by its name, non–ST-segment elevation MI (NSTEMI) is defined as presence of myocardial damage (typically detected by biochemical markers of myocardial necrosis) in the absence of ST segment elevation, true posterior MI, or new left bundle branch block on 12-lead ECG [3]. Its pathogenesis, clinical presentation, even angiographic appearance are virtually indistinguishable from those of unstable angina, save for evidence

of myocardial necrosis, which is usually not apparent at initial presentation [4,5]. Therefore, the combined entity of unstable angina/NSTEMI is often referred to as non–ST-segment elevation ACS (NSTE ACS). There are subtle but important differences in the pathogenesis of NSTE ACS and ST-segment elevation MI (STEMI); more crucial are differences in treatment, specifically in urgency of reperfusion therapy.

This article focuses on pathogenesis and early management of NSTE ACS. Because atherosclerotic coronary artery disease represents the typical substrate for NSTE ACS, the discussion would be incomplete without an overview of the development of the atherosclerotic plaque. The article then reviews the specific pathologic pathways leading to NSTE ACS, with particular attention to disruption of the vulnerable plaque and ensuing nonocclusive thrombosis. Finally, it addresses appropriate early management based on the current understanding of the underlying pathophysiology and on a review of available clinical data.

Pathogenesis of coronary artery disease

In 1986, Ross [6] proposed the "response to injury" hypothesis of atherogenesis implicating endothelial injury and subsequent intimal smooth muscle cell proliferation and inflammation as the initiating events in atherosclerosis. This article presents an overview of the proposed mechanisms of endothelial injury and the molecular and cellular responses to such injury that lead to plaque

---

* Corresponding author.
E-mail address: tayala@medicine.umaryland.edu (T.H. Ayala).

cardiology.theclinics.com

formation, progression, and ultimately rupture. It is useful, first, to review the histologic characteristics of the developing plaque at various stages.

Histology of atherosclerotic lesions

Stary and colleagues [7] have proposed a classification scheme of atherosclerotic lesions based on distinct morphologic characteristics. They describe two types of precursor or early lesions, two types of advanced lesions, and a linking stage between the two groups. The first three lesion types are characterized by being focal and lacking evidence of intimal disruption. More advanced lesions demonstrate intimal disruption and even modification of underlying media and adventitia.

Initial or type I lesions are microscopic collections of isolated macrophage foam cells (MFC)—macrophages containing lipid droplets—within arterial intima; these lesions have been found in as many as 45% of infants aged 8 months [8]. By the time of puberty, type II lesions are present [9]. These display a more organized pattern of MFC, arranged in adjacent layers and accompanied by smooth muscle cells that also contain lipid droplets, as well as small quantities of dispersed lipid droplets in the extracellular matrix (ECM) [7]. The preatheroma or type III lesion represents a transitional stage between early lesions and advanced atheroma. Its morphologic composition is marked by the presence of extracellular lipid pools between layers of smooth muscle cells. This lesion type still contains layers of MFC and non–lipid-containing macrophages [7]. The lipid pools eventually coalesce to form the lipid core that is characteristic of atheroma or type IV lesion [10]. In this lesion, the lipid core disrupts intimal structure but generally does not narrow the arterial lumen; instead there is compensatory eccentric expansion of the external boundary of the vessel, a process known as positive arterial remodeling (Fig. 1) [11,12]. Type V lesions also have a lipid core, now surrounded by layers of fibrous tissue [10]. These lesions are quite heterogeneous but generally are composed of varying proportions of collagen-rich ECM (also with proteoglycans and elastic fibers), a lipid core, smooth muscle cells, inflammatory cells (MFC and T lymphocytes), thrombi, and calcium deposits [10,13]. It is this advanced lesion that is generally prone to disruption.

Endothelium and endothelial injury

More than being simply a selectively permeable vascular inner layer, the endothelium is a dynamic organ with paracrine and autocrine functions that has a central role in regulating vascular hemodynamics and vascular hemostasis [14]. Endothelial regulation of vasomotion is performed by a balance in synthesis and release of vasodilators such as nitric oxide and prostacyclin, as well as vasoconstrictors such as endothclin-1 and platelet activating factor (PAF). The synthesis and release of these substances is controlled locally, modulated by a variety of biologically active molecules and mediators that allow an appropriate response to mechanical or chemical injury. In addition to their vasomotor effects, nitric oxide and prostacyclin are also central in inhibiting platelet activation, thereby preventing thrombosis. When disrupted, however, endothelial cells become procoagulant in an effort to stop blood flow and restore vascular integrity [14].

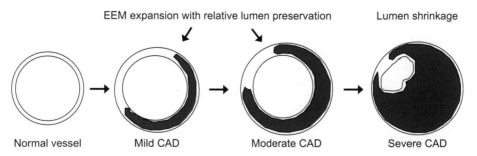

Fig. 1. Positive remodeling. In early atherosclerosis, plaque growth is compensated for by eccentric expansion of the external elastic membrane (EEM) with relative preservation of luminal area. As atherosclerosis progresses, the EEM does not expand further, and plaque growth results in luminal shrinkage. CAD, coronary artery disease. (*Adapted from* Glagov S, Weisenberg E, Zarins CK, et al. Compensatory enlargement of human atherosclerotic coronary arteries. N Eng J Med 1987;316:1371; with permission.)

A number of mechanisms of endothelial injury leading to dysfunction have been proposed. Chronic minimal injury caused by turbulent flow at bending points, chronic exposure to elevated low-density lipoprotein (LDL) cholesterol levels, smoking, diabetes, hypertension, oxidative stress, and infectious factors may all contribute to alterations in the function of endothelial cells (Fig. 2) [4,6]. This altered response includes a decrease in nitric oxide biosynthesis, increase in endothelin-1 production, and activation of the transcription factor nuclear factor κB [6,15]. This transcription factor has been implicated in the regulation of inflammatory cytokines such as tumor necrosis factor α (TNF-α), interleukin (IL)-1β, and macrophage colony-stimulating factor; chemokines such as macrophage chemoattractant protein 1 (MCP-1); and adhesion molecules such as intercellular adhesion molecule 1 and vascular cell adhesion molecule-1 [16]. These factors serve to attract blood monocytes [17], which migrate into the subendothelial space and transform into macrophages. In turn, these activated macrophages internalize oxidized LDL to become MFC and release mitogens that lead to smooth muscle cell proliferation [6]. They also amplify the effect of nuclear factor κB by releasing MCP-1, IL-1β,

TNF-α, and various other inflammatory cytokines, perpetuating the inflammatory cell recruitment process [17,18]. Plaque macrophages are stimulated to produce cytokines and collagen-degrading enzymes by a variety of factors, including angiotensin II [19], oxidized LDL [20], and the very inflammatory cytokines they express [21]. TNF-α, IL-1β (both expressed primarily by macrophages), and interferon gamma (IFN-γ) are overexpressed in atherosclerotic lesions but not in normal arteries [22]. IFN-γ is uniquely expressed by the activated T-helper type 1 lymphocyte, induced primarily by a combination of IL-18 and IL-12, both produced by macrophages [18,23]. These inflammatory cells and cytokines play a central role in the development of atherosclerosis and in the pathogenesis of ACS.

Pathogenesis of the acute coronary syndromes

Myocardial ischemia occurs when myocardial oxygen demand exceeds supply. In ACS this occurrence is typically because of a sudden reduction in coronary blood flow, and therefore of oxygen supply, relative to oxygen demand. Braunwald [24] recognizes five general circumstances in which this scenario can occur. The most common,

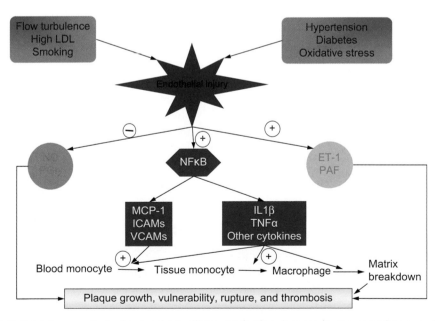

Fig. 2. Endothelial injury results in decreased vasodilator production, increase in vasoconstrictors, and increase in proinflammatory mediators that ultimately result in plaque growth and vulnerability. ET-1, endothelin-1; ICAMs, intercellular adhesion molecules; IL1β, interleukin 1 beta; MCP-1, macrophage chemoattractant protein-1; NO, nitric oxide; PAF, platelet-activating factor; PGI$_2$, prostacyclin; TNFα, tumor necrosis factor alpha; VCAMs, vascular cell adhesion molecules.

and most clinically important, involves disruption of the advanced atherosclerotic plaque with formation of a thrombus that partially or completely occludes the arterial lumen, thus reducing myocardial perfusion. A second cause is progressive narrowing of the arterial lumen caused by advancing chronic atherosclerosis. Vasospasm, or sudden contraction of vascular smooth muscle cells, results in a sudden narrowing of a focal segment of coronary artery, producing impaired myocardial perfusion. Arterial inflammation may lead to arterial narrowing or to plaque destabilization with ensuing plaque rupture and thrombosis. Finally, any systemic condition that increases myocardial oxygen demand (eg, fever, thyrotoxicosis), decreases overall coronary blood flow (eg, systemic hypotension), or decreases oxygen delivery (eg, profound anemia) can cause myocardial ischemia. Because of its clinical significance, plaque disruption and ensuing arterial thrombosis are the focus of this discussion.

The vulnerable plaque

Traditionally, the vulnerable plaque has been defined as one that is prone to rupture [25]. Recent pathologic findings suggest that, although rupture is the leading cause of arterial thrombosis, other processes can also result in thrombus formation. The comprehensive term of "high-risk plaque" provides a more complete description of the vulnerable plaque—one that may result in thrombus through rupture, cap erosion, or calcified nodules [26]. A significant limitation in the understanding of the pathology behind the ACS in humans is that histologic sections are available only after death. Most patients who have ACS do not die, and it is unclear if the pathologic process is identical in survivors.

Plaque rupture

Under appropriate circumstances the protective fibrous cap covering an atheromatous lesion can rupture, exposing the thrombogenic lipid core to coagulation factors and platelets in the bloodstream, which in turn leads to thrombosis [25,27]. Autopsy studies have shown that plaque rupture is associated with 60% to 80% of coronary thrombi in patients who have died of AMI [25,28]. Plaques prone to rupture seem to share common morphologic characteristics: a thin fibrous cap (<65 μm thick), an abundant population of macrophages, a relative scarcity of smooth muscle cells, and a soft extracellular lipid

core [22,29–31]. Plaques of this type are referred to as "thin-cap fibroatheromas." The clinical significance of thin-cap fibroatheromas was confirmed by an angioscopic study of coronary arteries in 63 patients demonstrating a relationship between yellow, lipid-rich plaques with thin fibrous caps and acute ischemic events [32]. Circumstances that lead to rupture are complex and are not completely understood; however, a combination of inflammatory factors and mechanical stress seems to be central in the development of plaque disruption.

Why does the fibrous cap fracture? Rather than being static, the fibrous cap is a metabolically active structure, constantly undergoing remodeling by means of synthesis and degradation of collagen and other ECM components (Fig. 3) [33]. Fibrillar interstitial collagen, synthesized by smooth muscle cells, is the principal determinant of the fibrous cap's biomechanical strength [27]. Inflammatory cytokines and inflammatory cells, specifically, macrophages and T lymphocytes, seem to exert significant control over the level of collagen and thus the cap's mechanical integrity. Dysregulation of normal ECM remodeling, mediated by inflammation, represents an attractive (although as yet unproven) hypothesis to explain aspects of fibrous cap rupture: an imbalance favoring breakdown of collagen over its synthesis results in structurally compromised areas of the fibrous cap.

Given that they play a central role in the progression of atherosclerosis, it is no surprise that macrophages and activated T lymphocytes have been found in abundance at the sites of plaque rupture [28,34]. These cells and the cytokines and enzymes they produce are responsible for detrimental effects to ECM composition. When appropriately activated by cytokines and other signals, macrophages degrade ECM through expression of a variety of matrix metalloproteinases (MMPs) that catalyze the critical initial steps of collagen breakdown. Certain MMPs, notably MMP-2 (also known as 72kD gelatinase), are present constitutively in nonatherosclerotic vessels and function in normal ECM metabolism; additionally, MMP-2 is secreted mainly in an inactive complex with its endogenous inhibitors (tissue inhibitor of metalloproteinase -1 and -2, TIMP-1 and -2) [35]. In contrast, atherosclerotic plaques demonstrate overexpression of activated MMP-1 (interstitial collagenase-1), MMP-3 (stromelysin), MMP-9 (92kD gelatinase), and MMP-13 (interstitial collagenase-3), especially at the shoulder

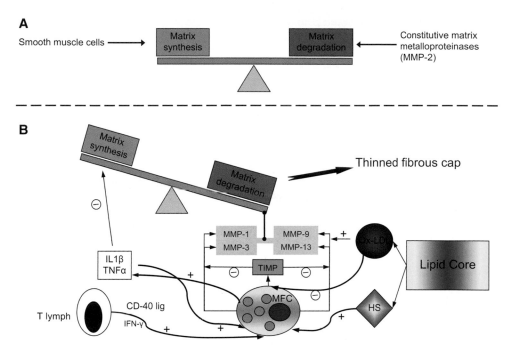

Fig. 3. (*A*). Balanced atherosclerotic cap homeostasis. (*B*) Activated macrophage foam cells (MFC) stimulated by T lymphocytes, inflammatory cytokines, oxidized LDL (ox-LDL), and circumferential hemodynamic stress (HS) overexpress matrix metalloproteinases (MMP) which leads to matrix degradation and cap thinning See text for details. IL1β, interleukin-1 beta; IFN-γ, interferon gamma; TIMP, tissue inhibitor of metalloproteinase.

region of the fibrous cap (the junction of the plaque with normal vessel) and surrounding the lipid core, where ruptures most often occur [22,35]. Macrophage expression of MMPs is induced by a variety of factors, including IL-1β, TNF-α, and IFN-γ [36], by activation by T lymphocytes through CD40 ligand [37], and by circumferential hemodynamic stress [38]. Induction of MMP is also accomplished by neutrophils and oxidized LDL. As is the case with macrophages and activated T lymphocytes, neutrophil infiltration has been noted in ruptured plaques [39]. Neutrophils express MMP-8, or neutrophil collagenase, which preferentially degrades type I collagen [40]. Oxidized LDL, present within the lipid core, stimulates the expression of MMP-9 by macrophages and inhibits the production of the MMP inhibitor TIMP-1 [41]. Even smooth muscle cells, when stimulated by IL-1β and IFN-γ, can degrade ECM by releasing activated MMPs [35] and the elastolytic proteases cathepsin S and K [42].

Protease-mediated degradation is complemented by reduced ECM production in the thin-cap fibroatheromas. IFN-γ has been shown to inhibit collagen gene expression in smooth muscle cells [27]. Additionally, the combination of IL-1β, TNF-α, and IFN-γ promotes smooth muscle cell apoptosis, which results in decreased collagen synthesis [43].

Inflammation in ACS may not be limited to a strictly local phenomenon. Evidence of neutrophil activation by reduced blood levels of neutrophil myeloperoxidase was found in samples from the aortic and great coronary veins of patients who had unstable angina [44]. This activation was found whether the culprit lesion was in the left anterior descending artery (which is drained selectively by the great coronary vein) or in the right coronary artery (which is not drained by the great coronary vein). Additionally, evidence of neutrophil activation was absent in patients who had chronic stable angina or variant angina. The presence of generalized coronary artery inflammation in the setting of ACS and the contribution of inflammation to the pathogenesis of ACS have led some to postulate that multiple unstable coronary lesions should be evident during an acute coronary event. In an intravascular ultrasound study of 24 patients who had initial ACS, there was evidence of multiple plaque ruptures at sites other than the culprit lesion, suggesting a generalized level of plaque instability [45]. Other evidence suggests that the extent of inflammation is not just regional but systemic. In a study of 36 patients admitted with AMI, the group that had preinfarction unstable angina had higher levels of the systemic inflammatory markers C-reactive protein, serum amyloid protein A, and IL-6, than did those with unheralded infarctions [46].

Mechanical factors can affect plaque's susceptibility to inflammatory assault. High circumferential stress has been associated with increased expression of MMP-1 [38]. A significant determinant of this stress is the eccentric, soft, lipid core, the presence of which has been shown to concentrate high circumferential stresses at the shoulder regions of the plaque [47]. Most plaques rupture at these regions of elevated tensile stress [48]. Shear stresses can also have an impact on plaque disruption. A study of carotid plaques at autopsy demonstrated that areas of plaque exposed to high flow and high shear forces had an abundance of plaque macrophages relative to the density of smooth muscle cells compared with areas of plaque exposed to low shear forces and low flow [49]. There seems to be increased susceptibility to rupture in areas with a higher concentration of inflammatory cells [50]. The thinness of the fibrous cap itself can have negative mechanical repercussions. A mathematical model of arterial vessels suggests that for a given luminal area, decreasing thickness of the fibrous cap is associated with increased circumferential stress [51]. Furthermore, repetitive exposure to pulsatile flow at these areas of high circumferential stress may result in plaque fatigue [51]. Another important aspect of the influence of mechanical stress on plaque rupture is positive arterial remodeling. Intravascular ultrasound studies in human coronaries have shown that positive remodeling is more common in patients who have unstable angina, whereas negative remodeling (in which the plaque encroaches on the lumen) is more common in patients who have chronic stable angina [52]. Positive remodeling also correlates with a larger lipid core and increased macrophage content, both of which promote plaque vulnerability [53]. Additionally, positive remodeling may influence plaque distensibility, that is, the softness of the plaque, which in turns makes it more prone to rupture [54]. Finally, positive arterial remodeling has been correlated with decreased density of collagen fibers [55]. The finding that positive arterial remodeling can increase plaque vulnerability while preserving luminal area may account for the observation that, in a majority of patients presenting with ACS, recent prior coronary angiography fails to demonstrate culprit lesion stenoses exceeding 70% [56,57].

The thin cap fibroatheroma is uniquely susceptible to rupture. In the setting of inflammation and matrix degradation, a structurally unstable fibrous cap exposed to both transient and steady mechanical disturbances leads to increases in tensile stress and ultimately to fracture. A variety of triggers of plaque rupture have been proposed, including air pollution [58], marijuana use [59], cocaine use [60], sexual activity, and emotional or physical stress [61], among others. The exact mechanism by which these activities prompt rupture in the susceptible plaque is not well understood.

Other mechanisms of plaque vulnerability

Although plaque rupture is the most important precipitating event for thrombosis in ACS, other mechanisms of thrombosis without rupture have been proposed. In one series of 125 cases of sudden coronary death caused by confirmed acute epicardial thrombosis, only 74 (59%) had histologic evidence of plaque rupture; 45 (36%) showed thrombus overlying a smooth muscle cell–rich, proteoglycan-rich plaque denuded of endothelial cells, and 6 (5%) showed a calcified nodule at the site of thrombus [26]. Additionally, compared with thrombosis associated with plaque rupture, cases with thrombosis caused by erosion were more likely to be younger than 50 years, women, and smokers [26,62]. These findings were confirmed in an autopsy series of 291 patients who died of AMI and had confirmed coronary thrombosis. In 25% of cases, thrombosis was caused by plaque erosion [63].

Although some have proposed repeated focal vasospasm as the underlying cause for the endothelial denudation seen in plaque erosion, this process has not been confirmed [26]. The observed absence of endothelial cells in these lesions has generated the attractive hypothesis that severe endothelial apoptosis as a response to mechanical or chemical injury leads to thrombosis. Cell membrane microparticles derived from apoptotic cells in atherosclerotic plaque have been shown to increase local levels of thrombogenic (TF) [64]. The same study showed, however, that most of these microparticles were derived from apoptotic macrophages and T lymphocytes, not from endothelial cells; it is unclear if endothelial apoptosis is always associated with thrombosis.

The most unusual lesion associated with thrombosis is the calcified nodule, a superficial fibrous-rich calcified lesion that erupts from the intima into the lumen [26]. The processes leading up to this lesion, or the way in which it induces thrombosis, are not known.

Arterial thrombosis

Plaque rupture or erosion both result in thrombus formation. This process is dynamic, and it is the balance of systemic and local procoagulant and fibrinolytic factors that ultimately determines the extent of thrombus formation and thus the clinical outcome [4].

Thrombus formation

The mechanisms behind thrombus formation associated with plaque disruption are better understood than those associated with plaque erosion. Davies [65] describes three stages of thrombosis. The first is characterized by platelet adhesion within the thrombogenic lipid core, the second by extension of the thrombus into the lumen with an increase in fibrin content and distal microembolization of activated platelets, and the third, by a growing thrombus composed of loose fibrin networks and entrapped red cells. This progression of stages is not deterministic and can be affected by host factors and clinical intervention.

Once plaque rupture occurs, the disrupted edges of the fibrous cap as well as the lipid core are exposed to blood-borne coagulation factors and platelets. Disruption of the normal endothelial layer transforms the endothelium from its constitutive antithrombotic state to a procoagulant state. It does so mainly by increased production of PAF and von Willebrand factor (vWF), a large multimeric protein with binding sites for subendothelial collagen [14]. Potentiated by arterial shear stress, platelets adhere to exposed subendothelium by platelet membrane glycoprotein Ib/IX-V complexed with vWF [66]. Adherent platelets then become activated under the influence of various mediators. Activation involves a shape change in the platelet, as well as release of alpha granules and dense granules containing potent platelet activation agents, including adenosine diphosphate and serotonin. Activation is also enhanced by circulating epinephrine and thrombin and by subendothelial collagen and vWF [67]. Additionally, activated platelets synthesize and release thromboxane A_2, a potent vasoconstrictor and platelet activator, which is increased in patients who have unstable angina [68]. The final step of activation is aggregation: expression of the platelet membrane Gp IIb/IIIa receptor allows platelet–platelet interactions whereby adherent platelets recruit circulating platelets to form an occlusive thrombus. Platelet aggregation is mediated by fibrinogen or vWF, either of which can bind to the Gp IIb/IIIa receptor, thus linking the platelets. The platelet thrombus is then stabilized by a fibrin mesh, the result of the simultaneously ongoing coagulation cascade [67].

Fernandez-Ortiz and colleagues [69] demonstrated that, at least in vitro, it is the lipid core that acts as the most significant substrate for the formation of the platelet thrombus. The exact source of the thrombogenic properties of the lipid core is not known. It has been suggested that lipids themselves and acellular debris found in the core may activate hemostasis [70]. This suggestion is an incomplete explanation and overlooks the significant role of TF. TF is a transmembrane glycoprotein that initiates the extrinsic clotting cascade. Its relationship to ACS was demonstrated in a study showing that TF is present in significantly greater amounts in the tissue of patients who have unstable angina than in those who have stable angina [71]. Despite its thrombogenicity, however, the lipid core is the source of surprisingly little TF. In fact, in patients who have unstable angina, TF is located predominantly in the cellular component of the plaque [71]. How can this apparent discrepancy be explained? Inflammatory cytokines, activated T cells, and oxidized LDL in the lipid core induce TF expression by plaque macrophages, smooth muscle cells, and endothelial cells [37,71,72]. At the time of plaque rupture, most TF seems to be associated with apoptotic cell fragments (mainly from macrophages and endothelial cells) that form part of the necrotic debris in the lipid core [64]. Thus, although there is no intrinsic TF expression within the lipid core, TF activity is found there in the setting of plaque rupture. Using an in vitro perfusion model, Toschi and colleagues [72] demonstrated the presence of active TF-VIIa complex within the lipid core, as well as a correlation between this complex and platelet adhesion.

TF, of course, is also responsible for initiating the plasma coagulation system that leads to the structural fibrin network of the thrombus. TF forms a high-affinity complex with coagulation factors VII and VIIa; this latter complex activates factors IX and X, and this activation in turn leads to thrombin generation and thrombosis [73]. Not only does thrombin serve to activate platelets, it converts fibrinogen to fibrin and activates factor XIII, which in turn stabilizes the fibrin clot [67].

Factors that mediate the extent of thrombosis

Not all thrombi or all plaque ruptures result in MI; they may, however, contribute to the progression of atherosclerotic disease. In his series of 25 cases of sudden cardiac death caused by acute coronary thrombosis, Falk [74] found that 81% of the thrombi had a layered appearance, suggesting alternating episodes of thrombus formation and fragmentation preceding the fatal infarction. Other investigators have suggested that healing of repeated plaque ruptures leads to progression of atherosclerosis: the thrombus organizes and heals by migration and proliferation of smooth muscle cells. This healing fibromuscular response incorporates the mural thrombus and worsens luminal stenosis [75]. Finally, even though fibrotic lesions lack a thrombogenic lipid core, erosion of these plaques has been associated with thrombus formation [26]. A number of factors, both local and systemic, have been implicated in determining the extent to which an arterial thrombus develops at the site of endothelial disruption.

Increased shear stress produces a conformational change in the platelet Gp Ib/IX-V receptor and vWF resulting in more avid platelet adhesion [66]. The clinical importance of this observation was demonstrated by a study that demonstrated increased platelet adhesion at the apex of a disrupted lesion; furthermore, it showed that the extent of platelet adhesion corresponded directly with the extent of stenosis following plaque rupture [76]. The same group also showed that increasing the extent of plaque disruption resulted in a larger, more stable, platelet thrombus [77]. This finding is hardly surprising, because more extensive plaque injury leads to greater exposure of blood to thrombogenic TF within the lipid core and to endothelial platelet activators such as PAF and vWF and thus results in more widespread activation of the coagulation cascade. Finally, the presence of a mural thrombus from prior plaque ruptures, such as those described by Falk [74], seems to contribute to extensive thrombosis. Not only does a mural thrombus increase the degree of luminal stenosis, it provides for a rich source of potent platelet activation in the form of thrombin. This scenario was observed in a pig model of vessel injury with mural thrombus in which the direct thrombin inhibitor hirudin prevented extension of thrombus, whereas aspirin

and heparin did not [78]. In summary, the extent of stenosis, plaque disruption, size of the lipid core, and the presence of a mural thrombus are local factors that seem to increase thrombogenicity in the disrupted plaque.

Several systemic factors, including elevated cholesterol levels, increased catecholamine levels, smoking, and hyperglycemia, have been associated with increased thrombogenicity [4]. LDL-lowering therapy with 3-hydroxy-3-methylglutaryl coenzyme A (HMG-CoA) reductase inhibitors (statins) has been shown to decrease blood thrombogenicity and thrombus growth [79]. Although some of this effect may be caused by pleiotropic effects of statins, it is clear that LDL, and in particular oxidized LDL, plays a role in increased thrombotic activity. LDL promotes TF expression in plaque macrophages and expression of prothrombotic plasminogen activator inhibitor-1 in endothelial cells [14,71]. Elevated catecholamines are associated with increased platelet activation; activities that increase circulating catecholamines, such as cigarette smoking, [80] cocaine use [60], and increased physical activity [61], have been associated with triggering acute cardiovascular events. Smoking seems to be of particular importance in young patients who have underlying plaque erosion, reflecting the significance of increased systemic thrombogenicity in these patients whose lesions lack a lipid core [62]. Hyperglycemia associated with poor diabetic control results in increased blood thrombogenicity, caused in part by increased platelet activation and also by activation of the TF pathway [81,82]. Other metabolic abnormalities may also increase blood thrombogenicity. Activation of the renin-angiotensin-aldosterone system increases activity of plasminogen activator inhibitor-1, mediated by angiotensin II [27]. Lipoprotein (a) is structurally similar to plasminogen and may competitively inhibit its fibrinolytic activity [4]. It is also likely that several proinflammatory cytokines promote both atherosclerosis and plaque rupture and thrombogenesis, suggesting a role for systemic inflammation in the development of ACS [27].

Early management of the non–ST-segment elevation acute cardiac syndromes

The most recent update of the American College of Cardiology/American Heart Association guidelines for NSTE ACS highlights several areas of management, including early risk stratification, early use of aspirin and clopidogrel, indications for early invasive strategy, and use of Gp IIb/IIIa inhibitors (abciximab, tirofiban, and eptifibatide) based on risk. Additionally, the guidelines recommend an algorithm for use of specialized chest pain units to manage patients who have possible and low-risk ACS while avoiding unnecessary hospitalizations [3]. This section discusses the early management of NSTE ACS, that is, management during the patient's initial stay in the chest pain unit.

Risk assessment

Patient management in ACS begins with risk stratification based on clinical history, physical examination, and ancillary data such as 12-lead ECG and biomarkers of cardiac injury. Based on this initial assessment, patients can be categorized into one of four groups: noncardiac chest pain, chronic stable angina, possible ACS, and definite ACS. Those who have possible or definite ACS are observed in a chest pain unit until the diagnosis is confirmed or discounted [3].

Given the wide range of presentations subsumed within ACS, risk assessment is essential in determining the choice of therapy, specifically the use of Gp IIb/IIIa inhibitors and of early invasive therapy. Gp IIb/IIIa inhibitors bind the platelet receptor and prevent platelet aggregation [83]. Their use has been shown to reduce the frequency and duration of ischemia [83] and the rate of the combined endpoint of death, reinfarction, or refractory angina in patients who have NSTE ACS [84]. Early invasive therapy consists of coronary angiography and angiographically guided revascularization within 48 hours of symptom onset. This approach, compared with conservative therapy of medical management and noninvasive evaluation of ischemia, has also been shown to reduce rates of the combined endpoint of death, reinfarction, or 6-month rehospitalization [85]. Although these trials suggest an overall benefit for aggressive therapy in NSTE ACS, there is such a wide range of clinical presentations that the risk–benefit ratio for these therapies may also vary greatly, depending on individual patient's risk.

Obviously, the presence of hemodynamic instability, pulmonary edema, prolonged rest chest pain, or sustained ventricular tachycardia portends a poor short-term outcome and should be addressed with early institution of aggressive therapy [3]. Many patients who do not have these clear high-risk features upon presentation may benefit from aggressive therapy, however. To predict risk in these patients a variety of schema has been proposed. Among the easiest to use and best-validated is the Thrombolysis in Myocardial Infarction (TIMI) risk score (Box 1) [86]. A score exceeding 4 in this equally weighted seven-item scale allows identification of the patients who benefit most from early invasive and Gp IIb/IIIa inhibitor therapies based on short- and long-term risks [87]. Many investigators, citing the direct relationship between rising cardiac troponin levels and poor outcomes, have suggested that elevated troponin levels alone should be considered markers of high risk [3].

Treatment

Initial treatment for NSTE ACS includes continuous ECG monitoring for ischemia and possibility of arrhythmia. Additionally, anti-ischemic therapy should be initiated promptly, tailored to the level of patient risk. Finally, the mainstay of initial therapy is directed at addressing arterial thrombus: antiplatelet and anticoagulant therapy (Table 1).

Box 1. Thrombolysis in Myocardial Infarction (TIMI) risk score prediction variables

Age greater than 65 years

Three or more risk factors for coronary artery disease

Known coronary artery stenosis greater than 50%

ST-segment deviation on presenting ECG

Two or more episodes of angina within the preceding 24 hours

Use of aspirin within the preceding 7 days

Elevated serum cardiac biomarker levels

Adapted from Gluckman TJ, Sachdev M, Schulman SP, et al. A simplified approach to the management of non-ST elevation acute coronary syndromes. JAMA 2005;293(3):349; with permission.

Table 1
Summary of cardiovascular disease management in NSTE ACS

Intervention	Agent(s)/Treatment Modalities	Comments
Antiplatelet therapy	Aspirin	All patients indefinitely Initially with 162–325 mg followed by 75–160 mg daily thereafter

	ADP receptor antagonist
	  (clopidogrel)
		All patients, unless anticipated need for
		  urgent CABG surgery or within
		  5 days of electively scheduled CABG surgery
		Duration up to 1 year

	GP IIb/IIIa inhibitor (abciximab,
	  eptifibatide, tirofiban)
		All patients with continuing ischemia, an
		  elevated troponin level, a TIMI risk
		  score > 4, or anticipated PCI
		Avoid abciximab if PCI is not planned

Anticoagulation	Unfractionated heparin	Alternative to LMWH for patients managed with early invasive strategy

	Low molecular weight heparin	Preferred anticoagulant if managed conservatively
		Alternative to unfractioned heparin for patients
		  managed with an early invasive strategy
		Avoid if creatinine clearance
		  < 60 mL/min (unless anti-Xa levels
		  are to be followed) or CABG
		  surgery within 24 hours

ACE inhibition	No clear preferred agent	All patients with left ventricular
		  systolic dysfunction (ejection
		  fraction < 40%), heart failure, hypertension,
		  or other high-risk features

Angiotensin receptor
  blockade
	No clear preferred agent	All patients intolerant to ACE inhibitors
		Avoid combination therapy with
		  ACE inhibitors acutely, but consider
		  in patients with chronic left
		  ventricular systolic dysfunction
		  (ejection fraction < 40%) and heart failure

Beta blockade	No clear preferred agent	All patients
Blood pressure control	ACE inhibitors and beta blockers first line	Goal BP at least < 130/85 mm Hg

Abbreviations: ACE, angiotensin-converting enzyme; ADP, adenosine diphosphate; BP, blood pressure; CABG, coronary artery bypass graft; LMWH, low molecular weight heparin; PCI, percutaenous coronary interventions.

Adapted from Gluckman TJ, Sachdev M, Schulman SP, et al. A simplified approach to the management of non-ST elevation acute coronary syndromes. JAMA 2005;293(3):349; with permission.

Anti-ischemic therapy

Beta blockade reduces cardiac workload and oxygen demand, and the use of beta-blockers in the acute setting has been associated with a 13% relative risk reduction in progression to AMI [87]. The current recommendation is for prompt initiation of beta-blocker therapy unless contraindicated (eg, by marked first-degree atrioventricular block, second- or third-degree atrioventricular block, history of asthma, left ventricular dysfunction with congestive heart failure) [3]. A recommended initial regimen for high-risk patients is intravenous metoprolol, 5 mg every 5 minutes to a total of 15 mg; if tolerated, 25 to 50 mg oral metoprolol should be administered 15 minutes after the last intravenous dose and given every 6 hours for the first 48 hours. Patients at lower risk may be managed with oral therapy [3]. For patients in whom beta-blockers are contraindicated, the nondihydropyridine calcium antagonists verapamil and diltiazem may be used. One trial using intravenous verapamil in 3447 patients who had suspected MI showed a trend toward lower risk of death or nonfatal MI [88]. Guidelines recommend the use of long-acting nondihydropyridine calcium antagonists either in the setting of beta-blocker intolerance or if ischemic pain persists despite full use of beta blockade and nitrate administration [3].

Nitroglycerin is an endothelium-independent arterial vasodilator that increases myocardial blood flow through coronary vasodilation and decreases myocardial oxygen demand through venodilation and reduced preload [89]. In the absence of contraindications such as hypotension or concurrent use of sildenafil, tadafil, or vardenafil within 24 hours, intravenous nitroglycerin is recommended for the patient who has ongoing chest pain despite three doses of sublingual nitroglycerin and administration of beta-blockers [3]. The purpose of nitroglycerin is to relieve ischemic pain, because it has not been demonstrated to improve survival [90,91]. American College of Cardiology guidelines currently recommend the use of intravenous morphine sulfate at doses of 1 to 5 mg if nitrate and beta-blocker therapy fail to relieve pain and in patients who have acute pulmonary edema, with care taken to avoid hypotension [3]. Recent registry data regarding 57,039 patients treated for NSTE ACS at 443 United States hospitals, however, showed that the 17,003 patients who received intravenous morphine within 24 hours of presentation had a higher adjusted risk of death (odds ratio, 1.48; 95% CI, 1.33–1.64), even though patients receiving morphine were also more likely to receive acute evidence-based therapies and to be treated by a cardiologist. These data suggest that morphine sulfate in acute NSTE ACS may not be as safe as previously thought and that randomized trials are needed [92].

HMG-CoA reductase inhibitors have been shown to decrease blood thrombogenicity [79], and early aggressive therapy with these agents in the setting of AMI reduced the risk of a combined endpoint of death, MI, unstable angina rehospitalization, revascularization, and stroke [93]. This therapy was instituted 10 days after presentation, however. It is unclear if administration of statins in the acute setting is of additional benefit.

Antiplatelet therapy

Given the central role of platelet activation and aggregation in thrombus formation, it is reasonable to expect that antiplatelet therapy would be at the core of NSTE ACS management. Recommended agents include aspirin, which inhibits platelet aggregation and activation primarily by inhibiting thromboxane A_2 synthesis, clopidogrel, which inhibits platelet activation by blocking the adenosine diphosphate receptor, and the Gp IIb/IIIa inhibitors.

Aspirin has been shown to reduce the rates of death or nonfatal MI by 51% (5% versus 10.1%; $P = .0005$) in patients who have unstable angina, without an increase in gastrointestinal symptoms [94]. Current guidelines recommend an initial dose of 162 to 325 mg followed by a daily dose of 75 to 160 mg [3].

In the Clopidogrel in Unstable Angina to Prevent Recurrent Ischemic Events (CURE) study, 12,562 patients who had NSTE ACS were randomly assigned to clopidogrel (300 mg loading dose followed by 75 mg daily for 9 months) and aspirin (75–325 mg daily) versus aspirin alone [95]. The group receiving clopidogrel had a relative risk reduction of 20% in the combined endpoint of cardiovascular death, nonfatal MI, or stroke (9.3% versus 11.4%; $P < .001$). The benefit was driven primarily by a reduction in risk of subsequent MI (5.2% versus 6.7%; relative risk, 0.77; 95% CI, 0.67–0.89). The benefit of clopidogrel also holds for patients undergoing percutaneous coronary interventions (PCI). The PCI-CURE study randomly assigned 2658 patients who had NSTE ACS and who were scheduled for PCI to pretreatment with clopidogrel plus aspirin versus aspirin alone; treatment was initiated a median of 6 days before PCI and continued for 8 months [96]. Patients who received clopidogrel experienced a 30% relative risk reduction in the combined endpoint of cardiovascular death, nonfatal MI, or urgent target vessel revascularization at 30 days and a 31% relative risk reduction of cardiovascular death or nonfatal MI at study end. Although clopidogrel is clearly beneficial in NSTE ACS, there are caveats to its use. In the CURE trial, major bleeding was significantly more common in the clopidogrel arm (3.7% versus 2.7%; $P = .001$), although there was no significant increase in life-threatening bleeding [95]. Additionally, use of clopidogrel within 5 days of surgery can increase bleeding risk [97]. Current guidelines recommend prompt initiation of clopidogrel, with use for at least 1 month and up to 9 months, withheld 5 to 7 days before coronary artery bypass grafting. Additionally, patients who have intolerance or hypersensitivity to aspirin should be given clopidogrel instead [3].

Benefit from Gp IIb/IIIa inhibitors is closely tied to patient risk and therefore to concomitant use of an early invasive strategy. A meta-analysis of six trials including 31,402 patients who had NSTE ACS and who were managed with conservative strategy found that benefit of Gp IIb/IIIa inhibitor use was limited to those who had elevated troponin levels or who needed early revascularization, that is, higher-risk patients [98]. Furthermore, in patients who had NSTE ACS and who were treated conservatively, the Gp IIb/IIIa inhibitor abciximab demonstrates no benefit and may be harmful [99]. In patients undergoing PCI, however, there is clear benefit to Gp IIb/IIIa inhibitor use. A meta-analysis of eight trials (14,644 patients) of any Gp IIb/IIIa inhibitor versus placebo in patients undergoing PCI showed a reduction of both MI rate (5% versus 7.8%; $P < .001$) and need for urgent revascularization (3.4% versus 5.9%; $P < .001$) [100]. Subgroup analysis in study showed that only abciximab resulted in a significant reduction in AMI after PCI. This effect may reflect the timing of PCI relative to drug administration. Data suggest that abciximab is the Gp IIb/IIIa inhibitor of choice for PCI within 4 hours of presentation, whereas tirofiban and eptifibatide should be used if PCI is deferred [87]. Based on these data, current guidelines recommend administration of eptifibatide or tirofiban (but not abciximab) to high-risk patients (ie, those who have elevated troponin levels, a TIMI risk score greater than 4, continuing ischemia) who have NSTE ACS and are undergoing conservative therapy [3,87]. Because the decision to proceed to PCI and the timing thereof are not always clear at the time of initial presentation, the choice of agent in this setting may be deferred until the time of PCI [3].

In summary, all patients who have NSTE ACS should receive aspirin and clopidogrel on presentation, unless there is anticipated need for urgent surgical revascularization. Gp IIb/IIIa inhibitors are clearly recommended in high-risk patients and those referred to PCI (ie, those with high-risk clinical features, TIMI score greater than 4, or elevated troponin levels). Unfortunately, there are no large-scale studies that evaluate the incremental benefit of combined use of all three proposed antiplatelet therapies versus strategies using only two agents.

Anticoagulation

Heparin potentiates thrombin inactivation by circulating antithrombin III, thus preventing thrombus extension [101]. In a meta-analysis of six trials of patients who had unstable angina treated with unfractionated heparin (UFH) for 2 to 5 days plus aspirin versus aspirin alone, there was a 33% relative risk reduction in the incidence of death or MI (7.9% versus 10.4%; $P = .06$) [102]. Unfortunately, UFH requires frequent monitoring

of the activated partial thromboplastin time (aPTT) and has been associated with delays in achieving appropriate anticoagulation, an aPTT 1.5 to 2.5 times control [103]. Low molecular weight heparin (LMWH) has more predictable pharmacokinetics, is more readily bioavailable, and is administered subcutaneously [103]. A recent meta-analysis of six trials encompassing 21,946 patients sought to compare the efficacy and safety of the LMWH enoxaparin at 1 mg/kg every 12 hours and UFH in patients who had NSTE ACS. At 30 days, there was no statistically significant difference in mortality and a small difference in the combined endpoint of death or MI favoring enoxaparin (10.1% versus 11.0%; 95% CI, 0.83–0.99), without significant difference in major bleeding [104]. The analysis showed benefit of LMWH over UFH in patients treated conservatively. Current guidelines recommend the use of LMWH in addition to aspirin in patients who have NSTE ACS unless coronary artery bypass grafting is planned within 24 hours [3]. For patients who have renal insufficiency or in whom early invasive strategy is planned, UFH is probably a better choice [87].

Another parenteral anticoagulant, the direct thrombin inhibitor hirudin, has been studied in NSTE ACS. In the trial by the Organisation to Assess Strategies for Ischemic Syndromes (OASIS-2), 10,141 patients who had NSTE ACS were randomly assigned to receive a 72-hour infusion of UFH or hirudin [105]. At 7 days those in the hirudin group had a lower (but not statistically significant) rate of the combined endpoint of death or new MI (3.6% versus 4.2%; relative risk, 0.84; 95% CI, 0.69–1.02, $P = .077$). Most of the benefit occurred during the drug infusion period, suggesting that the outcome of the therapies equalizes with time. A meta-analysis of 11 randomized trials consisting of 35,790 patients compared the use of any direct thrombin inhibitor (hirudin, bivalirudin, argatroban, efegatran, or inogatran) with UFH in patients who had ACS. At 30 days, there was a lower rate of death or MI in the group treated with direct thrombin inhibitors (7.4% versus 8.2%; relative risk, 0.91, 95% CI, 0.84–0.99, $P = .02$) [106]. The use of direct thrombin inhibitors along with aspirin and clopidogrel or Gp IIb/IIIa inhibitors in NSTE ACS has not been studied in large-scale trials; thus their incremental benefit is not known. Furthermore, hirudin has been shown to increase bleeding risks compared with heparin [105]. Although more studies are expected, routine use of direct thrombin inhibitors in NSTE ACS is not currently recommended [3].

Patients in the chest pain unit who have suspected NSTE ACS should be given UFH if early PCI is planned or if severe renal insufficiency (creatinine clearance < 60 mL/minute) is present. Otherwise, LMWH should be used in addition to aspirin and clopidogrel. The role for direct thrombin inhibitors is unclear at present.

Summary

NSTE ACS is a clinically significant problem. Endothelial dysfunction triggered by traditional cardiovascular risk factors (and perhaps by other as yet unidentified risks) in the susceptible host leads to the formation and development of atherosclerotic plaque. Inflammatory mediators and mechanical stresses contribute to plaque rupture by disrupting the protective fibrous cap. In about 25% of patients who have ACS, typically those who are younger, female, or smokers, plaque erosion seems to be the main underlying pathologic mechanism. Endothelial alteration, inflammation, or exposure of the lipid core results in the release of TF, vWF, and PAF. The release of these factors leads to platelet activation and aggregation as well as to the formation of a fibrin clot, resulting in arterial thrombosis that occludes the vessel. A variety of factors, including circulating catecholamines, LDL levels, blood glucose levels, and systemic thrombogenic factors, can affect the extent and stability of the thrombus, thereby determining whether the occlusion is complete and fixed, labile and nonocclusive (NSTE ACS), or clinically silent resulting in a mural thrombus and plaque growth. The acute treatment of NSTE ACS is directed at interrupting the prothrombotic environment surrounding the ruptured plaque; thus, antiplatelet agents such as aspirin, clopidogrel, and glycoprotein IIb/IIIa receptor antagonists, as well as anticoagulants such as heparin, are the mainstays of early therapy.

References

[1] McCaig LF, Burt CW. National Hospital Ambulatory Medical Care Survey: 2001 emergency department summary. Advance data from Vital and Health Statistics # 335. Hyattsville (MD): National Center for Health Statistics; 2003.

[2] Kozak LJ, Owings MF, Hall MJ. National Hospital Discharge Survey: 2001 annual summary with detailed diagnosis and procedure data. National Center for Health Statistics. Vital Health Stat 2004;13:156.

[3] Braunwald E, Antman EM, Beasley JW, et al. ACC/AHA 2002 guideline update for the management of patients with unstable angina and non–ST-segment elevation myocardial infarction: a report of the American College of Cardiology/American Heart Association Task Force on Practice Guidelines (Committee on the Management of Patients With Unstable Angina). 2002. Available at: http://www.acc.org/clinical/guidelines/unstable/unstable.pdf. Accessed February 1, 2005.

[4] Fuster V, Badimon L, Badimon JJ, et al. The pathogenesis of coronary artery disease and the acute coronary syndromes. N Engl J Med 1992;326 (4,5):242–50; 310–7.

[5] DeWood MA, Stifter WF, Simpson CS, et al. Coronary arteriographic findings soon after non-Q-wave myocardial infarction. N Engl J Med 1986; 315(7):417–23.

[6] Ross R. The pathogenesis of atherosclerosis—an update. N Engl J Med 1986;314(8):488–500.

[7] Stary HC, Chandler AB, Glagov S, et al. A definition of initial, fatty streak, and intermediate lesions of atherosclerosis. Circulation 1994;89(5):2462–78.

[8] Stary HC. Macrophages, macrophage foam cells, and eccentric intimal thickening in the coronary arteries of young children. Atherosclerosis 1987; 64(2–3):91–108.

[9] Stary HC. Evolution and progression of atherosclerotic lesions in coronary arteries of children and young adults. Arteriosclerosis 1989;9(Suppl I): I-19–32.

[10] Stary HC, Chandler AB, Dinsmore RE, et al. A definition of advanced types of atherosclerotic lesions and a histological classification of atherosclerosis. Circulation 1995;92(5):1355–74.

[11] Glagov S, Weisenberg E, Zarins CK, et al. Compensatory enlargement of human atherosclerotic coronary arteries. N Engl J Med 1987;316(22): 1371–5.

[12] Losordo DW, Rosenfield K, Kaufman J, et al. Focal compensatory enlargement of human arteries in response to progressive atherosclerosis. Circulation 1994;89(6):2570–7.

[13] Davies MJ. Stability and instability: two faces of coronary atherosclerosis. The Paul Dudley White Lecture 1995. Circulation 1996;94(8):2013–20.

[14] Cines DB, Pollak ES, Buck CA, et al. Endothelial cells in physiology and in the pathophysiology of vascular disorders. Blood 1998;91(10):3527–61.

[15] Kinlay S, Libby P, Ganz P. Endothelial function and coronary artery disease. Curr Opin Lipidol 2001;12(4):383–9.

[16] Barnes PJ, Karin M. Nuclear factor-kappa B: a pivotal transcription factor in chronic inflammatory diseases. N Engl J Med 1997;336(15):1066–71.

[17] Nelken NA, Coughlin SR, Gordon D, et al. Monocyte chemoattractant protein-1 in human atheromatous plaques. J Clin Invest 1991;88(4): 1121–7.

[18] Mallat Z, Corbaz A, Scoazec A, et al. Expression of interleukin-18 in human atherosclerotic plaques and relation to plaque instability. Circulation 2001;104(14):1598–603.

[19] Schieffer B, Schieffer E, Hilfiker-Kleiner D, et al. Expression of angiotensin II and interleukin 6 in human coronary atherosclerotic plaques: potential implications for inflammation and plaque instability. Circulation 2000;101(12):1372–8.

[20] Rosenfeld ME, Yla-Herttuala S, Lipton BA, et al. Macrophage colony-stimulating factor mRNA and protein in atherosclerotic lesions of rabbits and humans. Am J Pathol 1992;140(2):291–300.

[21] Uyemura K, Demer LL, Castle SC, et al. Cross-regulatory roles of interleukin (IL)-12 and IL-10 in atherosclerosis. J Clin Invest 1996;97(9):2130–8.

[22] Sukhova GK, Schonbeck U, Rabkin E, et al. Evidence for increased collagenolysis by interstitial collagenases-1 and -3 in vulnerable human atheromatous plaques. Circulation 1999;99(19):2503–9.

[23] Libby P. The molecular bases of the acute coronary syndromes. Circulation 1995;91(11):2844–50.

[24] Braunwald E. Unstable angina: an etiologic approach to management. Circulation 1998;98(21):2219–22.

[25] Davies MJ, Thomas A. Thrombosis and acute coronary artery lesions in sudden cardiac ischemic death. N Engl J Med 1984;310(18):1137–40.

[26] Virmani R, Kolodgie FD, Burke AP, et al. Lessons from sudden coronary death: a comprehensive morphological classification scheme for atherosclerotic lesions. Arterioscler Thromb Vasc Biol 2000;20(5):1262–75.

[27] Libby P. Current concepts of the pathogenesis of the acute coronary syndromes. Circulation 2001;104(3):365–72.

[28] van der Wal AC, Becker AE, van der Loos CM, et al. Site of intimal rupture or erosion of thrombosed coronary atherosclerotic plaques is characterized by an inflammatory process irrespective of the dominant plaque morphology. Circulation 1994;89(1):36–44.

[29] Burke AP, Farb A, Malcom GT, et al. Coronary risk factors and plaque morphology in men with coronary disease who died suddenly. N Engl J Med 1997;336(18):1276–82.

[30] Davies MJ, Richardson PD, Woolf N, et al. Risk of thrombosis in human atherosclerotic plaques: role of extracellular lipid, macrophage, and smooth muscle cell content. Br Heart J 1993;69(5):377–81.

[31] Kolodgie FD, Virmani R, Burke AP, et al. Pathologic assessment of the vulnerable human coronary plaque. Heart 2004;90(12):1385–91.

[32] Thieme T, Wernecke KD, Meyer R, et al. Angioscopic evaluation of atherosclerotic plaques: validation by histomorphologic analysis and association with stable and unstable coronary syndromes. J Am Coll Cardiol 1996;28(1):1–6.

[33] Libby P. The molecular bases of the acute coronary syndromes. Circulation 1995;91(11):2844–50.

[34] Moreno PR, Falk E, Palacios IF, et al. Macrophage infiltration in acute coronary syndromes: implications for plaque rupture. Circulation 1994;90(2):775–8.

[35] Galis ZS, Sukhova GK, Lark MW, et al. Increased expression of matrix metalloproteinases and matrix degrading activity in vulnerable regions of human atherosclerotic plaques. J Clin Invest 1994;94(6):2493–503.

[36] Libby P, Sukhova GK, Lee RT, et al. Cytokines regulate vascular functions related to stability of the atherosclerotic plaque. J Cardiovasc Pharmacol 1995;25(Suppl 2):S9–12.

[37] Mach F, Schonbeck U, Bonnefoy JY, et al. Activation of monocyte/macrophage functions related to acute atheroma complication by ligation of CD40. Circulation 1997;96(2):396–9.

[38] Lee RT, Schoen FJ, Loree HM, et al. Circumferential stress and matrix metalloproteinase 1 in human coronary atherosclerosis. Implications for plaque rupture. Arterioscler Thromb Vasc Biol 1996;16(8):1070–3.

[39] Naruko T, Ueda M, Haze K, et al. Neutrophil infiltration of culprit lesions in acute coronary syndromes. Circulation 2002;106(23):2894–900.

[40] Herman MP, Sukhova GK, Libby P, et al. Expression of neutrophil collagenase (matrix metalloproteinase-8) in human atheroma: a novel collagenolytic pathway suggested by transcriptional profiling. Circulation 2001;104(16):1899–904.

[41] Xu XP, Meisel SR, Ong JM, et al. Oxidized low-density lipoprotein regulates matrix metalloproteinase-9 and its tissue inhibitor in human monocyte-derived macrophages. Circulation 1999;99(8):993–8.

[42] Sukhova GK, Shi GP, Simon DI, et al. Expression of the elastolytic cathepsins S and K in human atheroma and regulation of their production in smooth muscle cells. J Clin Invest 1998;102(3):576–83.

[43] Geng YJ, Wu Q, Muszynski M, et al. Apoptosis of vascular smooth muscle cells induced by in vitro stimulation with interferon-gamma, tumor necrosis factor-alpha, and interleukin-1 beta. Arterioscler Thromb Vasc Biol 1996;16(1):19–27.

[44] Buffon A, Biasucci LM, Liuzzo G, et al. Widespread coronary inflammation in unstable angina. N Engl J Med 2002;347(1):5–12.

[45] Rioufol G, Finet G, Ginon I, et al. Multiple atherosclerotic plaque rupture in acute coronary syndrome: a three-vessel intravascular ultrasound study. Circulation 2002;106(7):804–8.

[46] Liuzzo G, Baisucci LM, Gallimore JR, et al. Enhanced inflammatory response in patients with preinfarction unstable angina. J Am Coll Cardiol 1999;34(6):1696–703.

[47] Richardson PD, Davies MJ, Born GV. Influence of plaque configuration and stress distribution on fissuring of coronary atherosclerotic plaques. Lancet 1989;2(8669):941–4.

[48] Cheng GC, Loree HM, Kamm RD, et al. Distribution of circumferential stress in ruptured and stable atherosclerotic lesions: a structural analysis with histopathological correlation. Circulation 1993; 87(4):1179–87.

[49] Dirksen MT, van der Wal AC, van den Berg FM, et al. Distribution of inflammatory cells in atherosclerotic plaques relates to the direction of flow. Circulation 1998;98(19):2000–3.

[50] Lendon CL, Davies MJ, Born GV, et al. Atherosclerotic plaque caps are locally weakened when macrophage density is increased. Atherosclerosis 1991;87(1):87–90.

[51] Loree HM, Kamm RD, Stringfellow RG, et al. Effects of fibrous cap thickness on peak circumferential stress in model atherosclerotic vessels. Circ Res 1992;71(4):850–8.

[52] Schoenhagen P, Ziada KM, Kapadia SR, et al. Extent and direction of arterial remodeling in stable versus unstable coronary syndromes: an intravascular ultrasound study. Circulation 2000;101(6): 598–603.

[53] Varnava AM, Mills PG, Davies MJ. Relationship between coronary artery remodeling and plaque vulnerability. Circulation 2002;105(8):939–43.

[54] Takano M, Mizuno K, Okamatsu K, et al. Mechanical and structural characteristics of vulnerable plaques: analysis by coronary angioscopy and intravascular ultrasound. J Am Coll Cardiol 2001;38(1):99–104.

[55] Lafont A, Durand E, Samuel JL, et al. Endothelial dysfunction and collagen accumulation: two independent factors for restenosis and constrictive remodeling after experimental angioplasty. Circulation 1999;100(10):1109–15.

[56] Giroud D, Li JM, Urban P, et al. Relation of the site of acute myocardial infarction to the most severe coronary arterial stenosis prior to angiography. Am J Cardiol 1992;69(8):729–32.

[57] Ambrose JA, Tannenbaum MA, Alexopoulos D, et al. Angiographic progression of coronary artery disease and the development of myocardial infarction. J Am Coll Cardiol 1988;12(1): 56–62.

[58] Peters A, Dockery DW, Muller JE, et al. Increased particulate air pollution and the triggering of myocardial infarction. Circulation 2001;103(23): 2810–5.

[59] Mittleman MA, Lewis RA, Maclure M, et al. Triggering myocardial infarction by marijuana. Circulation 2001;103(23):2805–9.

[60] Mittleman MA, Mintzer D, Maclure M, et al. Triggering of myocardial infarction by cocaine. Circulation 1999;99(21):2737–41.

[61] Muller JE. Circadian variation and triggering of acute coronary events. Am Heart J 1999;137(4 Pt 2):S1–8.

[62] Farb A, Burke AP, Tang AL, et al. Coronary plaque erosion without rupture into a lipid core: a frequent cause of coronary thrombosis in sudden coronary death. Circulation 1996;93(7): 1354–63.

[63] Arbustini E, Dal Bello B, Morbini P, et al. Plaque erosion is a major substrate for coronary thrombosis in acute myocardial infarction. Heart 1999; 82(3):269–72.

[64] Mallat Z, Hugel B, Ohan J, et al. Shed membrane microparticles with procoagulant potential in human atherosclerotic plaques: a role for apoptosis in plaque thrombogenicity. Circulation 1999; 99(3):348–53.

[65] Davies MJ. The pathophysiology of acute coronary syndromes. Heart 2000;83(3):361–6.

[66] Kroll MH, Hellums JD, McIntyre LV, et al. Platelets and shear stress. Blood 1996;88(5):1525–41.

[67] Shafer AI, Ali NM, Levine GN. Hemostasis, thrombosis, fibrinolysis, and cardiovascular disease. In: Braunwald E, Zipes DP, Libby P, editors. Heart disease: a textbook of cardiovascular medicine. 6th edition. Philadelphia: W.B. Saunders; 2001. p. 2099–107.

[68] Fitzgerald DJ, Roy L, Catella F, et al. Platelet activation in unstable coronary disease. N Engl J Med 1986;315(16):983–9.

[69] Fernandez-Ortiz A, Badimon JJ, Falk E, et al. Characterization of relative thrombogenicity of atherosclerotic plaque components: implications for consequences of plaque rupture. J Am Coll Cardiol 1994;23(7):1562–9.

[70] Guyton JR, Klemp KF. The lipid-rich core region of human atherosclerotic fibrous plaques: prevalence of small lipid droplets and vesicles by electron microscopy. Am J Pathol 1989;134(3): 705–17.

[71] Moreno PR, Bernardi VH, Lopez-Cuellar J, et al. Macrophages, smooth muscle cells, and tissue factor in unstable angina. Implications for cell-mediated thrombogenicity in acute coronary syndromes. Circulation 1996;94(12):3090–7.

[72] Toschi V, Gallo G, Lettino M, et al. Tissue factor modulates thrombogenicity of human atherosclerotic plaques. Circulation 1997;95(3):594–9.

[73] Nemerson Y. Tissue factor and hemostasis. Blood 1988;71(1):1–8.

[74] Falk E. Unstable angina with fatal outcome: dynamic coronary thrombosis leading to infarction and/or sudden death. Circulation 1985;71(4): 699–708.

[75] Burke AP, Kolodgie FD, Farb A, et al. Healed plaque ruptures and sudden coronary death: evidence that subclinical rupture has a role in plaque progression. Circulation 2001;103(7):934–40.

[76] Lassila R, Badimon JJ, Vallabhajosula S, et al. Dynamic monitoring of platelet deposition on severely damaged vessel wall in flowing blood: effects of different stenosis on thrombus growth. Arteriosclerosis 1990;10(2):306–15.

[77] Badimon L, Badimon JJ, Turitto VT, et al. Platelet thrombus formation on collagen type I: a model of deep vessel injury. Circulation 1988;78(6): 1431–42.

[78] Meyer BJ, Badimon JJ, Mahilac A, et al. Inhibition of growth of thrombus on fresh mural thrombus. Targeting optimal therapy. Circulation 1994; 90(5):2432–8.

[79] Rauch U, Osende JI, Chesboro JH, et al. Statins and cardiovascular diseases: the multiple effects of lipid-lowering therapy by statins. Atherosclerosis 2000;153(1):181–9.

[80] Narkiewicz K, van de Borne PJ, Hausber M, et al. Cigarette smoking increases sympathetic outflow in humans. Circulation 1998;98(6):528–34.

[81] Osende JI, Badimon JJ, Fuster V, et al. Thrombogenicity in type 2 diabetes mellitus patients is associated with glycemic control. J Am Coll Cardiol 2001;38(5):1307–12.

[82] Rao AK, Chouhan V, Chen X, et al. Activation of the tissue factor pathway of blood coagulation during prolonged hyperglycemia in young healthy men. Diabetes 1999;48(5):1156–61.

[83] Schulman SP, Goldschmidt-Clermont PJ, Topol EJ, et al. Effects of integrelin, a platelet glycoprotein IIb/IIIa receptor antagonist, in unstable angina. A randomized multicenter trial. Circulation 1996;94(9):2083–9.

[84] The platelet receptor inhibition in ischemic syndrome management in patients limited by unstable signs and symptoms (PRISM-PLUS) study investigators. Inhibition of the platelet glycoprotein IIb/IIIa receptor with tirofiban in unstable angina and non-Q wave myocardial infarction. N Engl J Med 1998;338(21):1488–97.

[85] Cannon CP, Weintraub WS, Demopoulos LA, et al. Comparison of early invasive and conservative strategies in patients with unstable coronary syndromes treated with the glycoprotein IIb/IIIa inhibitor tirofiban. N Engl J Med 2001;344(25): 1879–87.

[86] Antman EM, Cohen M, Bernink PJ, et al. The TIMI risk score for unstable angina/non-ST elevation MI: a method for prognostication and therapeutic decision making. JAMA 2000; 284(7):835–42.

[87] Gluckman TJ, Sachdev M, Schulman SP, et al. A simplified approach to the management of non-ST elevation acute coronary syndromes. JAMA 2005;293(3):349–57.

[88] The Danish Study Group on Verapamil in Myocardial Infarction. Effect of verapamil on mortality and major events after acute infarction. Am J Cardiol 1990;66(10):779–85.

[89] Cannon CP, Braunwald E. Unstable angina. In: Braunwald E, Zipes DP, Libby P, editors. Heart disease: a textbook of cardiovascular medicine. 6th edition. Philadelphia: W.B. Saunders; 2001. p. 1241–9.

[90] Fourth International Study of Infarct Survival Collaborative Group. ISIS-4: a randomised factorial trial assessing early oral captopril, oral mononitrate, and intravenous magnesium sulphate in 58,050 patients with suspected acute myocardial infarction. Lancet 1995;345(8951):669–85.

[91] Gruppo Italiano per lo Studio della Sopravvivenza nell'infarto Miocardico. Effects of lisinopril and transdermal glyceryl trinitrate singly and together on 6-week mortality and ventricular function after acute myocardial infarction. Lancet 1994; 343(8906):1115–22.

[92] Meine TJ, Roe MT, Chen AY, et al. Association of intravenous morphine use and outcomes in acute coronary syndromes: results from the CRUSADE quality improvement initiative. Am Heart J 2005; 149:1043–9.

[93] Cannon CP, Braunwald E, McCabe CH, et al. Intensive versus moderate lipid lowering with statins after acute coronary syndrome. N Engl J Med 2004;350(15):1495–504.

[94] Lewis HD Jr, Davis JW, Archibald DG, et al. Protective effects of aspirin against acute myocardial infarction and death in patients with unstable angina: results of a Veterans Administration Cooperative Study. N Engl J Med 1983;309(7): 396–403.

[95] The CURE investigators. Effects of clopidogrel in addition to aspirin in patients with acute coronary syndromes without ST-segment elevation. N Engl J Med 2001;345(7):494–502.

[96] Mehta SR, Yusuf S, Peters RJ, et al. Effects of pretreatment with clopidogrel and aspirin followed by long-term therapy in patients undergoing percutaneous coronary intervention: the PCI-CURE study. Lancet 2001;358(9281):527–33.

[97] Hongo RH, Ley J, Dick SE, et al. The effect of clopidogrel in combination with aspirin when given before coronary artery bypass grafting. J Am Coll Cardiol 2002;29(2):2271–5.

[98] Boersma E, Harrington RA, Moliterno DJ, et al. Platelet glycoprotein IIb/IIIa inhibitors in acute coronary syndromes: a meta-analysis of all major randomized clinical trials. Lancet 2002;359(9302): 189–98.

[99] Global use of strategies to open occluded in acute coronary syndromes (GUSTO IV-ACS) Investigators. Effect of glycoprotein IIb/IIIa receptor blocker abciximab on outcome in patients with acute coronary syndromes without early coronary revascularisation: the GUSTO IV-ACS randomised trial. Lancet 2001;357(9272):1915–24.

[100] Brown DL, Fann CS, Chang CJ. Meta-analysis of effectiveness and safety of abciximab versus

eptifibatide or tirofiban in percutaneous coronary intervention. Am J Cardiol 2001;87(5):537–41.

[101] Hirsh J. Heparin. N Engl J Med 1991;324(22): 1565–74.

[102] Oler A, Whooley MA, Oler J, et al. Adding heparin to aspirin reduces the incidence of myocardial infarction and death in patients with unstable angina. A meta-analysis. JAMA 1996;276(10):811–5.

[103] Cohen M, Demers C, Gurfinkel EP, et al for the Efficacy and Safety of Subcutaneous Enoxaparin in Non-Q Wave Coronary Events (ESSENCE) study group. A comparison of low molecular weight heparin with unfractionated heparin for unstable coronary artery disease. N Engl J Med 1997;337(7): 447–52.

[104] Petersen JL, Mahaffey KW, Hasselblad V, et al. Efficacy and bleeding complications among patients randomized to enoxaparin or unfractionated heparin for antithrombin therapy in non-ST-segment elevation acute coronary syndromes: a systematic overview. JAMA 2004;292(1):89–96.

[105] Organisation to Assess Strategies for Ischemic Syndromes. (OASIS-2) Investigators. Effects of recombinant hirudin (lepirudin) compared with heparin on death, myocardial infarction, refractory angina, and revascularisation procedures in patients with acute myocardial ischaemia without ST elevation: a randomised trial. Lancet 1999; 353(9151):429–38.

[106] Direct Thrombin Inhibitor Trialists' Collaborative Group. Direct thrombin inhibitors in acute coronary syndromes: principal results of a meta-analysis based on individual patients' data. Lancet 2002;359(9303):294–302.

ELSEVIER
SAUNDERS

CARDIOLOGY
CLINICS

Cardiol Clin 24 (2006) 37–51

Early Management of ST-segment Elevation Myocardial Infarction

Amish C. Sura, MD, Mark D. Kelemen, MD, MSc, FACC*

Division of Cardiology, University of Maryland School of Medicine, 22 South Greene Street, Baltimore, MD 21202, USA

The primary goal in treating ST-segment elevation myocardial infarction (STEMI), a condition caused by acute coronary occlusion, is rapid, early, complete, and sustained myocardial reperfusion. Animal models of coronary occlusion have demonstrated myocardial necrosis after 30 minutes, with 50% myocardial salvage if reperfusion is accomplished within 90 minutes [1]. Reperfusion in STEMI limits myocardial damage and reduces mortality by about 25% [2]. Various pharmacologic and mechanical reperfusion options are available that differ in efficacy based on time to treatment from symptom onset and hemodynamic status at presentation. Surgical approaches have limited utility as acute therapies for STEMI [3]. More important than the mode of reperfusion is the rapid initiation of a reperfusion strategy once a patient is identified as having a STEMI. The American College of Cardiology (ACC)/American Heart Association (AHA) guidelines suggest a maximum time from initial medical contact to initiation of thrombolytic therapy of 30 minutes and to balloon inflation of no more than 90 minutes if percutaneous coronary intervention (PCI) is chosen [3]. Several algorithms for identification of patients who have STEMI and choice of reperfusion therapy have been developed, each taking into account time to presentation, contraindications to therapy, and the hemodynamic status of the patient [4]. A realistic assessment of time required to initiate therapy must also factor in the choice of reperfusion strategy.

Pharmacologic reperfusion

Thrombolytic therapy with streptokinase was first attempted in 1958 [5]. Direct intracoronary administration was used briefly in the mid 1970s and early 1980s but was abandoned when intravenous administration was found to have similar efficacy [6–10]. Thrombolytic agents have a high specificity for the substrate plasminogen, hydrolyzing a peptide bond to yield the active enzyme plasmin. Free plasmin is rapidly neutralized by the serine proteinase inhibitor alpha-antiplasmin, whereas fibrin-bound plasmin is protected from rapid inhibition, thereby promoting clot lysis. Given its relative ease of administration and proven mortality benefit, intravenous thrombolytic therapy is the most common form of reperfusion therapy worldwide [11]. The benefits of reperfusion therapy are time related (Fig. 1), with decreasing benefits with increasing delays to therapy [2]. The beneficial effect of fibrinolytic therapy is substantially higher in patients presenting within 2 hours after symptom onset than in those presenting later [12]. Administration of thrombolytics primarily occurs upon patient presentation to the hospital, but prehospital thrombolysis reduces time to treatment by up to 1 hour and reduces mortality by 17% [13].

A 1994 meta-analysis from the Fibrinolytic Therapy Trialists' Collaborative Group found that the absolute mortality benefit at 5 weeks was 3% for those presenting within 6 hours from symptom onset, 2% for those presenting within 7 to 12 hours, and a nonsignificant benefit of 1% for those presenting within 13 to 18 hours [2]. The net effect in major thrombolytic trials has been an approximately 30% relative risk reduction in

* Corresponding author.

E-mail address: mkelemen@medicine.umaryland.edu (M.D. Kelemen).

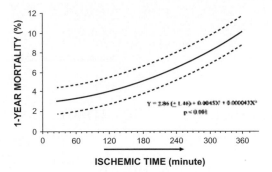

Fig. 1. There is a continuous relationship between time-to-treatment and mortality at 1 year, with increasing delays resulting in increased mortality. The relationship between time-to-treatment and 1-year mortality, as a continuous function, was assessed with a quadratic regression model. Dotted lines represent 95% CIs of predicted mortality. (*Modified from* Rogers WJCJ, Lambrew CT, et al. Temporal trends in the treatment of over 1.5 million patients who had myocardial infarction in the US from 1990 through 1999: the National Registry of Myocardial Infarction 1, 2 and 3. J Am Coll Cardiol 2000;36:2056–63; with permission.)

short-term mortality to an absolute value of 7% to 10%; the clinical advantage persists for at least 10 years [14,15]. A similar improvement in survival has been noted in community-based studies [16]. Several studies have demonstrated that the morbidity and mortality effects of thrombolytics are realized only if therapy is given within 12 hours of symptom onset [3,17,18]. Most patients, however, still do not receive thrombolytics within the recommended 30 minutes from presentation to the medical system [19].

Although time from symptom onset to initiation of therapy is a critical determinant of survival, many patients who have STEMI and are eligible for reperfusion receive delayed treatment or no treatment at all. Results from the multinational Global Registry of Acute Coronary Events (GRACE) show that approximately one third of patients who had STEMI and who had no known contraindications did not receive reperfusion therapy, and this finding was independent of geographic region [20–22]. Fear of bleeding complications from fibrinolytic drugs is the primary reason for underuse of these drugs [22].

Thrombolytic agents do have several limitations. There is failure to achieve patency in 15% to 20% of patients, failure to achieve normal (Thrombolysis in Myocardial Infarction trial [TIMI] grade III) flow in 40 to 50% of patients,

and a 10% to 15% rate of reocclusion [23]. There is also a 0.5% to 1% risk of intracranial hemorrhage [24,25]. As a result, there is an ongoing effort to develop newer agents that may overcome these limitations and enhance efficacy. The ideal thrombolytic agent should be fibrin specific and should be directed at newly formed fibrin (present within intravascular thrombus), while exerting a minimal effect on normal hemostasis [3,26]. The onset of fibrinolytic activity should be rapid, and the circulating half-life should be long enough to permit abbreviated dosing and wide-scale acceptance in clinical practice. It should not be antigenic, and it should be available at a cost that fosters its routine use. Although pharmacologic characteristics of newer thrombolytic agents have improved, large clinical trials have demonstrated only modest improvements in 30-day mortality [27]. The drugs currently approved for use in the United States are outlined in Table 1. There are several dosing regimens available for these drugs, consisting of single- or double-bolus administration or an accelerated front-loaded regimen consisting of a single bolus followed by continuous intravenous administration over 60 to 90 minutes. Double-bolus alteplase (tPA) was found to have an increased incidence of bleeding complications, stroke, and death as compared with front-loaded tPA [28]. Accelerated tPA has an approximately 1% survival advantage over streptokinase [23,29]. The benefit from tPA is greatest in patients less than 75 years old and in those who have anterior wall infarctions [23], but a consistent benefit is seen in virtually all subgroups, including patients who are older, have a nonanterior infarction or hypertension, or have had a prior myocardial infarction (MI) or coronary artery bypass grafting [29–31]. The benefit of tPA over streptokinase is thought to be caused by a significant increase in TIMI III (normal) blood flow in the infarct-related artery with tPA administration [32]. Compared with tPA, reteplase (rPA) is less fibrin selective and has a longer half-life. Several studies suggest similar clinical benefit with either tPA or rPA. The largest, trial, Global Use of Strategies to Open Occluded Coronary Arteries (GUSTO) III, compared 15,000 patients who had STEMI and found no significant difference between accelerated alteplase and double-bolus reteplase in 30-day and 1-year mortality or stroke incidence [33]. As with tPA, rPA has demonstrated a lower incidence of cardiogenic shock compared with streptokinase [34]. Tenecteplase (TNK-tPA) is a genetically modified variant

Table 1
Characteristics of currently approved thrombolytics in the United States

	Streptokinase	Alteplase (t-PA, activase)	Reteplase (r-PA, retevase)	Tenecteplase (TNK-tPA)
Dosing	1.5 million 30-60 min	15 mg bolus, 0.75 mg/kg (max 50 mg) Over 30 min, then 0.5 mg/kg (max 35 mg) Over 1 hour	10 U bolus ×2, 30 minutes apart	Weight based: 30 mg (<60 kg), 35 mg (60-69 kg), 40 mg (70-79 kg), 45 mg (80-89 kg), 50 mg (≥90 mg)
Systemic fibrinolytic state (fibrinogen depletion)	Marked	Mild	Moderate	Minimal to mild
Antigenic	Yes	No	No	No
Bolus administration	No	No	Yes (double bolus)	Yes
Approximate cost (US dollars, 2001)	300	2200	2200	2200
Intracranial hemorrhage (%)	0.5	0.8	0.9	0.9

of tPA which has a significantly longer half-life, more fibrin specificity, and less inhibition by plasminogen activation inhibitor than standard tPA. Single-bolus TNK-tPA is associated with less bleeding than tPA and with similar 30-day mortality [35,36]. Although there is no proven mortality benefit of TNK-tPA over tPA in patients presenting within 4 hours of symptom onset, these data favor TNK-tPA in patients who present later than 4 hours after the onset of symptoms [36]. Significantly, although the rates of intracranial hemorrhage are similar for the two drugs, TNK-tPA use is associated with fewer bleeding complications unrelated to intracranial hemorrhage and less need for blood product transfusion [35]. It is also easier and faster to use, because its longer half-life permits single-bolus administration. Although streptokinase is substantially less expensive than any of the newer thrombolytic agents, its potential antigenicity, short half-life, and lack of fibrin specificity led to a reduction in its use in the United States.

Indications and contraindications for pharmacologic reperfusion

The ACC/AHA class I indications for use of thrombolytic therapy in STEMI are patients who had symptom onset less than 12 hours previously and who have ST-segment elevation in at least two contiguous leads or new/presumably new left bundle branch block [3]. Thrombolytic therapy is most effective when applied to younger (<75 years) patients who do not have heart failure or

hemodynamic instability presenting early after symptom onset and in whom the risk of major bleeding is low [4]. Elderly patients (>75 years) who do not have contraindications for thrombolytic therapy also derive significant morbidity and mortality benefits, although the absolute mortality reduction is less than that for younger patients (Fig. 2) [37,38].

Indicators of successful reperfusion include relief of symptoms within 60 to 90 minutes of receiving thrombolytics or a ST-segment decrease of at least 50% [3,4]. Echocardiographic contrast perfusion is another marker of reperfusion. Angiographic evaluation of epicardial antegrade flow of the infarct related artery, as measured by the TIMI flow grade classification, is an important predictor of outcome. TIMI grade 0 refers to the absence of any antegrade flow beyond a coronary occlusion, whereas TIMI 1 flow is faint antegrade coronary flow beyond the occlusion with incomplete filling of the distal coronary bed. TIMI 2 flow is delayed or sluggish antegrade flow with complete filling of the distal territory, and TIMI 3 flow is defined as normal flow that fills the distal coronary bed completely [39]. Only restoration of normal epicardial flow (TIMI 3 flow) has been associated with improved left ventricular function and survival; the outcome of patients who have TIMI 2 flow is similar to those who have only TIMI 0 or 1 flow [29,40,41]. Other angiographic features of epicardial flow and myocardial perfusion also correlate with outcome after thrombolytic administration [42,43]. Patency of the infarct-related artery does not always result in cellular

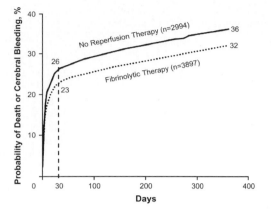

Fig. 2. Although there is increased risk, the probability of death or intracranial hemorrhage is not increased in patients older than 75 years who receive thrombolytic therapy. The figure shows the adjusted probability of death or cerebral bleeding in relation to fibrinolytic therapy in patients who had STEMI and who were 75 years old or older (*dotted line*) versus that among patients who had STEMI who did not receive fibrinolysis (*solid line*). At 30 days and 1 year, the probability was 23% and 32% versus 26% and 36%, respectively. (*Modified from* Stenestrand U, Wallentin L. Fibrinolytic therapy in patients 75 years and older with ST-segment-elevation myocardial infarction:one-year follow-up of a large prospective cohort. Arch Intern Med 2003;163:968.)

reperfusion, and a current of injury may persist. For this reason, early resolution of ST segment elevation is a better representation of complete reperfusion than angiographic criteria [17].

Several studies have demonstrated that the mortality benefits of thrombolytics are gender independent and are present regardless of blood pressure (if less than 180 mm Hg systolic), heart rate, presence of diabetes mellitus, or previous MI [2]. The greatest absolute mortality benefit is seen in patients who have anterior STEMI and significant myocardium at risk; the benefit is less in inferior STEMI, except in subgroups with associated right ventricular infarction or anterior ST segment depression [2].

Hemorrhage is the most severe risk of thrombolytic therapy, and most contraindications to thrombolytic therapy are based on the risk of bleeding after receiving thrombolytics. Absolute contraindications include any prior intracranial hemorrhage, recent face or head trauma (within 3 months), known central nervous system vascular malformation or neoplasm, ischemic stroke within 3 months (except acute ischemic stroke), and suspicion of aortic dissection [3]. Clinical predictors of intracranial bleeding with use of

thrombolytics are age (>65 years), female gender, systolic blood pressure higher than 180 mm Hg on presentation, and low (<70 kg) body weight [17]. The risk of bleeding with these drugs is, in part, related to relative fibrin specificity. The use of fibrinolytic drugs carries a category C (uncertain effect) rating in pregnancy, because there have been no well-controlled studies. Streptokinase is antigenic, and there is a risk of allergic reactions [17].

Mechanical reperfusion

In the TIMI and GUSTO trials, attempts at reperfusion using thrombolytics failed to restore full patency of the infarct-related arteries in up to 54% of cases [44,45]. Limitations of thrombolytics also included a risk of early recurrent ischemia of 10% to 15% and a 5% risk of reinfarction after thrombolytic therapy. Mechanical reperfusion with PCI has gradually replaced the used of lytics in many centers. Primary PCI is defined as mechanical reperfusion without prior thrombolytic therapy. Rescue PCI is emergent PCI after failed thrombolysis. Immediate and delayed (1–7 days) PCI refers to the timing of PCI after successful thrombolysis. Facilitated PCI is a newer concept referring to emergent PCI immediately after reduced-dose thrombolysis. Compared with thrombolysis, PCI restores normal epicardial blood flow (TIMI III) in 70% to 90% of cases [46]. Several studies have demonstrated that normal flow in the infarct-related artery is associated with a mortality of 3.7%, compared with 6.6% and 9.2% in patients who have impaired flow and an occluded or nearly occluded infarct-related artery [47,48]. PCI also allows early identification of patients who may benefit from surgical revascularization as well as the application of other mechanical interventions, such as the use of intra-arterial balloon counterpulsation therapy, thrombectomy, and distal protection devices, which may improve outcome.

Initial comparisons of PCI with thrombolytic therapy were conducted in the pre–coronary stent era and used percutaneous transluminal coronary angioplasty (PTCA). In the Primary Angioplasty in Myocardial Infarction trial of 395 patients who had STEMI presenting within 12 hours of symptom onset, PTCA therapy reduced the combined occurrence of in-hospital death or nonfatal reinfarction at 2-year follow-up, as compared with tPA therapy [46]. These benefits persisted although overall left ventricular systolic function did not differ in the two groups. Subgroup analysis revealed that location of the infarct affected outcome, with the mortality benefit in the PTCA group seen primarily in patients presenting with anterior wall MI [49]. Patients in the non–anterior wall MI group also derived benefit, however, having a lower rate of recurrent ischemia (9.7% versus 27.8%) and fewer urgent catheterizations and revascularization procedures [49].

A meta-analysis of 10 trials (Fig. 3) comparing use of streptokinase, tPA, and accelerated tPA with PTCA found that, at 30 days, primary angioplasty seemed to be superior to thrombolytic therapy for treatment of patients who had acute MI [50]. The rates of death or nonfatal reinfarction were 7.2% for angioplasty and 11.9% for thrombolytic therapy ($P < .001$). PTCA was also associated with a significant reduction in total stroke (0.7% versus 2.0%; $P = .007$) and hemorrhagic stroke (0.1% versus 1.1%; $P < .001$) when compared with the thrombolytics used in the trials. A potential limitation of these data is the limited use of newer, more effective thrombolytic regimens, stents, and adjunctive therapies. These issues were addressed in a subsequent meta-analysis of 23 trials comparing thrombolytics with PCI, 8 of which involved primary stenting of the infarct-related artery. PCI still reduced the combined endpoint of death, nonfatal reinfarction, recurrent ischemia, and stroke, and this benefit was maintained at 18 months [51]. The advantages of PCI in these meta-analyses should be viewed in light of several limitations of the studies, such as the relatively low numbers of patients and limited use of cardiac biomarkers in the PCI arms.

There was initial reluctance to use intracoronary stents in the setting of thrombus and an active coagulopathic state, but subsequent studies demonstrated improved outcomes of timely PCI

with stents over thrombolysis [52–54]. The Danish Acute Myocardial Infarction-2(DANAMI-2) trial randomly assigned 1572 patients to either frontloaded tPA or primary PCI with stents and was discontinued prematurely when PCI with stenting significantly reduced the primary combined endpoint of stroke, reinfarction, and mortality at 30 days [54]. The majority of this benefit was derived from a reduction in reinfarction rates. These results are independent of adjunctive glycoprotein (Gp) IIb/IIIa use [53]. Increasingly, drug-eluting stents are being used for primary PCI in STEMI, having been shown to reduce target-vessel revascularization at 300 days with no increase in stent thrombosis [55]. Comparison studies of primary stenting versus primary PTCA have shown that stenting results in a higher rate of successful reperfusion and lower rates of acute vessel closure and vessel restenosis [56–58]. These short-term benefits, however, have not translated into long-term reduction in recurrent MI or mortality benefit with stenting. Reductions in composite endpoints of death, stroke, reinfarction, and target-vessel revascularization have all been driven primarily by reductions in target-vessel revascularization [59,60]. Although most trials comparing PCI and thrombolytics have included patients eligible to receive thrombolytic therapy, studies have also shown benefits of PCI in thrombolytic-ineligible patients [61].

Analysis of PCI trials reveals that certain subgroups of STEMI patients derive particular benefit from a strategy of primary PCI over fibrinolysis. Several risk models (TIMI, GRACE, Gruppo Italiano per lo Studio della Sopravvivenza nell'Infarto-1 study [GISSI], prehospital risk index) identify a variety of individual patient

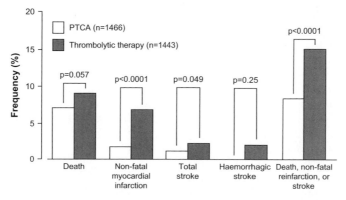

Fig. 3. PTCA is associated with significantly fewer complications than thrombolysis for patients presenting with STEMI. (*From* Keeley E, Boura J, Grines C. Primary angioplasty versus intravenous thrombolytic therapy for acute myocardial infarction: a quantitative review of 23 randomised trials. Lancet 2003;361:17; with permission.)

features, such as age, hemodynamic status, presence of comorbid conditions, infarct location, and time from onset of symptoms, to predict early mortality in patients presenting with STEMI [62–65]. These models allow rapid and early risk stratification and maintain predictive accuracy regardless of the reperfusion strategy chosen. In general, patients who have higher risk scores benefit from PCI instead of thrombolysis. Elderly patients (> 75 years old) presenting with STEMI more often have multivessel coronary disease and significantly increased mortality compared with younger patients. Data from thrombolytic trials shows that an age older than 65 years is an independent risk factor for mortality and increased incidence of stroke and intracranial hemorrhage with thrombolytic therapy [66]. Observational studies and trials comparing PCI and thrombolytics demonstrate a significant mortality benefit in elderly patients treated with PCI suggesting that primary PCI should be the preferred choice for revascularization in this patient group [37,67,68]. Another extremely high-risk group of patients who have STEMI are those presenting in cardiogenic shock, with mortality greater than 80% if left untreated. Both the GISSI-1 and the International Study Group trials demonstrated extremely high mortality rates in patients who had cardiogenic shock treated with thrombolytics; in some cases, results were no better than with placebo [15,69]. Results of the Should We Emergently Revascularize Occluded Coronaries for Cardiogenic Shock (SHOCK) trial, in which 302 patients were randomly assigned to emergent revascularization (64% PCI) or initial medical stabilization showed no difference in mortality at 30 days but a significant mortality reduction at 6 months in the revascularization arm [70]. Subsequent follow-up has also shown than emergent revascularization for patients who have cardiogenic shock produces improved functional status over time, with good quality of life and fewer symptoms of heart failure as compared with medical therapy. [71] The ACC/AHA has given a class I recommendation to a strategy of early reperfusion with intra-arterial balloon counter-pulsation support for all patients younger than 75 years who develop shock within 36 hours of MI and who can be treated within 18 hours from the onset of shock. Early revascularization for selected patients older than 75 years who have shock was given a class IIA recommendation [3]. There are also data to support use of PCI as the preferred reperfusion strategy in patients presenting with anterior MI or heart failure and in patients who have had prior coronary artery bypass grafting [70,72–74].

PCI involves risks and technical concerns that must be considered in determining the optimal reperfusion strategy for a patient. Mechanical complications associated with PCI include vessel dissection or rupture and are more frequent in elderly patients. The potential adverse effects of contrast medium must be considered. Resource availability, time of day, and expertise of medical personnel must also be taken into account and are a much more prominent concern than with use of thrombolytics. Data from the National Registry of Myocardial Infarction (NRMI) demonstrated that there are significantly longer door-to-balloon times when STEMI patients present outside the hours of 8 AM and 6 PM [75]. The NRMI study also showed no difference in outcome between thrombolytics and PCI for patients who had STEMI in low-volume centers (≤16 procedures/year), with lower volume centers having higher mortality rates. Intermediate-volume centers (17–48 procedures/year) and high-volume centers (≥49 procedures/year) had lower mortality rates with reperfusion by PCI [75]. A second NRMI analysis showed no significant relationship between hospital volume of thrombolytic interventions and mortality [76].

As with thrombolytic therapy, the time to reperfusion is critical. There is a positive linear relationship between duration of ischemic time and poor outcome. There are discordant data regarding time of symptom onset to PCI, however. Several studies claim no influence of time delay when PCI is performed within 2 to 3 hours of symptom onset [77,78]. These findings may result, at least in part, from discrepancies between time of symptom onset and presentation to hospital and exclusion of patients who died before reaching the hospital. Other studies, after adjusting for baseline characteristics, show a significant correlation between time from symptom onset to balloon inflation and 1-year mortality [79–81]. Data from a Dutch study showed a continuous relationship between symptom duration and mortality, with a relative risk of death of 1.08 for every 30-minute delay in reperfusion [80].

Adjunctive therapy in ST-segment elevation myocardial infarction

Adjunctive medical therapy is a critical component of therapy for STEMI and confers benefit in addition to that gained by reperfusion therapies, regardless of method of reperfusion (Table 2).

Ancillary therapy can be used to facilitate and enhance coronary reperfusion or to limit the consequences of myocardial ischemia. Early, aggressive use of antiplatelet therapies, such as aspirin, and clopidogrel, confers significant additional mortality benefit when given as adjuncts to thrombolysis or PCI [82].

Beta-blockers, angiotensin-converting enzyme inhibitors in appropriately selected patients, and 3-hydroxy-3-methylglutaryl CoA reductase inhibitors (statins) have all been shown to reduce the risk of cardiovascular events and mortality in patients who have STEMI. Therapies such as nitroglycerin and morphine have no mortality benefit but may improve symptoms and reduce ischemic burden. Calcium-channel blockers and prophylactic anti-arrhythmic drug therapy

(lidocaine) may increase mortality. The suggested benefit of metabolic modulation at the myocyte level with electrolytes, glucose, and insulin seen in small, early trials has not been reproduced in larger, randomized studies [83].

Thrombin inhibition enhances coronary thrombolysis and limits reocclusion. As a result, adjunctive anticoagulation is administered to most patients receiving thrombolytic therapy or PCI. Although it is extensively used, the benefit of heparin in the current era of antiplatelet therapy, advanced thrombolytics, and PCI is controversial. There are currently no data to support the routine administration of adjunctive unfractionated heparin in patients receiving earlier generation, non–fibrin-specific thrombolytic agents, providing aspirin is given [44,73]. Although streptokinase in

Table 2
Mechanisms and clinical effects of adjunctive therapies for patients who have ST elevation myocardial infarction

Agent	Mechanism	Clinical Effect
Adjunctive therapies for AMI		
Aspirin	Antiplatelet	Improve survival
		Decrease reinfarction, CVA
Thienopyridines (clopidogrel, ticlopidine)	Antiplatelet	Recommended in aspirin-allergic patients
		Decrease death, MI, CVA in NSTE ACS
Glycoprotein IIb/IIIa inhibitors	Antiplatelet	Decrease MI, ischemic complications following primary PCI
		Decrease death or MI in high-risk NSTE ACS
Unfractionated heparin	Antithrombin	Decrease death and MI in prefibrinolytic era
Low molecular weight heparins	Antithrombin	Reduce cardiac events in NSTE ACS versus unfractionated heparin
Direct thrombin inhibitors	Antithrombin	Recommended in heparin-induced thrombocytopenia
Beta-brockers	Decrease myocardial oxygen demand ($\downarrow$HR, $\downarrow$BP)	Improve survival
		Reduce infract size, ventricular arrhythmias, recurrent ischemia
Adjunctive therapies for AMI		
ACE Inhibitors	Vasodilator (BP)	Improve survival
	Prevent LV remodeling	Decrease heart failure. LV dysfunction
IV nitroglycerine	Venous, arterial, coronary vasodilator ($\downarrow$BP, $\downarrow$preload)	No effect on survival
		Decrease recurrent ischemia
HMG CoA Reductase Inhibitors	Lipid lowering	Decrease future CV death and MI
	Anti-inflammatory	May decrease early ischemic events
Magnesium	Myocardial protective	Therapy for torsades depointes
	Anti-arrhythmic	May improve reperfusion outcomes
Calcium-channel blocker	Decrease myocardial oxygen demand ($\downarrow$HR, $\downarrow$BP)	No survival benefit
		Possible use in beta-blocker–intolerant patients without CHF or LV dysfunction
Warfarin	Oral anticoagulant	Reduced embolic risk with atrial fibrilliation. LV thrombus or dysfunction
Glucose-insulin potassium infusion	Metabolic modulator	May improve intracellular myocardial energy stores and outcome

Abbreviations: ACS, acute coronary syndrome; BP, blood pressure; CHF, congestive heart failure; CV, cardiovascular; CVA, cerebrovascular accident; HR, heart rate; IV, intravenous; LV, left ventricular; MI, myocardial infarction; NSTE, non–ST-segment elevation; PCI, percutaneous coronary intervention.

combination with enoxaparin has been shown to have better ST-segment resolution and better angiographic patency at days 5 through 10, the possible benefit of enoxaparin on survival and long-term mortality with first-generation agents remains uncertain [84]. The 2004 ACC/AHA guidelines, however, did recommend unfractionated heparin therapy followed by long-term oral anticoagulation in patients who are at high risk for systemic thromboembolism (large or anterior MI, atrial fibrillation, previous embolus, or known left ventricular thrombus) [3]. Unlike older-generation agents, both unfractionated heparin and low molecular weight heparin have shown additional benefit when used with the newer agents tenecteplase, alteplase, and reteplase. Careful, monitored administration of intravenous unfractionated heparin in patients undergoing PCI has been shown to prevent acute vessel closure caused by thrombosis. Studies with Gp IIb/IIIa inhibitors as adjuvant therapy to thrombolysis have shown increased rates of moderate to severe bleeding without demonstrating significant reductions in 30-day and 1-year mortality rates, leading the Consensus Guideline Panel to give combination therapy a class IIB recommendation [3,85]. In contrast, Gp IIb/IIIa inhibitors have demonstrated early and sustained mortality benefit in patients undergoing PCI for reperfusion, with increasing benefit in higher-risk patients. Although thrombolytic therapy may be underused, realization of the benefits of adjunctive therapies has resulted in dramatic increases in their use over time.

Time to balloon inflation and mortality in primary percutaneous coronary intervention for ST-segment elevation myocardial infarction

In many of the studies comparing PCI and thrombolysis, PCI was performed within 3 hours of symptom onset. Registry data confirm that there is a significant difference in time from presentation to PCI depending on the need for transfer to a PCI-capable facility [19]. Several studies confirm the benefits of PCI even when there is some delay in therapy resulting from interhospital transfer and preparation for PCI [86–88]. As the time delay for PCI increases, however, the mortality benefit of PCI over thrombolytic therapy decreases, and thrombolysis may have a greater mortality benefit when there is a 60-minute or longer delay in performing PCI. In this meta-analysis, every 10-minute delay reduced the

absolute mortality benefit by approximately 1%, and the benefit in combined endpoint of stroke, reinfarction, and death was decreased by almost 2% [89].

The available data suggest that primary PCI is preferable to thrombolysis if PCI is performed within 90 minutes at the presenting institution by experienced interventionalists in a cardiac catheterization laboratory that performs more than 36 such procedures per year, even in community hospitals without surgical back-up [90]. Primary PCI is also preferable if transfer to a neighboring institution can be accomplished within 30 to 60 minutes. Compared with thrombolysis, primary PCI achieves a higher rate of TIMI 3 flow, does not carry the risk of intracranial hemorrhage, and is associated with improved outcomes. Primary PCI is not available at all institutions, however, there are often delays in implementation, and local expertise is an important determinant of outcome. As a result, the ACC/AHA task force gave a class I recommendation to the use of thrombolytic therapy for any patient who does not have contraindications and who presents to a facility without the capability for expert, prompt intervention with primary PCI within 90 minutes of first medical contact [3]. Thrombolytic therapy was also recommended if the relative delay necessary to perform primary PCI (the expected door-to-balloon time minus the expected door-to-needle time) is greater than 1 hour.

Combined reperfusion strategies

Although reperfusion with thrombolytics and PCI has demonstrated significant mortality and combined endpoint benefits in patients presenting with STEMI, there are limited data regarding combination therapy. The use of early, in some cases prehospital, thrombolytic therapy followed by early, planned PCI is known as facilitated PCI. This approach must be differentiated from PCI after thrombolytic failure, known as rescue PCI, and from urgent PCI for threatened reocclusion or hemodynamic instability. Initial data from the 1980s comparing PTCA immediately after administration of thrombolytics suggested no additional benefit and increased morbidity, primarily in the form of bleeding [91,92]. Advances in pharmacologic regimens, in PCI, and in adjunctive therapies, however, have led to re-examination of facilitated PCI. The Plasminogen-activator Angioplasty Compatibility trial examined the benefit

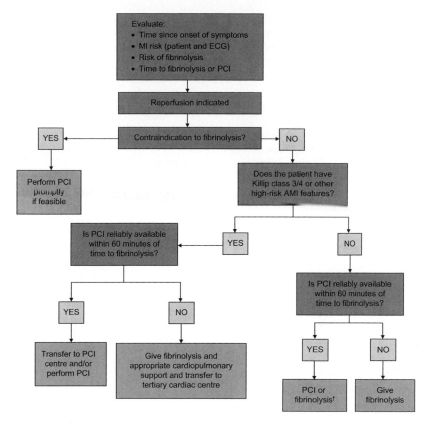

Fig. 4. A proposed model for the selection of reperfusion therapy for patients who have STEMI presenting within 12 hours of symptom onset. The figure shows the Canadian Cardiovascular Society Working Group algorithm for the selection of patients for reperfusion after STEMI. The algorithm applies to patients presenting within 12 hours of symptom onset. It assumes that the diagnosis of STEMI is not in doubt and indicates that, for most hospitals caring for patients who have STEMI who are not at high risk, fibrinolysis is the preferred option. AMI, acute myocardial infarction; PCI, percutaneous cardiac intervention. (*From* Canadian Cardiovascular Society Working Group. Applying the new STEMI guidelines: 1. Reperfusion in acute ST-segment elevation myocardial infarction. CMAJ 2004;171:10–41; with permission.)

of alteplase immediately before PCI in 606 patients who had STEMI. This study suggested that thrombolysis followed by immediate PCI led to more frequent early recanalization of the infarct-related artery, preservation of left ventricular function, and no increase in adverse events [93]. A synergistic approach offers the timeliness of thrombolytic therapy followed by early PCI to consolidate the reperfusion process and prevent reocclusion [94]. There are many issues to be resolved, such as timing of therapy (early versus delayed PCI after thrombolysis, timing of hybrid therapy with duration of symptoms), type of thrombolytic agent, need for adjuvant medical therapy, and appropriate patient selection. Several ongoing trials may provide insight into the role of combination therapy [95].

Future directions

Although improvements in the management of patients who have STEMI have led to a decline in acute and long-term fatality rates, reperfusion and ancillary therapies remain underused. Several initiatives (NMRI, Get With the Guidelines) are designed to improve adherence to guidelines and access to appropriate reperfusion therapies [22]. To date, clinical advancement is judged on achieving and maintaining epicardial artery patency. New fibrinolytics and combination therapies will continue to evolve. There will be technological advances and improvement in operator skills for PCI. There is increasing attention to improving outcome at the myocyte level, however, because an open artery does not equate to adequate tissue perfusion. Edema, inflammation, necrosis, micro-emboli, and microvascular constriction contribute to reperfusion injury and tissue death. Further advances for managing STEMI must focus on therapies that mitigate these factors. Initial studies have suggested benefit to anti-inflammatory and anti-complement therapies and suggest an expanding role for ancillary therapy [96]. The ultimate goal for the management of STEMI remains unchanged: to open occluded arteries quickly in carefully screened patients and in a cost-effective manner.

Current approach to initial treatment of ST-segment elevation myocardial infarction

Fig. 4 shows one suggested approach for the initial treatment of STEMI, taking into account symptom duration, hemodynamic status, local expertise, and transport systems to help make decisions regarding the choice of reperfusion therapy for patients presenting within 12 hours of symptom onset [4]. A directed history and physical examination, focusing on the time from onset of symptoms to presentation and hemodynamic status, should be completed quickly. If the history correlates with a 12-lead ECG demonstrating new or presumed new ST-segment elevation in two or more contiguous leads, or left bundle branch block the diagnosis of STEMI can be made, and focus can be directed to the appropriate mode of reperfusion. If there are no contraindications for thrombolysis, it is a reasonable option, especially if local PCI expertise is not on site or if transfer to a PCI-capable facility will add more than 60 minutes to the time to fibrinolysis. For patients in whom thrombolytics are contraindicated or who have high-risk STEMI features, such as cardiogenic shock, PCI is the preferred method of revascularization. In the worst-case scenario, a patient who has STEMI and high-risk features, contraindications to fibrinolysis, and for whom PCI is not readily available has an extremely high risk of dying. The approach to such patients is not well delineated, but it may be reasonable to try to obtain some level of reperfusion with thrombolytics and supportive measures before transfer to a tertiary level cardiac center. Although both thrombolytic therapy and PCI focus on epicardial artery patency, strategies to improve myocardial-level perfusion must also be employed. It is possible that near-maximal benefit has been obtained by modification of

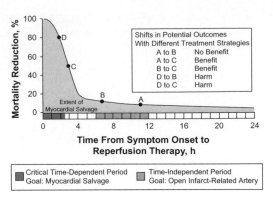

Fig. 5. A hypothetical model demonstrating the relationship of symptom duration, myocardial salvage, and mortality for patients presenting with STEMI. Mortality reduction as a benefit of reperfusion therapy is greatest in the first 2 to 3 hours after the onset of symptoms of acute myocardial infarction, most likely a consequence of myocardial salvage. The exact duration of this critical early period may be modified by several factors, including presence of functioning collateral coronary arteries, ischemic preconditioning, myocardial oxygen demands, and the duration of sustained ischemia. After this early period, the magnitude of the mortality benefit is much reduced, and as the mortality reduction curve flattens, time-to-reperfusion therapy is less critical. If a treatment strategy, such as facilitated PCI, is able to move patients back up the curve, a benefit would be expected. The magnitude of the benefit would depend on how far up the curve the patient can be shifted. The benefits of a shift from points A or B to point C would be substantial, but the benefit of a shift from point A to pint B would be small. A treatment strategy that delays treatment during the critical early period, such as patient transfer for PCI, would be harmful (shift from point D to point C or point B). Between 6 and 12 hours after the onset of symptoms, opening the infarct-related artery is the primary goal of reperfusion therapy, and primary PCI is preferred over fibrinolytic therapy. The possible contribution to mortality reduction of opening the infarct-related artery, independent of myocardial salvage, is not shown. Shaded boxes indicate the critical time-dependent period in which the goal is myocardial salvage; open boxes indicate the time-independent period in which the goal is to open the infarct-related artery. (*From* Gersh B, Stone G, White H, et al. Pharmacological facilitation of primary percutaneous coronary intervention for acute myocardial infarction: is the slope of the curve the shape of the future? JAMA 2005;298:980; with permission.)

thrombolytic agents, dosing regimens, and adjunctive treatments. Although developments in catheter, balloon, stent, and device design continue and make opening occluded arteries easier, current technology allows opening the infarct-related artery in more than 90% of cases, and the ability to improve clinical endpoints meaningfully with design advances seems limited.

Fig. 5 is a hypothetical construct of the relationship of duration of symptoms before reperfusion, mortality reduction, and extent of myocardial salvage [97]. It is a helpful way to judge future changes in MI care. In the example given, a reduction of time from 12 to 6 hours (from point A to B) results in only minimal clinical benefit. A high-cost solution, then, probably would not be cost effective. On the other hand, moving from point B to point C (or from C to D) would probably be associated with a substantial clinical benefit. Moving from point D to point C (or from C to B) represents a hazardous delay. In evaluating new therapies, whether in the process of delivering care, the drugs used, or the devices used in the catheterization, the goal remains rapid and complete reperfusion.

Significant mortality reductions can be realized if citizens are taught to activate emergency medical services immediately with the onset of chest pain, thereby reducing the all-important time from symptom onset to delivering therapy. Other process improvements are also possible, such as increased compliance with national guidelines and continued encouragement to deliver therapy to patients who qualify for it. As therapies become increasingly complex, the development of specialized MI hospitals built on the model of trauma centers may prove beneficial. Future treatment strategies must also attempt to provide earlier and sustained reperfusion at both the epicardial and tissue level. This advance may involve continued drug, device, and dosing developments as well as novel therapies to mitigate reperfusion injury and delay or limit myocyte necrosis. Ultimately, earlier patient presentation to the health care system followed by rapid, appropriately selected reperfusion therapy will result in more lives saved.

References

[1] Reimer K, Lowe J, Rasmussen M, et al. The wavefront phenomenon of ischemic cell death: 1. Myocardial infarct size vs duration of coronary occlusion in dogs. Circulation 1977;56:786–94.

[2] Fibrinolytic Therapy Trialists' (FTT) Collaborative Group. Indications for fibrinolytic therapy in suspected acute myocardial infarction: collaborative overview of early mortality and major morbidity results from all randomised trials of more than 1000 patients. Lancet 1994;343:311–22.

[3] Antman E, Anbe D, Armstrong P, et al. ACC/AHA guidelines for the management of patients with ST-elevation myocardial infarction—executive summary: a report of the American College of Cardiology/American Heart Association Task Force on Practice Guidelines (Writing Committee to Revise the 1999 Guidelines for the Management of Patients With Acute Myocardial Infarction). Circulation 2004; 110:588.

[4] Canadian Cardiovascular Society Working Group. Applying the new STEMI guidelines: 1. Reperfusion in acute ST-segment elevation myocardial infarction. CMAJ 2004;171:1039–41.

[5] Fletcher A, Alkjaersig N, Smyrniotis F, et al. Treatment of patients suffering from early myocardial infarction with massive and prolonged streptokinase therapy. Trans Assoc Am Physicians 1958;71: 287–96.

[6] Rentrop P, Blanke H, Karsch K, et al. Selective intracoronary thrombolysis in acute myocardial infarction and unstable angina pectoris. Circulation 1981;63:307–17.

[7] Chazov E, Mateeva L, Mazaev A, et al. Intracoronary administration of fibrinolysis in acute myocardial infarction. Ter Arkh 1976;48:8–19.

[8] Collen D, Topol E, Tiefenbrunn A, et al. Coronary thrombolysis with recombinant human tissue-type plasminogen activator. A prospective, randomized, placebo-controlled trial. Circulation 1984;70: 1012–7.

[9] Schroder R, Biamino G, Leitner E-R, et al. Intravenous short-term infusion of streptokinase in acute myocardial infarction. Circulation 1983;67:536–48.

[10] Ganz W, Geft I, Shah P, et al. Intravenous streptokinase in evolving acute myocardial infarction. Am J Cardiol 1984;53:1209–16.

[11] Waters R, Mahaffey K, Granger C, et al. Current perspectives on reperfusion therapy for acute ST-segment elevation myocardial infarction: integrating pharmacologic and mechanical reperfusion strategies. Am Heart J 2003;146:958–68.

[12] Boersma E, Maas A, Deckers J, et al. Early thrombolytic treatment in acute myocardial infarction: reappraisal of the golden hour. Lancet 1996;348: 771–5.

[13] Morrison L, Verbeek P, McDonald A, et al. Mortality and prehospital thrombolysis for acute myocardial infarction: a meta-analysis. JAMA 2000;283: 2686–92.

[14] Baigent C, Collins R, Appleby P, et al. ISIS-2: 10 year survival among patients with suspected acute myocardial infarction in randomised comparison of intravenous streptokinase, oral aspirin, both, or neither. The ISIS-2 (Second International Study of Infarct Survival) Collaborative Group. BMJ 1998; 316:1337–43.

[15] Franzosi M, Santoro E, De Vita C, et al. Ten-year follow-up of the first megatrial testing thrombolytic therapy in patients with acute myocardial infarction:

results of the Gruppo Italiano per lo Studio della Sopravvivenza nell'Infarto-1 study. The GISSI Investigators. Circulation 1998;98:2659–65.

[16] Furman M, Dauerman H, Goldberg R, Yarzebski J, et al. Twenty-two year (1975 to 1997) trends in the incidence, in-hospital and long-term case fatality rates from initial Q-wave and non-Q-wave myocardial infarction: a multi-hospital, community-wide perspective. J Am Coll Cardiol 2001;37:1571–80.

[17] Khan I, Gowda R. Clinical perspectives and therapeutics of thrombolysis. Int J Cardiolol 2003;91: 115–27.

[18] Late Assessment of Thrombolytic Efficacy (LATE) study with alteplase 6–24 hours after onset of acute myocardial infarction. Lancet 1993;342:759–66.

[19] Rogers WJCJ, Lambrew CT, et al. Temporal trends in the treatment of over 1.5 million patients with myocardial infarction in the US from 1990 through 1999: the National Registry of Myocardial Infarction 1, 2 and 3. J Am Coll Cardiol 2000;36: 2056–63.

[20] Fox KA. An international perspective on acute coronary syndrome care: Insights from the global registry of acute coronary events. Am Heart J 2004; 148(Suppl 5):S40–5.

[21] Fox K, Goodman S, Klein W, et al. Management of acute coronary syndromes. Variations in practice and outcome; findings from the Global Registry of Acute Coronary Events (GRACE). Eur Heart J 2002;23:1177–89.

[22] Eagle K, Goodman S, Avezum A, et al. Practice variation and missed opportunities for reperfusion in ST–segment-elevation myocardial infarction: findings from the Global Registry of Acute Coronary Events (GRACE). Lancet 2002;359:373–7.

[23] The GUSTO investigators. An international randomized trial comparing four thrombolytic strategies for acute myocardial infarction. N Engl J Med 1993;329:673–82.

[24] Gore J, Granger C, Simoons M, et al. Stroke after thrombolysis. Mortality and functional outcomes in the GUSTO-I trial. Global Use of Strategies to Open Occluded Coronary Arteries. Circulation 1995;92:2811–8.

[25] Berkowitz S, Granger C, Pieper K, et al. Incidence and predictors of bleeding after contemporary thrombolytic therapy for myocardial infarction. The Global Utilization of Streptokinase and Tissue Plasminogen activator for Occluded coronary arteries (GUSTO) I Investigators. Circulation 1997;95:2508–16.

[26] Giugliano R. Braunwald E, for the TTS Group. Selecting the best reperfusion strategy in ST-elevation myocardial infarction: it's all a matter of time. Circulation 2003;108:2828–30.

[27] Young JJ, Kereiakes DJ. Pharmacologic reperfusion strategies for the treatment of ST-segment elevation myocardial infarction. Rev Cardiovasc Med 2003;4: 216–27.

[28] The Continuous Infusion versus Double-Bolus Administration of Alteplase (COBALT) Investigators. A comparison of continuous infusion of alteplase with double-bolus administration for acute myocardial infarction. N Engl J Med 1997;337: 1124–30.

[29] Holmes DJ, Califf R, Topol E. Lessons we have learned from the GUSTO trial. Global Utilization of Streptokinase and Tissue Plasminogen Activator for Occluded Arteries. J Am Coll Cardiol 1995;25: 10S–7S.

[30] Labinaz M, Sketch MJ, Ellis S, et al. Outcome of acute ST-segment elevation myocardial infarction in patients with prior coronary artery bypass surgery receiving thrombolytic therapy. Am J Cardiol 2001; 141:469–77.

[31] Brieger D, Mak K, White H, et al. Benefit of early sustained reperfusion in patients with prior myocardial infarction (the GUSTO-I trial). Global Utilization of Streptokinase and TPA for occluded arteries. Am J Cardiol 1998;81:282–7.

[32] The GUSTO Angiographic Investigators. The effects of tissue plasminogen activator, streptokinase, or both on coronary-artery patency, ventricular function, and survival after acute myocardial infarction. N Engl J Med 1993;329:1615–22.

[33] The Global Use of Strategies to Open Occluded Coronary Arteries (GUSTO III) Investigators. A comparison of reteplase with alteplase for acute myocardial infarction. N Engl J Med 1997;337: 1118–23.

[34] International Joint Efficacy Comparison of Thrombolytics (INJECT). Randomised. double-blind comparison of reteplase double-bolus administration with streptokinase in acute myocardial infarction: trial to investigate equivalence. Lancet 1995;346: 329–36.

[35] Van de Werf F, Cannon C, Luyten A, et al. Safety assessment of single-bolus administration of TNK tissue-plasminogen activator in acute myocardial infarction: the ASSENT-1 trial. The ASSENT-1 Investigators. Am Heart J 1999;137: 786–91.

[36] Assessment of the Safety and Efficacy of a New Thrombolytic Investigators. Single-bolus tenecteplase compared with front-loaded alteplase in acute myocardial infarction: the ASSENT-2 double-blind randomised trial. Lancet 1999;354:716–22.

[37] Thiemann D, Coresh J, Schulman S. Lack of benefit for intravenous thrombolysis in patients with myocardial infarction who are older than 75 years. Circulation 2000;101:2239–46.

[38] White HD. Thrombolytic therapy in the elderly. Lancet 2000;356:2028–30.

[39] Gibson C, Murphy S, Menown I, et al. Determinants of coronary blood flow after thrombolytic administration. TIMI Study Group. Thrombolysis in Myocardial Infarction. J Am Coll Cardiol 1999; 34:1403–12.

[40] The GUSTO Investigators. An international randomized trial comparing four thrombolytic strategies for acute myocardial infarction. N Engl J Med 1993;329:673–82.

[41] Gibson C, Murphy S, Marble S, et al. Can we replace the 90-minute thrombolysis in myocardial infarction (TIMI) flow grades with those at 60 minutes as a primary end point in thrombolytic trials? Am J Cardiol 2001;87:450–3.

[42] French J, Ellis C, Webber B, et al. Abnormal coronary flow in infarct arteries 1 year after myocardial infarction is predicted at 4 weeks by corrected Thrombolysis in Myocardial Infarction (TIMI) frame count and stenosis severity. Am J Cardiol 1998;81:665–71.

[43] Gibson C, Cannon C, Murphy S, et al. Relationship of TIMI myocardial perfusion grade to mortality after administration of thrombolytic drugs. Circulation 2000;101:125–30.

[44] The GUSTO Investigators. The effects of tissue plasminogen activator, streptokinase, or both on coronary-artery patency, ventricular function, and survival after acute myocardial infarction. N Engl J Med 1993;329:1615–22.

[45] The TIMI Study Group. The Thrombolysis in Myocardial Infarction (TIMI) trial. N Engl J Med 1985; 312:932–6.

[46] Grines C, Browne K, Marco J. Primary Angioplasty in Myocardial Infarction Study Group (PAMI). A comparison of immediate angioplasty with thrombolytic therapy for acute myocardial infarction. N Engl J Med 1993;329:673–9.

[47] Fath-Ordoubadi F, Huehns T, Al-Mohammad A, et al. Significance of the thrombolysis in myocardial infarction scoring system in assessing infarct-related artery reperfusion and mortality rates after acute myocardial infarction. Am Heart J 1997;134:62–8.

[48] Smith D. For and against: primary angioplasty should be first line treatment for acute myocardial infarction. BMJ 2004;328:1254–8.

[49] Stone G, Grines C, Browne K, et al. Influence of acute myocardial infarction location on in-hospital and late outcome after primary percutaneous transluminal coronary angioplasty versus tissue plasminogen activator therapy. Am J Cardiol 1996;78: 19–25.

[50] Weaver W, Simes R, Betriu A, et al. Comparison of primary coronary angioplasty and intravenous thrombolytic therapy for acute myocardial infarction: a quantitative review. JAMA 1997;278:2093–8.

[51] Keeley E, Boura J, Grines C. Primary angioplasty versus intravenous thrombolytic therapy for acute myocardial infarction: a quantitative review of 23 randomised trials. Lancet 2003;361:13–20.

[52] Le May M, Labinaz M, Richard F, et al. Stenting versus thrombolysis in acute myocardial infarction trial (STAT). J Am Coll Cardiol 2001;37:985–91.

[53] Kastrati A, Mehilli J, Dirschinger J, et al. Myocardial salvage after coronary stenting plus abciximab versus fibrinolysis plus abciximab in patients with acute myocardial infarction: a randomised trial. Lancet 2002;359:920–5.

[54] Andersen H, Nielsen T, Rasmussen K, et al. A comparison of coronary angioplasty with fibrinolytic therapy in acute myocardial infarction. N Engl J Med 2003;349:733–42.

[55] Lemos P, Saia F, Hofma S, et al. Short- and long-term clinical benefit of sirolimus-eluting stents compared to conventional bare stents for patients with acute myocardial infarction. J Am Coll Cardiol 2004;43:704–8.

[56] Saito S, Hosokawa F, Kim K, et al. Primary stent implantation without Coumadin in acute myocardial infarction. J Am Coll Cardiol 1996;28:74–81.

[57] Bauters C, Lablanche J, Van Belle E, et al. Effects of coronary stenting on restenosis and occlusion after angioplasty of the culprit vessel in patients with recent myocardial infarction. Circulation 1997;96: 2854–8.

[58] Stone G, Brodie B, Griffin J, et al. Clinical and angiographic follow-up after primary stenting in acute myocardial infarction: the Primary Angioplasty in Myocardial Infarction (PAMI) stent pilot trial. Circulation 1999;99:1548–54.

[59] Nordmann A, Hengstler P, Harr T, et al. Clinical outcomes of primary stenting versus balloon angioplasty in patients with myocardial infarction: a meta-analysis of randomized controlled trials. Am J Med 2004;116:253–62.

[60] Zhu M, Feit A, Chadow H, Alam M, et al. Primary stent implantation compared with primary balloon angioplasty for acute myocardial infarction: a meta-analysis of randomized clinical trials. Am J Cardiol 2001;88:297–301.

[61] Grzybowski M, Clements E, Parsons L. Mortality benefit of immediate revascularization of acute ST-segment elevation myocardial infarction in patients with contraindications to thrombolytic therapy: a propensity analysis. JAMA 2003;290:1891–8.

[62] Morrow D, Antman E, Charlesworth A, et al. TIMI risk score for ST-elevation myocardial infarction: a convenient, bedside, clinical score for risk assessment at presentation: an Intravenous nPA for Treatment of Infarcting Myocardium Early II trial substudy. Circulation 2000;102:2031–7.

[63] Morrow D, Antman E, Giugliano R, et al. A simple risk index for rapid initial triage of patients with ST-elevation myocardial infarction: an InTIME II substudy. Lancet 2001;358:1571–5.

[64] Morrow DA, Antman EM, Parsons L, et al. Application of the TIMI risk score for ST-elevation MI in the National Registry of Myocardial Infarction 3. JAMA 2001;286:1356–9.

[65] Marchioli R, Avanzini F, Barzi F, et al. Assessment of absolute risk of death after myocardial infarction by use of multiple-risk-factor assessment equations: GISSI-Prevenzione mortality risk chart. Eur Heart J 2001;22:2085–103.

[66] Stone G, Grines C, Browne K. Predictors of in-hospital and 6-month outcome after acute myocardial infarction in the reperfusion era: the Primary Angioplasty in Myocardial Infarction (PAMI) trial. J Am Coll Cardiol 1995;25:370–7.

[67] O'Neill W, Menko J, Gibbons R. Lessons from the pooled outcome of the PAMI, ZWOLLE and Mayo Clinic randomized trials of primary angioplasty versus thrombolytic therapy of acute myocardial infarction. J Invest Cardiol 1998;10:4A–10A.

[68] Mehta R, Sadiq I, Goldberg R, et al. Effectiveness of primary percutaneous coronary intervention compared with that of thrombolytic therapy in elderly patients with acute myocardial infarction. Am Heart J 2004;147:253–9.

[69] Bates E, Topol E. Limitations of thrombolytic therapy for acute myocardial infarction complicated by congestive heart failure and cardiogenic shock. J Am Coll Cardiol 1991;18:1077–84.

[70] Hochman J, Sleeper L, Webb J, et al. Early revascularization in acute myocardial infarction complicated by cardiogenic shock. SHOCK Investigators. Should We Emergently Revascularize Occluded Coronaries for Cardiogenic Shock. N Engl J Med 1999;341:625–34.

[71] Sleeper L, Ramanathan K, Lejemtel T, et al. Functional status and quality of life after emergency revascularization for cardiogenic shock complicating acute myocardial infarction. SHOCK Investigators. J Am Coll Cardiol 2005;46:266–73.

[72] Garcia E, Elizaga J, Perez-Castellano N, et al. Primary angioplasty versus systemic thrombolysis in anterior myocardial infarction. J Am Coll Cardiol 1999;33:605–11.

[73] O'Keefe J, Bailey W, Rutherford B. Primary angioplasty for acute myocardial infarction in 1000 consecutive patients: results in an unselected population and high-risk subgroups. Am J Cardiol 1993;72:107G–15G.

[74] DeGeare V, Dangas G, Stone G, et al. Interventional procedures in acute myocardial infarction. Am Heart J 2001;141:15–24.

[75] Magid D, Calonge B, Rumsfeld J, et al. Relation between hospital primary angioplasty volume and mortality for patients with acute MI treated with primary angioplasty versus thrombolytic therapy. JAMA 2000;284:3131–8.

[76] Canto J, Every N, Magid D, et al. The volume of primary angioplasty procedures and survival after acute myocardial infarction. National Registry of Myocardial Infarction 2 Investigators. N Engl J Med 2000;342:1573–80.

[77] Cannon C, Gibson C, Lambrew C, et al. Relationship of symptom-onset-to-balloon time and door-to-balloon time with mortality in patients undergoing angioplasty for acute myocardial infarction. JAMA 2000;283:2941–7.

[78] Brodie B, Stuckey T, Wall T, et al. Importance of time to reperfusion for 30 day and late survival and recovery of left ventricular function after primary angioplasty for acute myocardial infarction. J Am Coll Cardiol 1998;32:1312–9.

[79] De Luca G, Suryapranata H, Zijlstra F, et al. Symptom-onset-to-balloon time and mortality in patients with acute myocardial infarction treated by primary angioplasty. J Am Coll Cardiol 2003;42:991–7.

[80] De Luca G, Suryapranata H, Ottervanger JP, et al. Time delay to treatment and mortality in primary angioplasty for acute myocardial infarction: every minute of delay counts. Circulation 2004;109: 1223–5.

[81] De Luca G, van't Hof AW, de Boer MJ, et al. Time-to-treatment significantly affects the extent of ST-segment resolution and myocardial blush in patients with acute myocardial infarction treated by primary angioplasty. Eur Heart J 2004;25: 1009–13.

[82] Sabatine M, Cannon C, Gibson C, et al. Addition of clopidogrel to aspirin and fibrinolytic therapy for myocardial infarction with ST-segment elevation. N Engl J Med 2005;352:1179–89.

[83] Mehta S, Yusuf S, Diaz R, et al. Effect of glucose-insulin-potassium infusion on mortality in patients with acute ST-segment elevation myocardial infarction: the CREATE-ECLA randomized controlled trial. JAMA 2005;293:437–46.

[84] Simoons M, Krzeminska-Pakula M, Alonso A, et al. Improved reperfusion and clinical outcome with enoxaparin as an adjunct to streptokinase thrombolysis in acute myocardial infarction. The AMI-SK study. Eur Heart J 2002;23:1282.

[85] Topol E. GUSTO V Investigators. Reperfusion therapy for acute myocardial infarction with fibrinolytic therapy or combination reduced fibrinolytic therapy and platelet glycoprotein IIb/IIIa inhibition: the GUSTO V randomised trial. Lancet 2001;357: 1905–14.

[86] Dalby M, Bouzamondo A, Lechat P, et al. Transfer for primary angioplasty versus immediate thrombolysis in acute myocardial infarction: a meta-analysis. Circulation 2003;108:1809–14.

[87] Widimsky P, Budesinsky T, Vorac D, et al. Long distance transport for primary angioplasty vs immediate thrombolysis in acute myocardial infarction. Final results of the randomized national multicentre trial–PRAGUE-2. Eur Heart J 2003;24:94–104.

[88] Grines C, Westerhausen DJ, Grines L, et al. A randomized trial of transfer for primary angioplasty versus on-site thrombolysis in patients with high-risk myocardial infarction: the Air Primary Angioplasty in Myocardial Infarction study. J Am Coll Cardiol 2002;39:1713–9.

[89] Nallamothu B, Bates E. Percutaneous coronary intervention versus fibrinolytic therapy in acute myocardial infarction: is timing (almost) everything? Am J Cardiol 2003;92:824–6.

[90] Aversano T, Aversano L, Passamani E, et al. Thrombolytic therapy vs primary percutaneous

coronary intervention for myocardial infarction in patients presenting to hospitals without on-site cardiac surgery: a randomized controlled trial. JAMA 2002;287:1943–51.

[91] TIMI Study Group. Comparison of invasive and conservative strategies after treatment with intravenous tissue plasminogen activator in acute myocardial infarction: results of the thrombolysis in myocardial infarction (TIMI) phase II trial. N Engl J Med 1989;320:618–27.

[92] The TIMI Research Group. Immediate vs delayed catheterization and angioplasty following thrombolytic therapy for acute myocardial infarction. TIMI II A results. JAMA 1988;260:2849–58.

[93] Ross A, Coyne KS, Reiner JS, et al. A randomized trial comparing primary angioplasty with a strategy of short-acting thrombolysis and immediate planned rescue angioplasty in acute myocardial infarction: the PACT trial. PACT investigators. Plasminogen-activator Angioplasty Compatibility Trial. J Am Coll Cardiol 1999;34:1954–62.

[94] Antman E, Van de Werf F. Pharmacoinvasive therapy: the future of treatment for ST-elevation myocardial infarction. Circulation 2004;109:2480–6.

[95] Ellis SGAP, Betriu A, Brodie B, et al. Facilitated Intervention with Enhanced Reperfusion Speed to Stop Events Investigators. Facilitated percutaneous coronary intervention versus primary percutaneous coronary intervention: design and rationale of the Facilitated Intervention with Enhanced Reperfusion Speed to Stop Events (FINESSE) trial. Am Heart J 2004;147:1–7.

[96] Mahaffey K, Granger C, Nicolau J, et al. Effect of pexelizumab, an anti-C5 complement antibody, as adjunctive therapy to fibrinolysis in acute myocardial infarction: the Complement Inhibition in Myocardial Infarction Treated with Thrombolytics (COMPLY) trial. Circulation 2003;108:1176–83.

[97] Gersh B, Stone G, White H, et al. Pharmacological facilitation of primary percutaneous coronary intervention for acute myocardial infarction: is the slope of the curve the shape of the future? JAMA 2005;293:979–86.

Cardiol Clin 24 (2006) 53–65

Emergency Cardiac Imaging: State of the Art

Dick Kuo, MD[a,b,*], Vasken Dilsizian, MD[a,b], Rajnish Prasad, MD[a,b],
Charles S. White, MD[a,b]

[a]University of Maryland School of Medicine, 655 West Baltimore Street, Baltimore, MD 21201, USA
[b]University of Maryland Medical System, 22 South Greene Street, Baltimore, MD 21201, USA

One of the most difficult challenges for emergency physicians is to determine whether chest pain is cardiac related and if the patient is at increased risk for a cardiac event (eg, nonfatal myocardial infarction or death). A certain group of high-risk patients can be identified readily based on history, ECG changes, and cardiac enzyme elevations. Based on recommendations by the American College of Cardiology (ACC) and American Heart Association (AHA), these patients usually undergo urgent coronary angiography [1]. A larger group of patients presenting with a less urgent clinical scenario and varying degrees of pretest likelihood for coronary artery disease require additional testing to evaluate their cardiac risk. Several noninvasive imaging modalities are helpful in this group of patients. Nuclear stress perfusion testing and stress echocardiography are useful in risk stratifying these patients, and new-generation CT scanners and MRI may soon develop their own roles.

Cardiac angiography remains the reference standard for imaging of the coronary vessels and provides an avenue for intervention, but cardiac catherization is an invasive procedure. An estimated 1.46 million cardiac catherizations were performed in 2002, although only 657,000 percutaneous transluminal coronary angioplasty procedures were performed [2]. Because most cardiac catherizations are diagnostic, there has been a long search for a noninvasive technique to diagnose coronary artery disease and visualize the coronary vessels, but until recently few techniques have been satisfactory.

Imaging of the heart in the emergency department begins with the plain chest radiograph. Although the plain chest radiograph states little about the coronary vessels, it provides important background information. Other options now available to visualize the coronary arteries without cardiac catherization include electron beam CT (EBCT), multidetector or multislice CT (MDCT) with CT angiography (CTA), and cardiac MR (CMR) with angiography. Provocative and nuclear testing can also provide much useful information in the evaluation of the patient who has suspected angina.

Plain chest radiograph

The plain chest radiograph has served for many years as a first-line imaging technique in the assessment of the cardiac patient in the emergency room. The chest radiograph is quite sensitive for diagnosis of some noncardiac causes of chest pain including pneumonia, pneumothorax, and rib fractures.

Direct evidence of myocardial ischemia is often absent on chest radiographs, but indirect evidence may be present in the form of atherosclerotic calcification of vessels. This calcification is usually most evident in the aorta but is more specific when found in the coronary arteries. The sensitivity for detection of coronary artery calcification on radiography is less than 50%. The usual location of visible coronary artery calcification is in the coronary triangle in the mid-upper part of the left heart corresponding to the proximal portions of the left coronary arteries [3]. Calcification may

---

* Corresponding author. 110 South Paca Street Sixth Floor, Suite 200, Baltimore, MD 21201.

E-mail address: dkuo@umaryland.edu (D. Kuo).

also be present on the lateral radiograph arising from the aortic root (Fig. 1). Data from a fluoroscopic study suggest that radiographically evident coronary calcification is associated with a higher likelihood of significant coronary artery stenosis [4].

A plain chest radiograph may also be useful for assessment of complications of early episodes of myocardial ischemia. An enlarged cardiac silhouette may be evidence of a previous myocardial event. Calcification along the left heart border is often an indication of a prior myocardial infarction (Fig. 2) [5]. The presumed mechanism is impaired wall motion followed by local thrombus formation, which may ultimately calcify. A focal bulge of the left heart border may represent a postinfarct myocardial aneurysm or pseudoaneurysm [6].

Other indirect signs of ischemic chest pain may be identified, including congestive heart failure. There is some correlation between the radiographic findings and the severity of congestive heart failure. In mild heart failure, cephalization may be present consisting of reduced flow to lower lobe vessels and diversion of flow to upper lobes. Cephalization requires a gravitational gradient and therefore is difficult to recognize on a supine or semierect radiograph. More severe heart failure is associated with interstitial and alveolar (airspace) pulmonary edema, respectively [7]. In a recent study of patients presenting to the emergency department with acute dyspnea, a plain chest radiograph showing enlarged heart size identified patients for whom a final diagnosis of heart failure was confirmed by two cardiologists with a sensitivity of 88% and a specificity of 72% [8].

The plain chest radiograph is unlikely to be replaced because it provides a large amount of useful information, and cardiac patients will almost uniformly require a chest radiograph to exclude other potential diagnoses associated with cardiac symptoms.

Electron beam CT

Current EBCT scanners deploy temporal resolutions of 50 to 100 milliseconds and ECG gating to evaluate the cardiac anatomy. For comparison, conventional angiography has a temporal resolution of less than 10 milliseconds. Multiple studies have evaluated the ability of EBCT to evaluate coronary stenosis and provide prognostic information for patients who have coronary calcifications. CT scanning, in particular EBCT, has been used to risk stratify patients who have suspected coronary artery disease by demonstrating coronary calcium. The presence of coronary calcium indicates coronary artery disease and is conventionally measured with the method described by Agatston and colleagues [9], in which the extent and density of coronary calcification are used to derive a global score. Coronary calcium is strongly associated with coronary artery disease and has been shown to have an odds ratio of 13.7 for any coronary artery disease and an odds ratio of 10.3 for obstructive coronary artery disease [10,11]. This association must be balanced with the results of a recent meta-analysis that found only a moderately increased risk for cardiac events (unstable angina, myocardial infarction, need for

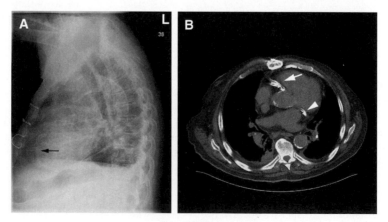

Fig. 1. Coronary calcification. (*A*) Lateral chest radiograph shows coronary artery calcification overlying the anterior cardiac silhouette (*arrow*). (*B*) Nonenhanced CT scan shows that the anterior calcification corresponds to the right coronary artery (*arrow*). The left circumflex artery is also calcified (*arrowhead*).

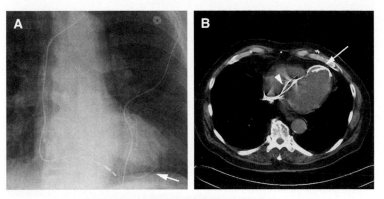

Fig. 2. Myocardial calcification. (*A*) Posteroanterior radiograph shows curvilinear calcification along the left heart border (*arrow*) in a patient with an implantable defibrillator. (*B*) Nonenhanced CT shows curvilinear myocardial calcification in the left ventricular apex (*arrow*). Defibrillator wires are also identified (*arrowhead*).

revascularization, cardiac death) associated with coronary calcifications in asymptomatic populations [12].

Several studies have also sought to evaluate coronary stenosis greater than 50% with EBCT. Reddy and colleagues [13] found an overall sensitivity of 88% and specificity of 79% in 23 patients although coronary artery calcifications resulted in decreased specificity. Budoff and colleagues [14] studied 52 patients and reported an overall sensitivity of 78% and a specificity of 91%. In this study 11% of the cardiac segments were noninterpretable, usually because of motion. The authors also noted difficulty in viewing the right coronary and circumflex arteries. Schmermund and colleagues [15] also reported increased false negatives secondary to segmental calcification with a sensitivity of 82% and a specificity of 88% in 28 patients. Another study by Achenbach and colleagues [16] discovered a sensitivity of 92% and a specificity of 94% in 125 patients although there 25% of segments were noninterpretable in this study. These studies illustrate the capabilities of EBCT but may not be applicable to patients in an emergency department where risk stratification and outcomes are more important measures of the success of a particular test, and where patients cannot be excluded secondary to their "noninterpretable segments."

A few studies have assessed the use of EBCT in the emergency department setting to evaluate patients who have angina-like chest pain [17–19]. Table 1 summarizes studies in which patients presenting to the emergency department with chest pain were evaluated by new techniques. Using the presence of coronary calcium as a marker,

these studies demonstrate a sensitivity ranging from 88% to 100% for coronary stenosis or cardiac events and negative predictive values of 97% to 100%. In addition, a high negative predictive value was found. In the study by Laudon and colleagues [17], no patient presenting with chest pain who had a negative EBCT had a cardiac event in the 4 months after presentation to the emergency department [17]. In the study by McLaughlin and colleagues [19], the 1-month cardiac event rate was 2%, compared with 8% in patients who had coronary artery calcium (CAC) scores greater than one. More recently Georgiou and colleagues [18] found a strong association between the age- and gender-adjusted CAC score and a subsequent cardiac event in a cohort of 192 patients who had undergone EBCT during the course of their emergency department evaluation for chest pain. Overall, the 1-year annualized rate for cardiac events was 0.6% for patients who had a CAC score of zero compared with a cardiac event rate of 13.9% in patients who had CAC scores greater than 400 (average follow-up after presentation in the emergency department was 50 ± 10 months with a range of 1–84 months). The results of this study are somewhat difficult to generalize, because follow-up time was not standard; instead, results were statistically annualized. This study, however, seems to confirm that a CAC score of zero has a high negative predictive value for cardiac events.

Other strategies for managing patients who have chest pain include EBCT replacement of stress testing, the combination of EBCT and stress testing [20], or EBCT scanning in patients who have indeterminate stress results [21].

Table 1
Studies evaluating patients presenting to the emergency department patients with chest pain

Study	n	Sensitivity	Specificity	PPV	NPV	Standards	FU period and outcome	Event Rate
EBCT								
Lauden [17] 1999	100	100	63	30	100	+ test, sten > 40 vs CAC > 0	4 mo CE	0% in neg EBCT
Georgiou [18] 2001	192	97	55	48	97	CAC > 0 vs CE	1 mo–84 mo (mean 50 mo) CE	1 yr annualized
		93	59	55	95	CAC > 4 vs CE		0.6% CAC = 0 13.9% CAC > 400
McLaughlin [19] 1999	134	88*	37*	8*	98%	CAC > 1	1 mo CE	2% versus 8%
MDCT								
White [31] 2005	69	83	96	83	96	CTA > 50% stenosis versus final diagnosis		not studied
CMR								
Kwong [36] 2003	161	84	85	ns	ns	ACS, NSTEMI, UA 70%sten or true + stress test		not studied
Takahashi [37] 2004	18	78	89	78	89	AMI and ultrasound		not studied

Abbreviations: ACS, acute coronary syndrome; AMI, acute myocardial infarction; CAC, coronary artery calcification score; CE, cardiac events; CMR, cardiac magnetic resonance imaging; EBCT, electron beam CT; FU, follow up; MDCT, multidetector CT; NPV, negative predictive value; NSTEMI, nonST elevation myocardial infarction; PPV, positive predictive value; UA, unstable angina.

* Value not provided in text but calculated using standard 2 × 2 table from which NPV was calculated.

The consensus statement on CAC and EBCT from the ACC/AHA can be summarized briefly. Negative tests occur in most patients who have angiographically normal coronaries and may be consistent with a low risk of cardiovascular risk in the next 2 to 5 years. A positive EBCT confirms the presence of atherosclerotic plaque and is best correlated with total amount of plaque burden. The greater the amount of calcium, the greater the likelihood of occlusive disease, and a high calcium score may be consistent with moderate to high cardiovascular risk in the next 2 to 5 years [22].

Multidetector CT

The latest generation of MDCT scanners features ECG gating, submillimeter spatial resolution, and relatively good temporal resolution that permits increasingly accurate assessment of coronary artery anatomy. Currently, scanners are available with 64 detectors, a spatial resolution of 0.5 to 0.6 mm, and temporal resolution of 50 to 100 milliseconds. CT scanners are increasingly being placed in the emergency suite, alleviating concerns about monitoring some patients who have chest pain. The improved technical parameters of MDCT allow determination of the extent of coronary calcification and acquisition of acceptable coronary CTA, ventricular function, and, perhaps myocardial perfusion.

The scanning protocol may be optimized to assess the heart alone or be acquired as a compromise between a coronary and lung CT protocol to assess for pulmonary emboli and aortic dissection also. Generally, 10 evenly spaced phases throughout the cardiac cycle are obtained. This approach permits selection of the phase with the least amount of coronary artery motion, typically in early or late diastole. Reconstructions centered along the curving centerline of the individual coronary arteries are produced and evaluated for hard and soft plaque and critical stenoses. Software exists for a quantitative assessment of the extent of the stenosis. Left ventricular ejection fraction can also be derived from determination of end-systolic and end-diastolic volumes. This postscan processing currently is labor-intensive, and much effort is being directed to streamlining this analysis.

MDCT technique requires intravenous contrast material and is usually done with an automatic triggering mechanism that times the contrast bolus so that opacification is optimized. Patients who have renal insufficiency or significant contrast allergies are thus not eligible. Beta-blockade, typically with metoprolol, can be used in patients who have a heart rate greater than 70 beats per minute. This strategy has been shown to improve image quality because of image degradation at higher rates [23].

As with EBCT, there have been multiple investigations with multidetector CTA to evaluate stenosis. A study by Nieman and colleagues [24] reported a sensitivity of 95% and a specificity of 86% in 59 patients and also reported higher accuracy for left main and left anterior descending arteries than for circumflex and right coronary arteries. This finding is thought to result from the increased motion of those vessels. Ropers and colleagues [25] conducted a study with 77 patients; with 12% excluded segments, sensitivity was 92% and specificity was 93%.

In a more recent study evaluating coronary arteries greater than 2 mm in patients undergoing elective evaluation for chest pain, coronary CTA has shown considerable potential, with sensitivity and specificity of 83% and 97%, respectively [26]. Thirty-seven percent of patients in this study had CAC scores of 400 or higher; if these patients were excluded, CTA sensitivity increased to 89% and specificity increased to 98%.

A PUB MED search (search terms: chest pain, multislice or multidetector, and emergency) found no studies using multislice CT for CTA of the coronary anatomy to evaluate patients presenting to the emergency department with chest pain, although there have been a couple of case reports showing acute myocardial infarction in patients presenting with chest pain [27,28]. Also, a couple of studies have used MDCT in acute coronary syndrome (ACS). Although it may be assumed that these patients presented to the emergency department initially, this information is not confirmed in the text of the articles. One study evaluated ejection fraction and stenosis with a 4-slice scanner [29], and another study used a predictive model to determine if a use of a 16-slice MDCT could decrease the number of diagnostic cardiac angiographies [30].

Currently, the appropriate use and timing of the MDCT in the emergency setting is unclear, and the authors have devised a protocol to test one scenario [31]. The authors have proposed that the examination be obtained in patients who have chest pain and an intermediate probability of angina, as initially assessed by the emergency physician by examination and ECG. Patients who have a high probability would be taken for emergent coronary angiography; those with low probability are unlikely to benefit from MDCT. In the authors' protocol, patients were brought to the emergency suite scanner between 30 minutes and 1 hour after initial assessment. The 16-slice CT scan using a dual heart–lung protocol was intended to provide a comprehensive evaluation of both coronary and noncoronary causes of chest pain.

In this study, 69 patients met all criteria for enrollment, 45 (65%) of whom otherwise would not have undergone CT scanning [29]. Fifty-two patients (75%) had no significant CT findings and a final diagnosis of clinically insignificant chest pain. Thirteen patients (18%) had significant CT findings concordant with the final diagnosis (10 cardiac, 3 noncardiac). Fig. 3 shows an example of a curved planar reconstruction used to visualize the coronary vessels. CT failed to suggest a diagnosis in two patients (3%), both of whom proved to have clinically significant coronary artery stenoses. In two patients (3%), CT overdiagnosed a coronary stenosis. Sensitivity and specificity for the establishment of a cardiac cause of chest pain were 83% and 96%, respectively. Overall sensitivity and specificity for all cardiac and noncardiac causes of chest pain were 87% and 96%, respectively. The cardiac assessment was done several hours or more after acquisition of the CT scan because of software limitations. The study suggests that MDCT is logistically

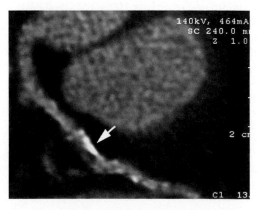

Fig. 3. CT scanning in the emergency room. A curved planar reconstructed image of a diagonal branch shows calcification and narrowing (*arrow*).

feasible and may prove useful if hardware and software improvements continue. Current technology involves the use of 40- and 64-slice scanners; studies evaluating their use in patients presenting to the emergency department with chest pain have yet to be published.

Cardiac MR and angiography

MRI is effective in evaluating myocardial ischemia and thus has potential applications in the emergency room setting. After intravenous infusion of gadolinium chelate, myocardial perfusion can be assessed with rapid temporal imaging. Wall-motion abnormalities can be delineated with bright blood cine imaging. Delayed images after gadolinium enhancement are valuable to depict myocardial viability. Delayed hyper-enhancement 10 to 20 minutes after injection is a strong indicator of myocardial infarction (Fig. 4) [32].

In one of the earlier studies evaluating CMR for detection of coronary stenoses, Regenfus and colleagues [33] reported sensitivity of 94.4% and specificity of 57.1% on a patient basis with 50 patients in the study. Only 76.6% of segments could be evaluated, and the left circumflex could be evaluated in only 50% of cases. In a larger study of 109 patients, coronary magnetic resonance angiography was performed before elective radiographic coronary angiography, and the results of the two diagnostic procedures were compared. Six hundred thirty-six of 759 proximal and middle segments were interpretable on magnetic resonance angiography (84%). In these segments, the sensitivity, specificity, and accuracy for patients who had disease of the left main coronary artery or three-vessel disease were 100%, 85%, and 87%, respectively. The negative predictive values for any coronary artery disease and for left main artery or three-vessel disease were 81% and 100%, respectively [34]. In a recent brief report by van Geuns and colleagues [35], CMR was found to have only 46% sensitivity but 90% specificity for stenosis that was greater than 50% in a small study of 27 patients.

Again, fewer studies have examined the usefulness in emergency department patients. Kwong and colleagues [36] assessed the use of CMR in a prospective study of 161 patients who presented to the emergency room with suspected ACS. Inclusion criteria were an episode of chest pain lasting more than 30 minutes and an abnormal but nondiagnostic ECG. Resting CMR was

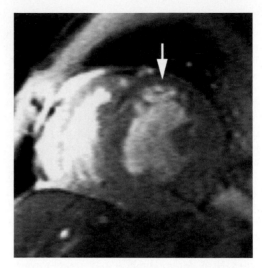

Fig. 4. CMR of myocardial infarction. Short-axis image from CMR viability study shows an area of hyper enhancement in the anterior wall, indicating myocardial infarction (*arrow*).

performed within 12 hours of presentation. The image protocol consisted of perfusion, wall motion, and viability sequences. CMR demonstrated a sensitivity of 84% and specificity of 85%, respectively, for ACS.

Another small study of 18 patients in 2004 by Takahashi and colleagues [37] also evaluated CMR in patients who had ACS as defined by acute myocardial infarction and ultrasound. Because the majority of patients in this study actually were classified as having acute myocardial infarction, this study probably more accurately appraises the utility of CMR in acute myocardial infarction and than in true ACS.

CMR has the advantage of good spatial and excellent temporal resolution, and Gadolinium contrast agent is widely available. Nevertheless, CMR is limited by the need for specialized, often expensive equipment that may not be located near the emergency room. Other issues that potentially make CMR unfeasible for many emergency department patients are patient claustrophobia and the need to monitor an acutely ill patient appropriately in the bore of the MR imager.

Other techniques

Although there are other new techniques available to evaluate patients who have chest pain that better establish plaque composition, these new techniques are invasive and investigational and have little if any application in the emergency department or in the initial evaluation of the patient who has potential cardiac disease. These techniques include intravascular ultrasound, optical coherence tomography, thermography, and angioscopy and are beyond the scope of this discussion.

Stress echocardiography

Stress echocardiography is readily available, is relatively low in cost, and can assess cardiac anatomy and function during stress. It also has the advantage of providing incremental information of value by evaluating baseline ventricular function, valvular function, aortic root morphology, and pericardial anatomy. Such information can provide further insight into the possible causes of the chest pain. Regional wall-motion abnormalities are early signs of myocardial ischemia and provide an indirect evaluation of abnormal myocardial perfusion [1] and coronary blood flow. Wal-motion abnormalities at rest identify patients who have had ischemic injury. The number of abnormal wall-motion segments is quantified by the wall-motion score index (Fig. 5). The higher the wall-motion score index, the greater the number of abnormal segments and, thus, the higher risk for the patient [38].

The decision to perform either an exercise or pharmacologic stress echocardiogram depends on the functional status of the patient. Ideally, an exercise stress test should be performed because it provides valuable physiologic information including functional capacity. A normal exercise stress echocardiogram confers an excellent prognosis. The overall cardiac event rate (cardiac death, nonfatal myocardial infarction) ranges from 0.9% to 1.1% per year. An abnormal study increases the risk of a cardiac event by three to four times [39–42].

Other factors may affect prognosis as well. Exercise stress–induced wall-motion abnormalities in the left anterior descending distribution predict a fivefold higher cardiac event rate at 5 years than wall-motion abnormalities in other regions [43]. Even with a normal stress echocardiogram, patients who have diabetes mellitus have significantly higher cardiac event rates (6% per year) than nondiabetics (2.7% per year) [44], and hypertensive patients who have a normal

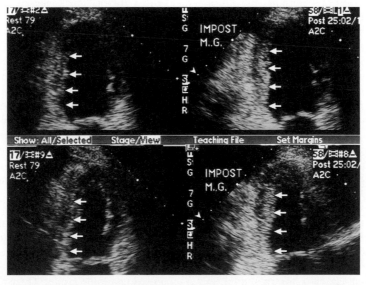

Fig. 5. Exercise echocardiogram recorded in a patient with a disease of the right coronary artery. The two left panels were recorded at rest and the two right panels immediately after treadmill exercise; the top panels show diastole, and the bottom panels show systole. In each panel the arrows note the location of the inferior wall endocardium at end-diastole. At rest there is appropriate thickening and inward motion of the inferior wall that can be seen to move inward through the body of the arrows. Immediately after exercise the proximal inferior wall (*lower two arrows*) becomes frankly dyskinetic, and the mid and diastole portion of the inferior wall is akinetic. There is no incursion of the endocardium into the previously placed arrows. (*From* Braunwald E. Heart disease: a textbook of cardiovascular medicine. 6th edition. Philadelphia: Elsevier Inc.; 2001. p. 214; with permission.)

dobutamine stress echocardiogram have an over-all higher cardiac event rate (1.8% per year) than the general population (approximately 1% per year) but a significantly lower rate than those who have an abnormal study (3.8% per year) [45].

When the patient is unable to exercise, pharmacologic testing provides a valuable alternative and provides similar prognostic information. The most common drug used for a pharmacologic stress test is dobutamine. The infusion begins at 5 μg/kg/min and is increased by 5- to 10-μg/kg/min increments until target heart rate is achieved. Frequently, atropine may be required if the dobutamine infusion does not achieve the target heart rate. Continuous ECG monitoring is performed throughout the stress test and the recovery period. Echocardiogram images are obtained during the pre-infusion period (resting state), at low-dose stress, at peak stress (when target heart rate is achieved), and then in recovery.

Several studies have found death and nonfatal myocardial infarction rates of approximately 1.1% per year for a normal test [46,47]. The death and nonfatal myocardial infarction rates for abnormal studies are about 7% per year [46–51]. In studies evaluating exercise and dobutamine stress echocardiography, a normal study translates into a low cardiac event rate (0.8%–0.9% per year) [52,53]. Abnormal studies could be further stratified into intermediate (3.1% per year cardiac event rate) and high (5.2% per year cardiac event rate) risk groups based on the wall-motion score index [52].

Because regional wall-motion abnormalities usually precede the onset of definitive echocardiographic signs of ischemia, echocardiographic detection of regional left ventricular dysfunction has been assessed as a tool to improve the diagnosis of acute cardiac ischemia in the emergency room. Among patients undergoing echocardiographic study during active chest pain in the emergency room, Peels and colleagues [54] found echocardiography to be highly sensitive for the detection of myocardial infarction and acute ischemia (92% and 88%, respectively). The specificity of this approach was limited, at 53% for infarction and 78% for ischemia. In the absence of ongoing symptoms, the sensitivity of echocardiography was limited [55]. Echocardiographic analysis in these studies was limited to patients exhibiting normal conduction systems and no prior myocardial infarction, because both conduction disturbances and prior areas of infarction can cause regional wall-motion abnormalities in the absence of acute ischemia.

Sabia and colleagues [56] examined the value of regional wall-motion abnormality for the diagnosis of acute myocardial infarction in the emergency room. The sensitivity for echocardiographically detected regional wall-motion abnormalities to identify acute ischemic heart disease presenting as myocardial infarction was 93%. The specificity, however, was modest (57%). These investigators estimated that the use of echocardiography in the emergency room could result in a 32% reduction in hospital admissions, but this estimate was not demonstrated in a prospective manner. In a small subset of patients ultimately diagnosed as having non-Q wave infarction, echocardiography failed to demonstrate regional wall-motion abnormality. False-negative findings by echocardiography have also been observed by other investigators [57,58].

Recently, Kontos and colleagues [59] demonstrated a high negative predictive value of normal echocardiographic studies in patients who had chest pain, which correlated with a benign prognosis at 10 months. In a subsequent study [60], these authors also compared myocardial perfusion imaging with single-photon emission CT (SPECT) and echocardiography in 185 patients who presented to the emergency room with chest pain and who were considered to have low to moderate risk of coronary ischemia based on history and echocardiography. In 90% of the patients, acute rest sestamibi perfusion and echocardiographic studies were performed within 1 hour of each other. The two techniques had similar sensitivities and specificities for the detection of acute myocardial infarction or acute myocardial ischemia. Further confirmatory studies are needed to determine the impact of symptom resolution on this comparison, because the earlier studies of echocardiography demonstrated that optimal sensitivity is dependent on the presence of symptoms during the emergency room evaluation [54–58]. The most recent studies evaluating the role of dobutamine tele-echocardiography [61] and contrast echocardiography [62] for patients presenting to the emergency room with chest pain have also reported favorable results. These techniques or technologies are not in widespread clinical use, however.

These studies suggest that regional wall-motion assessment by echocardiography to determine early signs of ischemia in patients presenting to the emergency room with chest pain is feasible. For optimal sensitivity this approach requires ongoing symptoms during the study. The sub-optimal specificity suggests this technique has limited use in decreasing the number of false-positive admissions for patients presenting to the emergency department with chest pain. Moreover, no study has evaluated the actual impact of the use of echocardiography on triage from the emergency room.

Stress echocardiography has been shown to be comparable with nuclear stress perfusion scanning for detecting coronary disease and for predicting short- and long-term cardiac events [63–65]. Exercise stress testing and pharmacologic stress testing seem to provide comparable short- and long-term prognostic information. Dobutamine stress echocardiography is equal to dipyridamole Technetium sestamibi scanning in sensitivity and has greater specificity for detecting single-vessel and multivessel disease [64]. An abnormal exercise stress echocardiography or Thallium perfusion study predicted a 4.1-fold and 4.9-fold increase, respectively, in the risk of all cardiac events over an almost 4-year follow-up [65]. For even a longer follow-up period (mean, 7.3 years), a normal dobutamine stress echocardiogram predicted a cardiac event rate of 3.6% per year, whereas a normal dobutamine stress Technetium sestamibi scan predicted a cardiac event rate of 2.8% per year. Abnormal stress echocardiograms predicted a cardiac event rate of 6.5%, whereas abnormal Technetium sestamibi scans predicted a rate of 6.9% per year [63]. Therefore, exercise stress echocardiography and pharmacologic stress echocardiography provide similar detection and prognostic information when compared with nuclear stress studies.

Application of single-photon emission CT myocardial perfusion imaging in the emergency department

In patients who present in the emergency departments with chest pain and are suspected to be experiencing ACS, radionuclide myocardial perfusion imaging techniques can provide both diagnostic and prognostic information. Evidence from controlled, randomized trials suggests that incorporating SPECT myocardial perfusion imaging in emergency department patients who have suspected ACS but no definitive ECG changes can improve triage decisions. The ACC/AHA/American Society of Nuclear Cardiology Radionuclide Imaging Guidelines classify myocardial perfusion imaging in this setting as a class I, level A indication [66] for patients in whom the diagnosis is uncertain.

Among ACS patients who present with ST segment elevation myocardial infarction or non-ST segment elevation myocardial infarction/unstable angina, the typical role for imaging in the stabilized patient is to provide risk-stratification information to drive a management strategy aimed at improving natural history. Thus, the role of myocardial perfusion SPECT early during ST segment elevation myocardial infarction or non-ST segment elevation myocardial infarction/unstable angina is to identify the location and extent of myocardial injury. After therapeutic intervention a follow-up study is compared with the earlier study to identify the extent of myocardial salvage and final infarct size (Fig. 6).

The role of myocardial perfusion imaging in patients presenting with chest pain and nondiagnostic ECG changes

In patients presenting with chest pain and non-diagnostic ECG changes, myocardial perfusion SPECT data have been shown to have an incremental risk stratification value over clinical data for predicting unfavorable cardiac events [67]. The injection of Technetium-99m–based perfusion tracer in a patient during chest pain and imaging 45 to 60 minutes later allows the assessment of myocardial blood flow at the time of injection. In all observational studies, the negative predictive value for ruling out myocardial infarction has equaled or exceeded 99% in this setting. This finding suggests that a normal myocardial perfusion study in this setting portends very small risk of myocardial infarction or ischemic event [68]. In contrast, patients exhibiting abnormal regional perfusion defect have a higher risk of cardiac events during the index hospitalization as well as during follow-up. One study by Kontos and colleagues [69] found the sensitivity of SPECT sestamibi performed in the emergency department to be 92% for detecting acute myocardial infarction, whereas initial troponin I values drawn at the same time had a sensitivity of only 39%. The maximum troponin I over the first 24 hours had sensitivity similar to rest sestamibi imaging, but at a distinctly later time point. Thus, acute myocardial perfusion imaging has the potential to identify ACS earlier than biomarkers, thereby providing assistance in patient triage decisions (admit or discharge) in the emergency department.

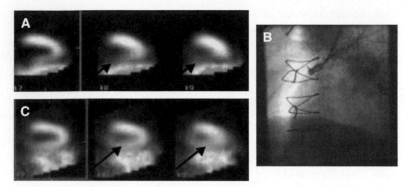

Fig. 6. Inferior myocardial perfusion defect in a patient with chest pain but no ischemic ECG abnormalities. (*A*) Vertical long-axis resting SPECT myocardial perfusion images of a 67-year-old-man who presented to the emergency room with chest pain and no ischemic ECG changes. His troponin T was negative and troponin I was less than 0.1. He was injected with Technetium-99m sestamibi at rest in the emergency room and underwent SPECT imaging soon thereafter. The images show severely reduced inferior perfusion defect (*arrows*), which in the setting of ongoing symptoms was suggestive of acute coronary syndrome. (*B*) Cardiac catheterization showed totally occluded right coronary artery and graft. (*C*) A prior myocardial perfusion SPECT study performed showed normal perfusion in all myocardial regions, including the inferior region (*arrows*).

Although these observational studies emphasize the importance of myocardial perfusion imaging for ruling out ACS, in none of those studies were the imaging data allowed to affect patient triage decisions in the emergency department. In a prospective study by Stowers and colleagues [70], 46 patients who had ongoing chest pain and a nondiagnostic ECG were randomly assigned to an image-guided strategy (in which patient management was based on the SPECT results) or a conventional strategy (in which imaging results were kept blinded, and patient management was independent of the SPECT data). The results showed that an image-guided strategy incurred approximately 50% lower costs and resulted in shorter lengths of hospital stay. In a larger prospective trial (the ERASE Chest Pain Trial) [71], 2475 patients who had symptoms suggestive of ACS and a normal or nondiagnostic ECG were randomly assigned to a usual emergency department evaluation strategy or a strategy including acute rest SPECT myocardial perfusion information. The results showed that the imaging data were among the most powerful factors associated with the appropriate decision to discharge the patient from the emergency department. For patients ultimately determined not to have ACS as the presenting syndrome, SPECT myocardial imaging was associated with a 32% reduction in the odds of being admitted unnecessarily to the hospital for treatment or observation [71]. On 30-day follow-up of all patients, there were no differences in outcomes between the usual emergency

department evaluation strategy and SPECT image-guidance. These findings suggest that the incorporation of SPECT perfusion imaging into the emergency department triage decision-making process reduces unnecessary hospital admissions without inappropriately reducing admission for patients who have ACS. In the future, metabolic imaging with a fatty acid tracer called methyl-[123I]-iodophenyl-pentadecanoic acid (BMIPP) may extend the time window for identifying myocardial ischemia in the emergency room up to 30 hours after the cessation of chest pain [72].

The chest pain center protocol: stress myocardial perfusion single-proton emission CT

Another strategy that has been proposed for patients who have suspected ACS but a nondiagnostic ECG is serial evaluation of cardiac specific enzymes over 6 to 24 hours, followed by stress testing if the enzymes are negative. Among patients who are considered clinically to be at very low risk, however, stress myocardial perfusion SPECT study can be performed rather early. SPECT myocardial perfusion imaging in this setting can potentially allow earlier patient triage decisions than serial enzyme evaluation. The current data suggest that if stress myocardial perfusion studies are normal, the risk of ACS or unfavorable cardiac events is low, and therefore early discharge from the emergency department may be considered. On the other hand, if the stress imaging results are abnormal (ischemia or infarction), rapid admission and entry into an appropriate evidence-based treatment pathway for ACS are in order.

Summary

Multiple strategies and testing modalities are available to evaluate patients presenting to the emergency department with cardiac complaints. Many provide anatomic and prognostic information about coronary stenosis and long-term outcomes. Although nuclear and stress echo imaging have the ability to predict outcomes in patients in the emergency department population, the newer modalities of cardiac imaging (EBCT, MDCT, and CMR) continue to show promising results and may soon be incorporated into emergency department chest pain centers. Protocols can be developed within an institution to meet the needs of the patient population while minimizing risk and improving outcomes for all patients.

References

[1] Braunwald E, Antman EM, Beasley JW, et al. ACC/AHA 2002 guideline update for the management of patients with unstable angina and non-ST-segment elevation myocardial infarction—summary article: a report of the American College of Cardiology/American Heart Association task force on practice guidelines (Committee on the Management of Patients With Unstable Angina). J Am Coll Cardiol 2002;40(7):1366–74.

[2] American Heart Association. 2005 heart disease and stroke statistics—2005 update. Dallas (TX): American Heart Association; 2005.

[3] Souza AS, Bream PR, Elliott LP. Chest film detection of coronary artery calcification. The value of the CAC triangle. Radiology 1978;129:7–10.

[4] Margolis JR, Chen JT, Kong Y, et al. The diagnostic and prognostic significance of coronary artery calcification. A report of 800 cases. Radiology 1980;137:609–16.

[5] MacGregor JH, Chen JT, Chiles C, et al. The radiographic distinction between pericardial and myocardial calcifications. AJR Am J Roentgenol 1987;148:675–7.

[6] Higgins CB, Lipton MJ, Johnson AD, et al. False aneurysms of the left ventricle. Identification of distinctive clinical, radiographic, and angiographic features. Radiology 1978;127:21–7.

[7] Higgins CB, Lipton MJ. Radiography of acute myocardial infarction. Radiol Clin North Am 1980;18:359–68.

[8] Dao Q, Krishnaswamy P, Kazanegra R, et al. Utility of B-type natriuretic peptide in the diagnosis of congestive heart failure in an urgent-care setting. J Am Coll Cardiol 2001;37(2):379–85.

[9] Agatston AS, Janowitz WR, Hildner FJ, et al. Quantification of coronary artery calcium using ultrafast computed tomography. J Am Coll Cardiol 1990;15:827–32.

[10] Rich S, McLaughlin VV. Detection of subclinical cardiovascular disease: the emerging role of electron beam computed tomography. Prev Med 2002;34(1):1–10.

[11] Rumberger JA, Sheedy PF II, Breen JF, et al. Electron beam computed tomography and coronary artery disease: scanning for coronary artery calcification. Mayo Clin Proc 1996;71(4):369–77.

[12] O'Malley PG, Taylor AJ, Jackson JL, et al. Prognostic value of coronary electron-beam computed tomography for coronary heart disease events in asymptomatic populations. Am J Cardiol 2000;85(8):945–8.

[13] Reddy GP, Chernoff DM, Adams JR, et al. Coronary artery stenoses: assessment with contrast-enhanced electron-beam CT and axial reconstructions. Radiology 1998;208(1):167–72.

[14] Budoff MJ, Oudiz RJ, Zalace CP, et al. Intravenous three-dimensional coronary angiography using contrast enhanced electron beam computed tomography. Am J Cardiol 1999;83(6):840–5.

[15] Schmermund A, Rensing BJ, Sheedy PF, et al. Intravenous electron-beam computed tomographic coronary angiography for segmental analysis of coronary artery stenoses. J Am Coll Cardiol 1998;31(7):1547–54.

[16] Achenbach S, Moshage W, Ropers D, et al. Value of electron-beam computed tomography for the noninvasive detection of high-grade coronary-artery stenoses and occlusions. N Engl J Med 1998;339(27):1964–71.

[17] Lauden DA, Vukov LF, Breen JF, et al. Use of electron-beam computed tomography in the evaluation of chest pain patients in the emergency department. Ann Emerg Med 1999;33(1):15–21.

[18] Georgiou D, Budoff MJ, Kaufer E, et al. Screening patients with chest pain in the emergency department using electron beam tomography: a follow-up study. J Am Coll Cardiol 2001;38:105–10.

[19] McLaughlin VV, Balogh T, Rich S. Utility of electron beam computed tomography to stratify patients presenting to the emergency room with chest pain. Am J Cardiol 1999;84:327–8.

[20] Shavelle DM, Budoff MJ, LaMont DH, et al. Exercise testing and electron beam computed tomography in the evaluation of coronary artery disease. J Am Coll Cardiol 2000;36(1):32–8.

[21] Schmermund A, Baumgart D, Sack S, et al. Assessment of coronary calcification by electron-beam computed tomography in symptomatic patients with normal, abnormal or equivocal exercise stress test. Eur Heart J 2000;21(20):1674–82.

[22] O'Rourke RA, Brundage BH, Froelicher VF, et al. American College of Cardiology/American Heart Association Expert Consensus Document on electron-beam computed tomography for the diagnosis and prognosis of coronary artery disease. J Am Coll Cardiol 2000;36(1):326–40.

[23] Hoffmann MH, Shi H, Manzke R, et al. Noninvasive coronary angiography with 16-detector row CT: effect of heart rate. Radiology 2005;234(1):86–97.

[24] Nieman K, Cademartiri F, Lemos PA, et al. Reliable noninvasive coronary angiography with fast submillimeter multislice spiral computed tomography. Circulation 2002;106(16):2051–4.

[25] Ropers D, Baum U, Pohle K, et al. Detection of coronary artery stenoses with thin-slice multi-detector row spiral computed tomography and multiplanar reconstruction. Circulation 2003;107(5):664–6.

[26] Morgan-Hughes GJ, Roobottom CA, Owens PE, et al. Highly accurate coronary angiography with submillimetre, 16 slice computed tomography. Heart 2005;91:308–13.

[27] Silberman S, Dambrin G, Ghostine S, et al. [Diagnosis of acute myocardial infarction using multislice computed tomography in emergency room.] Arch Mal Coeur Vaiss 2004;97(4):366–9 [in French].

[28] Hastreiter D, Lewis D, Dubinsky TJ. Acute myocardial infarction demonstrated by multidetector CT scanning. Emerg Radiol 2004;11(2):104–6.

[29] Dirksen MS, Jukema JW, Bax JJ, et al. Cardiac multidetector-row computed tomography in patients with unstable angina. Am J Cardiol 2005; 95(4):457–61.

[30] Dorgelo J, Willems TP, Geluk CA, et al. Multidetector computed tomography-guided treatment strategy in patients with non-ST elevation acute coronary syndromes: a pilot study. Eur Radiol 2005; 15(4):708–13.

[31] White CS, Kuo D, Keleman M, et al. Chest pain evaluation in the emergency room: can multi-slice CT provide a comprehensive evaluation? AJR Am J Roentgenol, 2005;185(2):533–40.

[32] Wagner A, Mahrholdt H, Sechtem U, et al. MR imaging of myocardial perfusion and viability. Magn Reson Imaging Clin N Am 2003;11(1):49–66.

[33] Regenfus M, Ropers D, Achenbach S, et al. Noninvasive detection of coronary artery stenosis using contrast-enhanced three-dimensional breath-hold magnetic resonance coronary angiography. J Am Coll Cardiol 2000;36(1):44–50.

[34] Kim WY, Danias PG, Stuber M, et al. Coronary magnetic resonance angiography for the detection of coronary stenoses. N Engl J Med 2001;345(26): 1863–9.

[35] van Geuns RJ, Oudkerk M, Rensing BJ, et al. Comparison of coronary imaging between magnetic resonance imaging and electron beam computed tomography. Am J Cardiol 2002;90(1):58–63.

[36] Kwong RY, Schussheim AE, Rekhraj S, et al. Detecting acute coronary syndrome in the emergency department with cardiac magnetic resonance imaging. Circulation 2003;107:531–7.

[37] Takahashi N, Inoue T, Oka T, et al. Diagnostic use of T2-weighted inversion-recovery magnetic resonance imaging in acute coronary syndromes compared with 99mTc-Pyrophosphate, 123I-BMIPP and 201TlCl single photon emission computed tomography. Circ J 2004;68(11):1023–9.

[38] Gottdiener JS. Overview of stress echocardiography: uses, advantages, and limitations. Prog Cardiovasc Dis 2001;43(4):315–34.

[39] McCully RB, Roger VL, Mahoney DW, et al. Outcome after abnormal exercise echocardiography for patients with good exercise capacity: prognostic importance of the extent and severity of exercise-related left ventricular dysfunction. J Am Coll Cardiol 2002;39(8):1345–52.

[40] Elhendy A, Mahoney DW, Burger KN, et al. Prognostic value of exercise echocardiography in patients with classic angina pectoris. Am J Cardiol 2004; 94(5):559–63.

[41] Arruda-Olson AM, Juracan EM, Mahoney DW, et al. Prognostic value of exercise echocardiography in 5,798 patients: is there a gender difference? J Am Coll Cardiol 2002;39(4):625–31.

[42] Marwick TH, Case C, Short L, et al. Prediction of mortality in patients without angina: use of an exercise score and exercise echocardiography. Eur Heart J 2003;24(13):1223–30.

[43] Elhendy A, Mahoney DW, Khandheria BK, et al. Prognostic significance of the location of wall motion abnormalities during exercise echocardiography. J Am Coll Cardiol 2002;40(9):1623–9.

[44] Kamalesh M, Matorin R, Sawada S. Prognostic value of a negative stress echocardiographic study in diabetic patients. Am Heart J 2002;143(1):163–8.

[45] Sozzi FB, Elhendy A, Rizzello V, et al. Prognostic value of dobutamine stress echocardiography in patients with systemic hypertension and known or suspected coronary artery disease. Am J Cardiol 2004;94(6):733–9.

[46] Chuah SC, Pellikka PA, Roger VL, et al. Role of dobutamine stress echocardiography in predicting outcome in 860 patients with known or suspected coronary artery disease. Circulation 1998;97(15): 1474–80.

[47] Amici E, Cortigiani L, Coletta C, et al. Usefulness of pharmacologic stress echocardiography for the long-term prognostic assessment of patients with typical versus atypical chest pain. Am J Cardiol 2003; 91(4):440–2.

[48] Steinberg EH, Madmon L, Patel CP, et al. Long-term prognostic significance of dobutamine echocardiography in patients with suspected coronary artery disease: results of a 5-year follow-up study. J Am Coll Cardiol 1997;29(5):969–73.

[49] Marwick TH, Case C, Sawada S, et al. Prediction of mortality using dobutamine echocardiography. J Am Coll Cardiol 2001;37(3):754–60.

[50] Bholasingh R, Cornel JH, Kamp O, et al. Prognostic value of predischarge dobutamine stress echocardiography in chest pain patients with a negative cardiac troponin T. J Am Coll Cardiol 2003;41(4):596–602.

[51] Biagini E, Elhendy A, Bax JJ, et al. Seven-year follow-up after dobutamine stress echocardiography: impact of gender on prognosis. J Am Coll Cardiol 2005;45(1):93–7.

[52] Yao SS, Qureshi E, Sherrid MV, et al. Practical applications in stress echocardiography: risk stratification and prognosis in patients with known or suspected ischemic heart disease. J Am Coll Cardiol 2003;42(6):1084–90.

[53] Chung G, Krishnamani R, Senior R. Prognostic value of normal stress echocardiogram in patients with suspected coronary artery disease–a British general hospital experience. Int J Cardiol 2004; 94(2–3):181–6.

[54] Peels CH, Visser CA, Kupper AJF, et al. Usefulness of two-dimensional echocardiography for immediate detection of myocardial ischemia in the emergency room. Am J Cardiol 1990;65:687–91.

[55] Sasaki H, Charuzi Y, Beeder C, et al. Utility of echocardiography for the early assessment of patients with non-diagnostic chest pain. Am Heart J 1986; 112:494–7.

[56] Sabia P, Afrookteh A, Touchstone D, et al. Value of regional wall motion abnormality in the emergency room diagnosis of acute myocardial infarction. Circulation 1991;84:I-85–92.

[57] Villanueva FS, Sabia PJ, Afrookteh A, et al. Value and limitations of current methods of evaluating patients presenting to the emergency room with cardiac-related symptoms for determining long-term prognosis. Am J Cardiol 1992;69:746–50.

[58] Loh IK, Charuzi Y, Beeder C, et al. Early diagnosis of non-transmural myocardial infarction by two-dimensional echocardiography. Am Heart J 1982;104: 963–8.

[59] Kontos MC, Arrowood JA, Paulsen WHJ, et al. Early echocardiography can predict cardiac events in emergency department patients with chest pain. Ann Emerg Med 1998;31:550–7.

[60] Kontos MC, Arrowood JA, Jesse RL, et al. Comparison between 2-dimensional echocardiography and myocardial perfusion imaging in the emergency department in patients with possible myocardial ischemia. Am Heart J 1998;136:724–33.

[61] Trippi JA, Lee KS, Kopp G, et al. Dobutamine stress tele-echocardiography for evaluation of emergency department patients with chest pain. J Am Coll Cardiol 1997;30:627–32.

[62] Kaul S, Senior R, Firschke C, et al. Incremental value of cardiac imaging in patients presenting to the emergency department with chest pain and without ST-segment elevation: a multicenter study. Am Heart J 2004;148:129–36.

[63] Schinkel AF, Bax JJ, Elhendy A, et al. Long-term prognostic value of dobutamine stress echocardiography compared with myocardial perfusion scanning in patients unable to perform exercise tests. Am J Med 2004;117(1):1–9.

[64] Smart SC, Bhatia A, Hellman R, et al. Dobutamine-atropine stress echocardiography and dipyridamole sestamibi scintigraphy for the detection of coronary artery disease: limitations and concordance. J Am Coll Cardiol 2000;36(4):1265–73.

[65] Olmos LI, Dakik H, Gordon R, et al. Long-term prognostic value of exercise echocardiography compared with exercise 201Tl, ECG, and clinical variables in patients evaluated for coronary artery disease. Circulation 1998;98(24):2679–86.

[66] Klocke FJ, Baird MG, Lorell BH, et al. ACC/AHA/ASNC guidelines for the clinical use of cardiac radionuclide imaging-executive summary: a report of the American College of Cardiology/American Heart Association Task Force on Practice Guidelines (ACC/AHH/ASNC Committee to revise the 1995 Guidelines for the clinical use of cardiac radionuclide imaging). Circulation;108(11): 1404–18. 2003.

[67] Heller GV, Stowers SA, Hendel RC, et al. Clinical value of acute rest technetium-99m tetrofosmin tomographic myocardial perfusion imaging in patients with acute chest pain and non diagnostic electrocardiogram. J Am Coll Cardiol 1998;31:1011.

[68] Wackers FJ, Brown KA, Heller GV, et al. American Society of Nuclear Cardiology position statement on radionuclide imaging in patients with suspected acute ischemic syndrome in the emergency department or chest pain center. J Nucl Cardiol 2002;9: 246.

[69] Kontos MC, Jesse RL, Anderson P, et al. Comparison of myocardial perfusion imaging and cardiac troponin I in patients admitted to the emergency department with chest pain. Circulation 1999;99: 2073.

[70] Stowers SA, Eisenstein EL, Wackers FJ, et al. An economic analysis of an aggressive diagnostic strategy with single photon emission computed tomography myocardial perfusion imaging and early exercise stress testing in emergency department patients who present with chest pain but nondiagnostic electrocardiograms. Ann Emerg Med 2000; 35:17.

[71] Udelson JE, Beshansky JR, Ballin DS, et al. Myocardial perfusion imaging for evaluation and triage of patients with suspected acute cardiac ischemia: a randomized controlled trial. JAMA 2002;288:2693.

[72] Dilsizian V, Bateman TM, Bergmann SR, et al. Metabolic imaging with methyl-[123I]-iodophenylpentadecanoic acid (BMIPP) identifies ischemic memory following demand ischemia. Circulation 2005;112(14):2169–74.

ELSEVIER
SAUNDERS

Cardiol Clin 24 (2006) 67–78

CARDIOLOGY
CLINICS

Cardiac Risk Assessment: Matching Intensity of Therapy to Risk

Mark R. Vesely, MD, Mark D. Kelemen, MD, MSc, FACC*

*Division of Cardiology, University of Maryland School of Medicine, 22 South Greene Street,
Baltimore, MD 21202, USA*

The concept of cardiac risk assessment is applicable to many settings, from primary prevention and preoperative evaluation to post–myocardial infarction (MI) management. In the context of emergency cardiac care, cardiac risk assessment is typically focused on the evaluation of acute coronary syndrome (ACS): ST-segment elevation MI (STEMI), non–ST-segment elevation MI (NSTEMI), and unstable angina (UA). The likelihood of cardiac death and significant morbidity guides management decisions, including the need for further diagnostic evaluation, specific treatment, and the degree of monitoring for complications. Risk scores of varying complexity are available to guide early management. This article briefly describes the clinical spectrum of NSTE ACS, which encompasses NSTEMI and UA, and focuses on the use of scoring systems in tandem with clinical guidelines to determine the intensity and timing of early therapy. Discussion then focuses on the process of developing these tools and potential future developments in risk assessment.

The rationale of a risk stratification system

The goal of risk assessment is to predict the likelihood of occurrence of a clinically significant outcome, given a complex initial presentation. Risk models can be used in stratification within clinical trials, in quality of care evaluation based on expected outcomes, and, as described here, in medical decision making [1]. Once a risk model is

developed and validated, the frequency of clinical outcomes (beneficial and adverse) following a specific therapy can be determined within the risk levels. The high risk of morbidity and mortality from ACS must be balanced with the degree of benefit and risk of adverse events inherent in the various therapeutic options available for ACS. For instance, antiplatelet therapy with a platelet glycoprotein (Gp) IIb/IIIa receptor antagonist improves outcome in many patients who have ACS but is associated with increased rates of thrombocytopenia and bleeding. A risk stratification system (RSS), through a standardized assessment scheme, allows a concise and simplified method for characterizing this risk. Once derived and validated, risk models can be tested prospectively to assess their predictive capacity. If effective, they can help the clinician make the risk benefit calculation. Optimal risk stratification and delivery of care remains a moving target, however. The understanding of the pathophysiology of ACS and available treatment options constantly evolve. As additional risk factors and therapies arise, an RSS can become outdated because these new features are not included in the model. Therefore, the optimal use of an RSS depends on an understanding of the strengths and weaknesses of the RSS, including the setting in which it was developed.

Mortality from acute ischemic heart disease has fallen considerably during the past 2 decades because of advances in prevention, diagnosis, and treatment. Despite well-established consensus guidelines, however, many patients do not receive recommended treatments or are given medications that may actually increase risk. Observational studies from the early 1990s (Thrombolysis In

---

* Corresponding author.

E-mail address: mkelemen@medicine.umaryland.edu (M.D. Kelemen).

Myocardial Infarction [TIMI] 3 registry) [2] to 2002 (Can Rapid Risk Stratification of Unstable Angina Patients Suppress Adverse Outcomes with Early Implementation of the ACC/AHA Guidelines [CRUSADE]) [3] confirm the increased use of aspirin (from 82% to 90%) and beta-blockers (from 45% to 76%) but demonstrate low rates of use of heparin (53%) and, recently, Gp IIb/IIIa inhibitors (31%).

RSSs may improve compliance with the national guidelines, however, they have the potential for being very complicated. The measurement of the biomarkers including troponin, C-reactive peptide, and B-type natriuretic peptide (BNP), each give independent and additive prognostic information [4]. Table 1 provides a more complete list of variables that have been associated with increased mortality in NSTE ACS. A scoring system that incorporates all of them would be time-consuming; and time-to-treatment itself is an important risk factor. While some variables can be determined quickly, others require improvements in the speed of laboratory testing or in computer processing. Furthermore, certain predictors are strong and consistently associated with risk, such as the peak level of cardiac troponin I (or T) [2]. The peak level is not known for several days in NSTE ACS, however, so therapy cannot be guided in the first few hours of presentation.

The consensus guidelines for NSTE ACS introduce the concept of matching intensity of therapy to risk identified during a hospitalization, but no randomized controlled trials have focused on a strategy based entirely on risk scoring. According to the class I recommendations from the guidelines, high-risk and low-risk patients have clearly identified pathways with different treatment strategies. Patients at intermediate risk typically 30% to 40% of all patients, probably account for much of the variability in treatment prescription.

Interaction of consensus guidelines and quality improvement studies

An individual's risk during an episode of ACS is determined by factors unique to that patient and factors related to the pathophysiology of ACS. Patient factors include age, known prior ischemic heart disease, and evidence of heart failure on presentation. Angina pectoris can be classified as unstable in three scenarios: rest angina (angina occurring at rest and continuing for longer than 20 minutes), new-onset angina (new onset with slight limitation of ordinary activity), and increasing angina (previously present but now more frequent, longer in duration, and with decreased exertional threshold) [14]. The Canadian Cardiovascular Society [15] classification system differentiates symptoms into four grades based on exertional tolerance, but descriptive classification of angina pectoris based on severity of symptoms has been found to be unreliable in providing prognostic information [15,16].

There are five mechanisms underlying myocardial ischemia in NSTE ACS, resulting in disproportionate supply and demand of myocardial oxygen [17]. Decreased myocardial perfusion and oxygen delivery are common to four mechanisms; nonocclusive thrombus and microembolization are the most common. Dynamic obstruction from epicardial vasospasm, progressive severe narrowing without spasm, and localized inflammation also decrease oxygen delivery. Secondary UA is caused by either decreased supply (anemia and hypoxemia) or increased demand (fever and hypotension), typically in the setting of underlying CAD. These mechanisms are nonexclusive and do not offer reliable prognostic information within the initial evaluation period.

When facing an ACS presentation, the clinician's first critical decision point is excluding STEMI. An ECG should be obtained within the first 10 minutes of arrival (or sooner if possible). The first set of biomarkers should be available within 60 minutes [18]. This inherent delay results in reduced efficiency in identifying and treating high-risk patients; therefore risk assessment tools were developed. Aspirin, heparin (unfractionated or low molecular weight) and beta-blockers are given to all patients who do not have contraindications, and Gp IIb/IIIa inhibitors are used in high-risk patients for whom early cardiac catheterization is also recommended. Although patients who have ACS are, as a group, at increased risk of death and nonfatal ischemic complications, the spectrum of disease severity and subsequent outcomes remains wide. Initial evaluation should focus on immediate management of hemodynamic instability and identifying patients at significant risk for death, recurrent MI, stroke, heart failure, and recurrent ischemic symptoms. Because the intensity of therapy typically depends on this prognostic information, risk assessment facilitates further decisions on the type of antithrombin and antiplatelet therapy, the indications for and timing of invasive angiographic evaluation, and the appropriate level of further monitoring

Table 1
Variables associated with increased mortality in acute coronary syndrome

	TIMI [5]	PURSUIT [6]	GRACE [7]	Other
Demographics				
Age ≥65 y	+	.	.	.
Latin American race	.	+	.	.
Female gender	.	.	+	.
Medical history				
≥3 CAD risk factors*	+	.	.	.
Diabetes mellitus	*	+	+	.
Hypertension	*	.	+	.
Hyperlipidemia	*	+	+	.
Current smoking	*	+	-	.
Family history of CAD	*	+	.	.
Congestive Heart Failure	.	+	+	.
Stroke	.	+	+	.
Peripheral vascular disease	.	+	+	.
Renal dysfunction	.	.	+	+ [8]
Angina	.	.	-	.
Atrial fibrillation	.	.	+	.
Prior (+) exercise stress test	.	.	+	.
Bleeding	.	.	+	.
CAD history				
Coronary stenosis ≥50%	+	.	.	.
Prior angioplasty	+	+	-	.
Coronary artery bypass	.	+	+	.
Myocardial infarction	.	+	.	.
Presentation				
Cardiac arrest	.	.	+	.
Severe angina	+	+	.	.
Enrolled as MI, not UA	.	+	.	.
Rales (≥1/3 of lung fields)	.	+	.	.
ECG changes				
ST deviation	+	.	+	.
ST depression	.	+	+	.
Anterior ST depression	.	.	+	.
Inferior ST depression	.	.	+	.
T-wave inversion	.	+	-	.
Significant Q-wave	.	.	+	.
Left bundle branch block	.	.	+	.
Right bundle branch block	.	.	+	.
Prior medication use				
Aspirin	+	+	-	.
Statin	.	.	-	.
β-blocker	.	+	.	.
Calcium channel blocker	.	+	.	.
Nitrates	.	+	.	.
ACE inhibitor	.	+	.	.
Biomarkers				
Troponin I (or T)	+	.	+	+ [9]
CK-MB	+	.	+	.
Myoglobin	.	.	.	+ [10]
NT-proBNP	.	.	.	+ [9]
C-reactive protein	.	.	.	+ [11]
Hemoglobin	.	.	.	+ [12]
White blood cell count	.	.	.	+ [13]

Abbreviations: ACE, angiotensin-converting enzyme; CAD, coronary artery disease; CK-MD, MB isoenzyme of creatine kinase; GRACE, Global Registry of Acute Coronary Events; NT-proBNP, N-terminal probrain natriuretic peptide; PURSUIT, Platelet Glycoprotein IIb/IIIa in Unstable Angina: Receptor Suppression Using Integrilin Therapy Trail.

(ranging from evaluation in the chest pain unit and outpatient follow-up to critical care admission).

What makes a risk stratification system useful?

As a clinical tool, the usefulness of an RSS depends on its accuracy (ie, predictive capacity) and applicability (ie, ease of use). The number and type of variables used in the system, the endpoints for which the system is meant to predict, and the populations in which a system is tested and to which a system is applied are important for the success of an RSS. Ideally, an RSS can be used at the bedside to provide highly accurate and relevant prognostic information within a short time frame. The clinical variables should be informative and obtained easily and quickly. Intuitively, the more variables there are within a risk stratification model, the more informative it is likely to be. As knowledge of the pathophysiology of ACS continues to expand, so do the number and complexity of the potential variables available for use within an RSS. As additional factors are used to provide more predictive capacity, each additional variable can add potential time and difficulty for use, making the system more cumbersome and thus less applicable.

A typical RSS design is based on a point system, in which points are assigned for the presence (or absence) of specific clinical factors. The sum of these points correlates to a specific risk level. An RSS with absolute discriminatory capacity would account for all of the variables influencing a particular outcome. If such a system were composed of five independent risk factors (A, B, C, D, and E) of equal impact to the overall risk, each factor would account for 20% of the overall risk burden. If, however, factor A portrays twice the level of risk as the others A would represent 33.3% of the overall risk burden, and each of the remaining four factors would represent 16.6% of the overall risk. This variability in attributable risk must be accounted for in risk stratification to maximize accuracy. In point-system risk models, accuracy is maximized by weighing each factor by the percentage of its contribution to total risk of the outcome (eg, factor A, 2 points; factors B, C, D, and E, 1 point each) [1]. As additional, appropriately weighted factors are added to a system for improved accuracy, the system's complexity expands and can potentially become a hindrance to its quick and appropriate use.

ACS has many potential adverse outcomes, including need for urgent revascularization, recurrent MI, and death. To provide clinically useful prognostic information, an RSS may be developed with these relevant outcomes combined into a composite endpoint, with the perspective that the risk of any one of the outcomes is pertinent to optimizing management. A composite endpoint such as a major adverse cardiac event (MACE), is easier to use clinically, in that a therapeutic option can be provided if the risk of MACE (any one of the many outcomes included in MACE) is not too high. If a health care provider is attempting to avoid any and all of these outcomes, combining them in one RSS is simpler than having an RSS for each of the individual outcomes. Specific factors within an RSS, however, may be predictive only of certain events within a composite endpoint (ie, urgent revascularization but not death). If the practitioner is primarily concerned about mortality, a scale with an accurate predictor of risk of death should be chosen.

Finally, the practitioner using the RSS should be aware of the patient population in which the scale was derived. An RSS is best developed in a diverse patient population to allow applicability to a similarly wide population. If an RSS is developed in a selective population, significant factors may exist within that population that are not accounted for but that uniformly add risk to the general population. If those factors do not exist in a subsequent patient, the predicted risk may be less accurate. For example, if the derivation cohort of an RSS for ACS outcomes contains a high prevalence of smoking, then smoking may not add predictive capacity to the RSS and may not be included in the final model. If that RSS is then applied to a nonsmoking patient, the RSS may suggest higher risk than the patient really has. The application of an RSS to a patient not similar to the derivation cohort or subsequently verified population may thus provide inaccurate information. The responsibility for the appropriate use of an RSS thus falls on the user, who must maintain this perspective when relying on an RSS to assist in medical decision making.

Anatomy of a risk stratification system: the Thrombolysis In Myocardial Infarction risk score for unstable angina/non–ST-segment elevation myocardial infarction

Among the types of RSS available for clinical use, models developed through multivariable regression are frequently employed [19]. Multiple clinical characteristics are first identified as associated with the likelihood for the event. These characteristics are then compiled into a composite score that functions as a mathematical representation of the probability of the clinical event's occurrence [1].

As an example of an RSS, the development of the TIMI risk score (TIMI RSS) for UA/NSTEMI is discussed. The purpose of the TIMI RSS is to assist in the identification of the patients at highest risk for further adverse events such as death and recurrent ischemia or infarction. Given the variability of potential adverse outcomes, the primary endpoint (within follow up for 14 days) was chosen as a composite of all-cause mortality, new or recurrent MI, or recurrent ischemia leading to urgent revascularization. The creation of the TIMI RSS included two stages of production, the initial development of the system using one cohort of patients and a subsequent validation of the system with a different set of patients. The initial patient population used for the development of the system, defined as the "derivation cohort," consisted of the 1957 patients in the TIMI 11B trial who were randomly assigned to receive standard treatment including aspirin and unfractionated heparin (UFH) [20]. Study subjects were enrolled between August 1996 and March 1998, with an adjustment in inclusion criteria after the first 10 months. Initial parameters for enrollment included the presence of ischemic discomfort at rest for at least 5 minutes and additional evidence of ischemic heart disease including history of CAD, ST-segment deviation, or elevated serum cardiac markers. After 10 months of enrollment, the criteria were adjusted to focus on higher-risk patients who have evidence of ischemic heart disease and was limited to only those with ST-segment deviation or elevated serum cardiac markers. The study subjects had a mean age of 66 years, and 64% were male. CAD risk factors within the patient population included family history (34%), hypertension (50%), hypercholesterolemia (32%), diabetes mellitus (20%), and current smoking (27%). Prior cardiac history was also present in many patients, such as previous MI (32%), history of coronary artery bypass graft surgery (CABG) (13%), and history of percutaneous transluminal coronary angioplasty (12%). ECG abnormality, including ST-segment deviations or T-wave inversion, was present in 83% of the patients, and elevated serum cardiac markers were present at enrollment in 40% of

the patients. The majority of patients were ultimately diagnosed as having UA (58%), but 34.5% of the patients had a non–Q-wave MI, and 3.8% had a Q-wave MI. Through the full 14-day follow-up period, 16.7% of the patients experienced the composite endpoint.

The choice of potential predictor variables was completed with the goal of producing an easily applicable stratification system with useful predictive capacity. The number of predictors for the model was thus critical, because too few variables might limit predictive capacity, but too many variables would make the system cumbersome and hamper clinical utility. Thus the potential predictor variables selected were those that were easily identifiable as a baseline characteristic and previously demonstrated to be predictive of outcome. Twelve variables were chosen as potential contributors to the scoring system:

1. Age greater than 65 years
2. Presence of more than three CAD risk factors (including family history of CAD, hypertension, hypercholesterolemia, diabetes, current smoking)
3. Prior coronary stenosis greater than 50%
4. Prior MI
5. Prior CABG
6. Prior percutaneous transluminal coronary angioplasty
7. ST-segment deviation greater than 0.5 mV
8. Severe anginal symptoms (two anginal events in the prior 24 hours)
9. Use of aspirin in last 7 days,
10. Use of intravenous UFH within 24 hours of enrollment
11. Elevated serum cardiac markers (creatine kinase myocardial band or troponin)
12. Prior history of congestive heart failure

These 12 variables were then analyzed by univariate logistic regression, and the variables with a significant correlation ($P < .20$) were subjected to multivariate logistic regression analysis. The seven variables found to correlate significantly with the endpoint were chosen subsequently for the risk stratification model (Fig. 1) [21].

Two additional statistical tests, the C-statistic and the Hosmer-Lemeshow statistic, were applied to the final variable set to assess the model's performance in terms of discrimination and calibration. The C-statistic measures a stratification model's predictive capacity by assessing discriminative ability to classify an individual to the

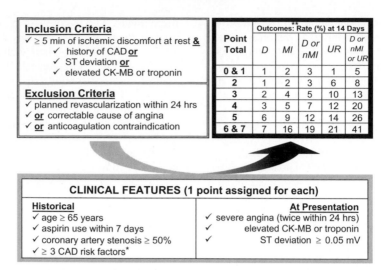

Inclusion Criteria	Point Total	Outcomes: Rate (%) at 14 Days				
✓ ≥ 5 min of ischemic discomfort at rest **&**		D	MI	D or nMI	UR	D or nMI or UR
0 & 1	1	2	3	1	5

Fig. 1. The TIMI risk score for UA/NSTEMI was derived from the TIMI 11B patient cohort. Multivariate logistic regression identified seven clinical features, which provide equally weighted prognostic information. One point is assigned for each present feature, and points are summed to derive the patient's TIMI risk score. The risk scores of 0 and 1 and the risk scores of 6 and 7 are combined to derive six TIMI risk levels. Rates of individual events and composite outcomes were determined from the entire TIMI 11B patient population, including both the unfractionated heparin and enoxaparin arms. Likelihood of death, MI, or urgent revascularization increases with each risk level ($P < .001$). Risk factors for coronary artery disease are a family history of coronary artery disease, hypertension, hypercholesterolemia, diabetes mellitus, active smoking. D, all-cause mortality; MI, myocardial infarction; nMI, nonfatal myocardial infarction; UR, urgent revitalization. (*From* Antman EM, Cohen M, Bernink PJ, et al. The TIMI risk score for unstable angina/non-ST elevation MI: a method for prognostication and therapeutic decision making. JAMA 2000;284:835.)

appropriate risk level. The Hosmer-Lemeshow statistic assesses a model's "goodness of fit" or calibration by comparing rates of actual events with predicted events within each risk group. The C-statistic and Hosmer-Lemeshow statistic showed the TIMI RSS to be well balanced for discriminatory capacity and calibration (Hosmer-Lemeshow statistic: 3.56, 8 degrees of freedom, $P = 0.89$; C-statistic: 0.65 with 0.83 the best balance of discrimination and calibration) [21].

Although a multivariate logistic regression model could provide a weighted score for each variable to be used in predicting a risk score, it would require complex calculations probably requiring computer assistance. Given the desire to produce an easily applicable bedside tool, each of the seven significant variables was weighted equally because the seven variables had similar prognostic significance (odds ratio). Thus the TIMI RSS was produced as a summed score of one point for each of the seven variables, making eight possible scores, ranging from 0 to 7. The summed scores of 0 and 1 were combined, as were those of 6 and 7, to make a final total of six levels of risk (Fig. 1).

When examining the clinical applicability of the TIMI RSS, several favorable characteristics

were identified, each adding to the overall utility of the model. The six risk levels were found to have a normal distribution within the derivation cohort. In addition, each subsequent risk level correlated with significantly increased rates of clinical endpoints, producing a wide range of risk across the six levels. The risk of experiencing death (from any cause), new or recurrent MI, or urgent revascularization secondary to recurrent ischemia within 14 days of presentation ranged from 4.7% (at the 0–1 risk level) to 40.9% (at the 6–7 risk level.) Finally, the trend of 14-day risk for each of the individual components of the composite endpoint increased in parallel with the composite endpoint.

Once set in its final form, the risk stratification model was retrospectively applied to three additional cohorts for validation, including the patients receiving enoxaparin in TIMI 11B (n = 1953) [11] and both the UFH (n = 1564) and enoxaparin (n = 1564) arms of the Efficacy and Safety of Subcutaneous Enoxaparin in Non-Q-wave Coronary Events (ESSENCE) trial [22]. Both discriminatory capacity and calibration were maintained within these additional patient cohorts.

Application of the Thrombolysis In Myocardial Infarction risk score for unstable angina/non–ST-segment elevation myocardial infarction

The purpose of identifying high-risk patients is to alter management to mitigate risk. The TIMI RSS was assessed for the ability to predict which patients gained benefit from the choice of enoxaparin over UFH. Patients within the TIMI 11B and ESSENCE trials were stratified by their TIMI RSS to test retrospectively for improved outcome with enoxaparin (Fig. 2). When assessing patients within each TRS, enoxaparin was shown to provide greater benefit than UFH to patients who had a TRS of 4 or higher. A superior outcome in the high-risk groups with enoxaparin is conceptually plausible, because bolus subcutaneous dosing may reach therapeutic levels faster than the slowly titrated UFH continuous intravenous infusion. Unlike UFH, however, the degree of anticoagulation with enoxaparin is not monitored. If the presence of low molecular weight heparin delays a needed cardiac catheterization and revascularization, the benefit for high-risk patients may not

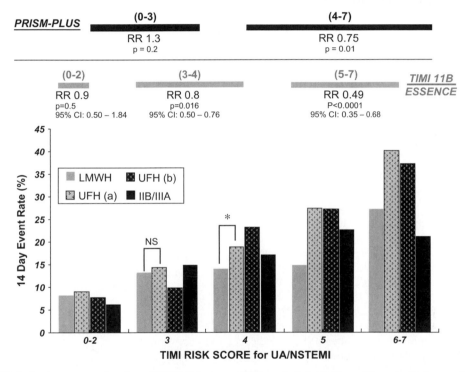

Fig. 2. Clinical outcomes as a function of TIMI risk scores. Efficacy of strategies for antithrombotic therapy in patients with NSTE ACS following stratification with the TIMI risk score (TRS) for UA/NSTEMI. All strategies included aspirin and determined composite endpoint event rates at 14 days. LMWH, patients receiving enoxaparin in the TIMI 11B and ESSENCE trials; UFH (a), patients receiving unfractionated heparin in the TIMI 11B and ESSENCE trials; UFH (b), patients receiving unfractionated heparin in the PRISM-PLUS trial; IIb/IIIa, patients receiving unfractionated heparin and the glycoprotein IIb/IIIa receptor antagonist tirofiban in the PRISM-PLUS trial. Compared with UFH alone, patients receive greater benefit with UFH and tirofiban if their TRS is 4 or higher (TRS 0–3: relative risk [RR], 1.3; $P = .2$; TRS 4–7: RR, 0.75; $P = .01$). When risk scores are further grouped into low-risk (TRS 0–2), intermediate-risk (TRS 3–4), and high-risk (TRS 5–7) groups, patients with intermediate or high risk have greater benefit with enoxaparin (TRS 0–2: RR, 0.91; 95% CI, 0.67–1.22; $P = .5$; TRS 3–4: RR, 0.8; 95% CI 0.67–0.96; $P = .016$; TRS 5–7: RR, 0.49; 95% CI 0.35–0.68; $P < 0.0001$). In analysis of clinical benefit within individual TIMI risk scores, however, there is greater benefit with enoxaparin than with UFH if the TRS is 4 or higher (TRS 3: RR, 0.91; 95% CI, 0.71–1.16; $P = .43$; TRS 4: RR, 0.71; 95% CI, 0.54–0.93; $P = .009$). (*Data from* Antman EM, Cohen M, Bernink PJ, et al. The TIMI risk score for unstable angina/non-ST elevation MI: a method for prognostication and therapeutic decision making. JAMA 2000;284:835; Morrow DA, Antman EM, Snapinn SM, et al. An integrated clinical approach to predicting the benefit of tirofiban in non-ST elevation acute coronary syndromes. Application of the TIMI Risk Score for UA/NSTEMI in PRISM-PLUS. Eur Heart J 2002;23:223.)

be fully realized. Since the publication of the consensus guidelines, no randomized clinical trial has prospectively assessed the relative benefit of enoxaparin over UFH in high-risk patients. On the other end of the risk spectrum, therapeutic anticoagulation with heparin (UFH or enoxaparin) can increase the risk of hemorrhage, stroke, and thrombocytopenia [22,23]. No randomized clinical trial has examined the benefit of heparin (UFH or enoxaparin) anticoagulation in low-risk NSTE ACS.

In addition to medical management of NSTE ACS with antianginal and antithrombotic therapy, the treating clinician must decide whether invasive cardiac catheterization is indicated. Two general strategies for approaching cardiac catheterization are generally used: an invasive approach in which patients routinely undergo catheterization within 48 hours of admission, or a conservative approach in which catheterization is completed if recurrent ischemia occurs spontaneously or is provoked through noninvasive testing. Between December 1997 and December 1999, 2220 patients were enrolled into the Treat Angina with Aggrastat and Determine Cost of Therapy with an Invasive or Conservative Strategy (TACTICS)-TIMI 18 trial and were randomly assigned to one of these two strategies [24]. Medical antithrombotic therapy consisted of aspirin, UFH, and tirofiban. Over a 6-month follow-up period, patients who underwent routine early catheterization experienced significantly less recurrent ischemia but suffered higher rates of protocol-defined bleeding (5.5% versus 3.3%; $P < .01$). Stratification with the TIMI RSS demonstrated patients who have intermediate risk (3–4) or high risk (5–7) benefited from the routine early catheterization. Patients at low risk (0–2) did not obtain greater benefit from one strategy over the other (Fig. 3). The benefit of routine early catheterization in the intermediate-risk group of patients was barely significant ($P = .048$; upper bound of 95% CI, .999). Whether analysis of patient groups within individual scores (3 versus 4; Fig. 2) or redefining the bounds of the intermediate risk group would enhance predictive capacity remains unclear. Current consensus guideline class I recommendations call for an early invasive strategy if any of the following high-risk indicators are present:

1. Recurrent angina/ischemia with rest or low-level exertion in setting of intense anti-ischemic therapy

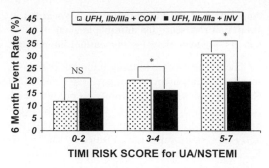

Fig. 3. Assessment of cardiac catheterization strategies in addition to aspirin, unfractionated heparin (UFH), and tirofiban (IIb/IIIa) in the TACTICS-TIMI 18 trial. Rates of a composite endpoint (death, nonfatal MI, or rehospitalization for ACS) at 6 months were compared between conservative (CON: selective catheterization) and invasive (INV: routine catheterization) strategies. Risk levels were stratified as low (TIMI risk score 0–2), intermediate (TIMI risk score 3–4) and high (TIMI risk score 5–7). Although there was no difference between strategies in the low-risk group, routine catheterization was beneficial in the intermediate-risk ($P = .048$) and high-risk ($P = .018$) groups. (*From* Cannon CP, Weintraub WS, Demopoulos LA, et al. Comparison of early invasive and conservative strategies in patients with unstable coronary syndromes treated with the glycoprotein IIb/IIIa inhibitor tirofiban. N Engl J Med 2001;344:1879.)

2. Elevated troponin (I or T)
3. New ST-segment depression
4. Recurrent angina/ischemia with signs or symptoms of congestive heart failure
5. High-risk results from noninvasive stress testing
6. Left ventricular ejection fraction less than 0.40
7. Hemodynamic instability
8. Sustained ventricular tachycardia
9. PCI within 6 months
10. Prior CABG

Either the early invasive strategy or early conservative strategy is recommended if none of these findings are present. Risk stratification by multivariate RSS has not yet been addressed in consensus guidelines. Likewise, the best combination of medical and invasive management for NSTE ACS is likely to remain undetermined. As new therapies and equipment continue to arise, the time required to complete a clinical trial to assess a specific combination of therapies will persist as a barrier to this goal. Nonetheless, stratified trials to assess benefit from routine early catheterization with drug-eluting stents, a different antithrombotic regimen (enoxaparin in place of UFH), or additional therapeutic agents such clopidogrel [25] have not been completed.

Other risk stratification systems

Because risk stratification is a multivariable issue with continuously evolving risk factors and management options, current consensus guidelines describe specific clinical features independently associated with various risk levels rather than endorsing one single RSS. Multiple tables are used to illustrate how specific factors derived from the Duke Cardiovascular Databank are associated with risk of clinical events such as true ACS from CAD, death, and nonfatal MI [26]. With this system, patients are assessed as being at high, intermediate, or low risk with the presence of any one factor in that risk level grouping [27].

In efforts to maximize the predictive capacity in risk stratification during the initial time period of an ACS presentation, the Platelet Glycoprotein IIb/IIIa in Unstable Angina: Receptor Suppression Using Integrilin Therapy Trial (PURSUIT) investigators examined both dichotomous and continuous baseline characteristics for prognostic utility [6]. Outcomes (30-day rates of mortality and nonfatal MI) were assessed in 9461 patients randomly assigned to receive the Gp IIb/IIIa inhibitor eptifibatide or placebo upon presentation with NSTE ACS. After univariate and subsequent multivariate logistic regression analysis, an equation was derived to calculate the probability of 30-day mortality, including 23 weighted clinical variables. Because information on all 23 variables and use of a computer would be required to complete this calculation, this model is not easily applicable at the bedside. A simplified model was then developed by removal of the 16 least informative features and subsequent placement of the remaining seven variables into a weighted point system. To estimate risk of 30-day mortality or nonfatal MI, or mortality alone, the sum of points is then applied against a curve. Although the discriminatory capacity of the mortality model is excellent (C-statistic 0.814), the complexity of the model reduces its applicability at the bedside.

To assess the risk of death across the entire ACS spectrum (UA, NSTEMI, and STEMI) and to allow application to a more generalized patient population, the Global Registry of Acute Coronary Events (GRACE) RSS was more recently developed from patients who had ACS sampled

from 94 hospitals located in 14 different countries [7]. A nomogram was developed to facilitate risk assessment by summing eight weighted variables, including Killip class, systolic blood pressure, heart rate, age, creatinine level, presence of cardiac arrest at admission, ST-segment deviation, and elevated cardiac enzyme levels. Discriminatory ability was again demonstrated to be excellent (C-statistic 0.83). A comparison of the GRACE RSS and the PURSUIT RSS was recently completed with application to the Canadian ACS Registry, comprising 4627 patients who had ACS enrolled between September 1999 and June 2001 [28]. Again, both models were found to have excellent predictive capacity (C statistic: 0.84 for PURSUIT, 0.83 for GRACE). Although the GRACE RSS was found to be well calibrated (Hosmer Lemeshow $P = .40$), the PURSUIT RSS calibration was suboptimal (Hosmer Lemeshow $P < .001$). This observation demonstrates the potential for differences between clinical trial populations and real-world patients and reinforces the appropriateness of validation among diverse patient populations before widespread use of an RSS. In an effort to maximize predictive capacity, large numbers of variables with associated weighting for attributable risk are employed in the PURSUIT and GRACE systems. These systems, however, are too complex to be used easily straight from memory, and their complexity detracts from their clinical applicability. Alternatively, the TIMI RSS employs seven equally weighted variables to allow improved applicability but at the cost of predictive capacity (C statistic 0.65). With greater ease of use, the TIMI RSS has been more routinely tested for ability to assist in medical decision making, but as hand-held computers become more available to clinicians, the more complicated systems are likely to be more useful.

Future developments in risk stratification

The goal of developing optimal management for NSTE ACS will remain a moving target. Improvements in risk stratification tools and their appropriate use are needed to guide clinicians through the complicated options for management. As such, methods and tools for risk stratification will continue to evolve. Since the development of the RSS discussed here, additional variables have been recognized as prognostically important and subsequently have been shown to provide additional stratification potential. These new risk factors are likely to be spliced into existing systems or used in the creation of new scoring systems. As one example of an attempt to improve stratification beyond that by existing systems, Bazzino and colleagues [9] assessed numerous molecular markers in conjunction with clinical features for predictive capacity, including N-terminal probrain natriuretic peptide (NT-proBNP), high sensitivity C-reactive protein, troponin T, and myoglobin. Predictive capacity for 6-month mortality improved with additional stratification with NT-proBNP level, beyond that provided by the TIMI risk score for UA/NSTEMI (Fig. 4) and the American College of Cardiology/American Heart Association classification system. Other clinical variables are frequently examined for independent prognostic utility and hence qualify for future RSS. Features associated with the pathophysiologic processes involved in ACS, including markers of inflammation (white blood cell count) [13] and myocardial injury (myoglobin) [10], as well as comorbidities such as anemia (hemoglobin) [12] and renal insufficiency (creatinine clearance) [29], have been shown to predict adverse clinical outcomes independently. How to best use this additional information within the perspective of clinical decision making and future risk models remains to be determined.

Although molecular markers that are directly reflective of cardiomyocyte death, such as troponin I (and T), provide prognostic information, the delay in achieving elevated levels significant enough for detection can be prevent their use as a variable for early risk stratification. Biomarkers of underlying processes leading to cellular death have potential for providing early prognostic information, because they will potentially reach clinically significant elevated levels earlier within the course of an ACS presentation. Some potential upstream biomarkers with early promise include myeloperoxidase, metalloproteinase-9, soluble CD-40 ligand, pregnancy-associated plasma protein A, choline, ischemia-modified unbound free fatty acids, placental growth factor, and glycogen phosphorylase isoenzyme BB [30]. Although the many clinical and biomarker factors currently used in stratification systems account for the majority of variance in outcomes, molecular markers have potential to differentiate risk more quickly and accurately. As this field continues to develop with newly recognized biomarkers and organization of biomarker panels, more precise stratification within the intermediate-risk group may allow improved delivery of optimized care.

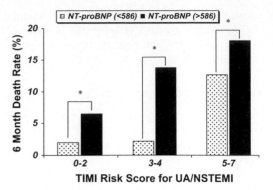

Fig. 4. Risk stratification for 6-month mortality is enhanced when N-terminal probrain natriuretic peptide (NT-proBNP levels) are checked within 7 hours of admission for NSTE ACS. Within each TIMI risk level, likelihood of the composite death or nonfatal MI, or of death alone, was higher with the NT-proBNP level greater than 586 pg/mL ($P < .001$ for interaction test). (*From* Bazzino O, Fuselli JJ, Botto F, et al. Relative value of N-terminal probrain natriuretic peptide, TIMI risk score, ACC/AHA prognostic classification and other risk markers in patients with non-ST-elevation acute coronary syndromes. Eur Heart J 2004;25:859.)

Summary

Simple RSS allow for rapid decision making in the emergency department. The data presented in this article suggest that for patients at the highest risk and the lowest risk for complications of NSTE ACS, the scoring systems work well and allow effective triage and treatment. For patients at intermediate risk (30%–40% of all patients who have ACS), however, it is not clear whether early aggressive treatment with cardiac catheterization or routine conservative management should be the standard of care. The consensus guidelines are vague, and the scoring systems discriminate less well for these patients. The authors think that patients at intermediate risk are best served by initial screening with an RSS like the TRS (with risk scores of 3–4), followed by a multimarker strategy to define risk better. They also think that the next step is to design clinical trials to test strategies of care defined prospectively by risk. This step would, in the authors' opinion, begin the next round of the cycle of clinical therapeutics [31]. The treatment of patients who have NSTE ACS has been characterized in the past 2 decades by care based on evidence from many excellent clinical trials. The consensus panels have convened and guide patient management. Quality-improvement initiatives such as CRUSADE and GRACE give feedback to improve compliance with guidelines. The understanding of risk is developing with the help of these scoring systems. Discovery is ongoing. The next decade of acute cardiac care will focus on early identification of patients at high risk and on matching the most intensive treatments to the patients most in need. Excessive testing and care promotes cost inefficiency and, perhaps, increased hazard for some patients. New trials are needed to move these new hypotheses back into practice.

References

[1] Mourouga PGC, Rowan KM. Does it fit? Is it good? Assessment of scoring systems. Curr Opin Crit Care 2000;6:176.

[2] Stone PH, Thompson B, Anderson HV, et al. Influence of race, sex, and age on management of unstable angina and non-Q-wave myocardial infarction: The TIMI III registry. JAMA 1996;275:1104.

[3] Bhatt DL, Roe MT, Peterson ED, et al. Utilization of early invasive management strategies for high-risk patients with non-ST-segment elevation acute coronary syndromes: results from the CRUSADE Quality Improvement Initiative. JAMA 2004;292: 2096.

[4] Sabatine MS, Morrow DA, de Lemos JA, et al. Multimarker approach to risk stratification in non-ST elevation acute coronary syndromes: simultaneous assessment of troponin I, C-reactive protein, and B-type natriuretic peptide. Circulation 2002;105: 1760.

[5] Antman EM, Cohen M, Bernink PJ, et al. The TIMI risk score for unstable angina/non-st elevation MI: A method for prognostication and therapeutic decision making. JAMA 2000;284:835–42.

[6] Boersma E, Pieper KS, Steyerberg EW, et al. Predictors of outcome in patients with acute coronary syndromes without persistent ST-segment elevation. Results from an international trial of 9461 patients. The PURSUIT Investigators. Circulation 2000;101: 2557.

[7] Granger CB, Goldberg RJ, Dabbous O, et al. Predictors of hospital mortality in the global registry of acute coronary events. Arch Intern Med 2003; 163:2345.

[8] Gibson CM, Pinto DS, Murphy SA, et al. Association of creatinine and creatinine clearance on presentation in acute myocardial infarction with subsequent mortality. J Am Coll Cardiol 2003;42: 1535–43.

[9] Bazzino O, Fuselli JJ, Botto F, et al. Relative value of N-terminal probrain natriuretic peptide, TIMI risk score, ACC/AHA prognostic classification and other risk markers in patients with non-ST-elevation acute coronary syndromes. Eur Heart J 2004;25:859.

[10] de Lemos JA, Morrow DA, Gibson CM, et al. The prognostic value of serum myoglobin in patients with non-ST-segment elevation acute coronary syndromes. Results from the TIMI 11B and TACTICS-TIMI 18 studies. J Am Coll Cardiol 2002;40:238.

[11] Morrow DA, Rifai N, Antman EM, et al. C-reactive protein is a potent predictor of mortality independently of and in combination with troponin T in acute coronary syndromes: A TIMI 11a substudy. Thrombolysis in myocardial infarction. J Am Coll Cardiol 1998;31:1460–5.

[12] Sabatine MS, Morrow DA, Giugliano RP, et al. Association of hemoglobin levels with clinical outcomes in acute coronary syndromes. Circulation 2005;111:2042.

[13] Bhatt DL, Chew DP, Lincoff AM, et al. Effect of revascularization on mortality associated with an elevated white blood cell count in acute coronary syndromes. Am J Cardiol 2003;92:136.

[14] Braunwald E. Unstable angina. A classification. Circulation 1989;80:410.

[15] Campeau L. Grading of angina pectoris [letter]. Circulation 1976;54:522.

[16] Campeau L. The Canadian Cardiovascular Society grading of angina pectoris revisited 30 years later. Can J Cardiol 2002;18:371.

[17] Braunwald E. Unstable angina: an etiologic approach to management. Circulation 1998;90:2219.

[18] Wu AH, Apple FS, Gibler WB, et al. National Academy of Clinical Biochemistry Standards of Laboratory Practice: recommendations for the use of cardiac markers in coronary artery diseases. Clin Chem 1999;45:1104.

[19] Harrell FE Jr, Lee KL, Mark DB. Multivariable prognostic models: issues in developing models, evaluating assumptions and adequacy, and measuring and reducing errors. Stat Med 1996;15:361.

[20] Antman EM, McCabe CH, Gurfinkel EP, et al. Enoxaparin prevents death and cardiac ischemic events in unstable angina/non-Q-wave myocardial infarction. Results of the thrombolysis in myocardial infarcion (TIMI) 11B trial. Circulation 1999; 100:1593.

[21] Sabatine MS, Antman EM. The thrombolysis in myocardial infarction risk score in unstable angina/non-ST-segment elevation myocardial infarction. J Am Coll Cardiol 2003;41:89S.

[22] Cohen M, Demers C, Gurfinkel EP, et al. A comparison of low-molecular-weight heparin with unfractionated heparin for unstable coronary artery disease. Efficacy and Safety of Subcutaneous Enoxaparin in Non-Q-Wave Coronary Events Study Group. N Engl J Med 1997;337:447.

[23] Theroux P, Ouimet H, McCans J, et al. Aspirin, heparin, or both to treat acute unstable angina. N Engl J Med 1988;319:1105.

[24] Cannon CP, Weintraub WS, Demopoulos LA, et al. Comparison of early invasive and conservative

strategies in patients with unstable coronary syndromes treated with the glycoprotein IIb/IIIa inhibitor tirofiban. N Engl J Med 2001;344:1879.

[25] Mitka M. Results of CURE trial for acute coronary syndrome. JAMA 2001;285:1828.

[26] Antiplatelet Trialists' Collaboration. Collaborative overview of randomised trials of antiplatelet therapy. I: prevention of death, myocardial infarction, and stroke by prolonged antiplatelet therapy in various categories of patients. BMJ 1994;308:81.

[27] Braunwald E, Antman EM, Beasley JW, et al. ACC/AHA 2002 guideline update for the management of patients with unstable angina and non-ST-segment elevation myocardial infarction–summary article: a report of the American College of Cardiology/American Heart Association Task Force on Practice Guidelines (Committee on the Management of Patients With Unstable Angina). J Am Coll Cardiol 2002;40:1366.

[28] Yan AT, Jong P, Yan RT, et al. Clinical trial–derived risk model may not generalize to real-world patients with acute coronary syndrome. Am Heart J 2004;148:1020.

[29] Gibson CM, Dumaine RL, Gelfand EV, et al. Association of glomerular filtration rate on presentation with subsequent mortality in non-ST-segment elevation acute coronary syndrome; observations in 13,307 patients in five TIMI trials. Eur Heart J 2004;25:1998.

[30] Apple FS, Wu AH, Mair J, et al. Future biomarkers for detection of ischemia and risk stratification in acute coronary syndrome. Clin Chem 2005;51:810.

[31] Califf RM, Peterson ED, Gibbons RJ, et al. Integrating quality into the cycle of therapeutic development. J Am Coll Cardiol 2002;40:1895.

ELSEVIER
SAUNDERS

Cardiol Clin 24 (2006) 79–85

Improving Systems of Care in Primary Angioplasty

Stanley Watkins, MD, MHS[a], Lynnet Tirabassi, RN, BSN[b],
Thomas Aversano, MD[b],*

[a]Division of Cardiology, 600 North Wolfe Street, Johns Hopkins Hospital, Baltimore, MD 21287, USA
[b]Division of Cardiology, Johns Hopkins School of Medicine, 5501 Hopkins Bayview Circle,
Baltimore, MD 21224, USA

The authors have had the honor and unique opportunity to develop primary angioplasty programs at more than 40 hospitals in the United States as part of the Cardiovascular Patient Outcomes Research Team (C-PORT) projects. C-PORT projects have included a completed randomized trial and an on-going primary angioplasty registry.

The idea that simply providing appropriate equipment and expert physicians to use it results in a good or even adequate primary angioplasty program, although commonly held, is deeply naive. Expert interventionalists and state-of-the-art equipment are necessary but far from sufficient conditions for the appropriate, prompt, safe, and effective application of this therapy for acute myocardial infarction (AMI).

Primary percutaneous coronary intervention (PPCI) is not simply a procedure that occurs in the cardiac catheterization laboratory. Rather, it is a strategy of care that at a minimum involves the emergency room, coronary care unit (CCU), and the step-down unit as well as the catheterization laboratory. In certain circumstances, PPCI may importantly involve prehospital care, as well. Failure to recognize PPCI as a strategy of care, not simply a procedure, is the most common and most dangerous misconception about this form of therapy.

What follows is not a manual, guideline, or prescription for development of a PPCI program.

Program development is an immensely detailed undertaking whose description is far beyond the scope of this report. Furthermore, because each institution is unique in its resources, requirements, and culture, development procedures and specifics are peculiar to each institution. There is no cookbook for PPCI development. Nevertheless, there are elements of program development and issues that must be addressed that are common to all or many institutions. This report provides a general description of the process of PPCI program development.

Program elements

The original C-PORT PPCI development program is divided arbitrarily into four main components: (1) the setting of standards, (2) training of staff, (3) development of logistics, and (4) implementation of a quality and error management program. This program has been incorporated into the American College of Cardiology (ACC)/American Heart Association guidelines for both AMI and PCI [1,2].

Standards

"Standards" refer to those for physicians, facilities, equipment, treatment guidelines and the nurses and technicians caring for the PPCI patient. Interventional physician and treatment guidelines (eg, ACC guidelines) are provided by national organizations; facilities standards are typically set by state regulation. Balloons, stents, and rheolytic or suction thrombectomy devices are the main devices used. Various forms of atherectomy or ablating devices are specifically

* Corresponding author. Johns Hopkins Medical Institutions JHAAC 1B.40, 5501 Hopkins Bayview Circle, Baltimore, MD 21224.
E-mail address: taversan@jhmi.edu (T. Aversano).

excluded; otherwise, equipment standards are set by the physicians performing intervention. Competency standards for nurses and technicians caring for the PPCI patient in the catheterization laboratory and postprocedure units do not exist. The training of these staff members is an important part of program development.

Training

No amount of training can take the place of actual experience. Nevertheless, training in the elements of care specifically related to PPCI can be useful for catheterization laboratory nurses and technicians who are already expert at caring for patients undergoing diagnostic catheterization and for CCU nurses already expert at caring for patients who have AMI.

Training can be didactic, observational, or hands-on, depending on need and expectation. Didactic training takes the form of lectures given by experts in a particular area (eg, postprocedure care discussed by an experienced postprocedure nurse, drugs used in PPCI discusses by practitioners or pharmacists) and in-services given by vendors of devices and drugs used in PPCI. These programs are extremely useful but are limited by their nature as lectures. Supplementing didactic teaching with observational training in the staff member's area of care is extremely helpful. Thus the catheterization laboratory nurse and technician staff can spend anywhere from 1 day to a week or more observing elective PCI procedures at an affiliated tertiary hospital, and the CCU and step-down unit nursing staff may spend a similar amount of time in the postprocedure care area of the same tertiary hospital. Having this experience in an affiliated tertiary hospital (one in which the interventionalists practice) has the added benefit of allowing community hospital staff to become acquainted with the policies, procedures, and methods of care to which their interventionalists are accustomed and also allows personal contact with highly experienced individuals (other nurses and other technicians) who may be resources in the future.

If an individual in the catheterization laboratory is to be a second operator, experience in the elective setting is important before being involved in a procedure during an AMI. This hands-on training is best accomplished in the affiliated tertiary hospital.

Although this program development is necessary, it is not sufficient for development of a PPCI program, because it fails to provide a mechanism for sustaining program excellence.

Logistics

"Logistics" refers to the policies and procedures that allow delivery of excellent PPCI treatment. Literally scores of issues must be addressed in development of logistics within a community hospital, and they tend to be peculiar to that hospital. Again, there is no cookbook. Despite the unique nature of specific logistical elements, there are nevertheless logistical goals common to all institutions. These are (1) immediate aspirin administration, (2) door-to-balloon time of 90 minutes or less, and (3) door-to-needle (or transfer) time of 30 minutes or less. The first two elements need no explanation. The goal of thrombolytic administration within 30 minutes of arrival at the emergency department recognizes that, no matter how well a system for performing PPCI is developed, it will fail. A formal plan for the fallback therapy (whether thrombolytics or transfer) needs to be in place. The 30-minute timeframe is justified because that is the national standard for door-to-needle time. When transfer for PCI elsewhere is the fallback plan, to this 30 minutes must be added the time to recall an ambulance for interhospital transport, pick up of the patient, delivery to the transfer hospital, removal to the cardiac catheterization laboratory, diagnostic catheterization, and then balloon inflation if appropriate. This process will probably take at least 1 hour and much longer in most instances.

It is impossible to detail logistics here. But attention to detail is critical. The authors can highlight several important steps in the acute care of the patient who has AMI.

Emergency medical services

Prehospital care

Multiple therapies have been proven to limit infarct size and improve mortality associated with myocardial infarction (MI). All of these therapies are time dependant, having significantly more efficacy when applied earlier than later. In most cases of acute myocardial infraction, a large portion of the delay arises from delay in the patient's activating emergency medical services (EMS). This delay from the time from onset of signs and symptoms of AMI to seeking medical assistance is termed "patient delay." "Transfer delay" describes the amount of time it takes for a patient to arrive at a care center once EMS has been activated. "Prehospital delay" refers to the total of patient delay plus transfer delay. The average prehospital delay in the United States is several hours, and the majority of this delay comes from the patient's delaying seeking medical attention [3].

Several studies have attempted to improve the prehospital delay using community-based interventions such as direct mail, radio, newspaper, and television advertising. This advertising is an attempt to educate the populace about the signs and symptoms of AMI and about the need for rapid diagnosis and treatment. In summary, the data regarding the effect of these community-based interventions are inconsistent. Earlier non-randomized trials had suggested a significant decline in patient delay following an education campaign [4–6]. A large prospective, randomized controlled trial was undertaken to address this issue in the late 1990s. The Rapid Early Action for Coronary Treatment trial randomly assigned 20 communities in the United States to an aggressive, multifaceted education campaign versus no intervention for an 18-month period. The intervention communities did decrease their prehospital delay time by 4.7% per year, but this change was significantly different from that of the control communities, which decreased 6.7% per year. EMS use increased by 20% in the intervention communities compared with the reference communities, but this increased use did not translate into an increase in emergency department visits or hospital discharges for acute cardiac care [7]. Thus it seems that aggressive community education does not directly affect prehospital delay and that new strategies are needed to improve patient delay significantly. The authors' group is conducting research to identify a group of high-risk patients who take and transmit a 12-lead ECG at the initial onset of symptoms.

Emergency medical services

Once the patient activates EMS, the blame for delays in care falls on the efficiency of the health care system. The delay from EMS activation to EMS arrival on the scene is largely a function of EMS availability and is beyond the scope of this discussion. Researchers have examined multiple ways to improve the transfer delay, which results from post-EMS arrival delays.

It is standard of care to do a brief assessment and administer chewed aspirin immediately upon arrival at the scene of a chest pain victim. Currently, the standard of care is to apply a three-lead rhythm monitor upon initial assessment of the patient and to have immediate access to external defibrillation. Although adequate to identify most rhythm disturbances, the rhythm strip does not give reliable information regarding acute ischemia. Furthermore, most of these devices are unable to transfer data electronically for physician interpretation. In experienced hands, performing a prehospital 12-lead ECG adds only 2 to 3 minutes to the initial assessment and can significantly affect downstream management. Less than 25% of patients who have chest pain transported by EMS have a final diagnosis of MI, and the non-ECG clinical predictors (diaphoresis, heart block) are insensitive [8,9]. Some have suggested that prehospital ECGs may result in further transport delay. A study examining on-scene times for paramedics using 12-lead ECGs compared with standard three-lead monitors found an on-scene time of 21.9 minutes for the ECG group and 22 minutes for the 3-lead group [10].

Issues have also been raised regarding the ability of EMS personnel to interpret a 12-lead ECG. EMS staff have been shown to diagnose 94% to 97% of physician-confirmed AMI correctly with prehospital ECGs after only 4 to 8 hours of training [11,12]. The legal issues remain an obstacle, in that nonphysician interpretation of the ECG is an off-label use of this device. Most EMS systems that routinely employ prehospital ECG testing transmit the ECG to an emergency department–based physician who confirms the interpretation and aids in guiding therapy. The ECG data can be transmitted by cellular telephone (in transit) or landline (on site). The former is less time-consuming but more prone to failed transmission.

Several studies have examined the downstream impact of the prehospital ECG. The Cincinnati Heart Project documented a reduction in prehospital treatment delay from 50 minutes in patients who were transported by EMS but did not receive a prehospital ECG to 30 minutes in patients who were transported by EMS but did receive a prehospital ECG [13]. The Myocardial Infarction Triage and Intervention Trial demonstrated a reduction in prehospital delay from 102 minutes to 46 minutes after the institution of system-wide prehospital ECGs [14].

Following initial assessment, EMS personnel routinely administer aspirin, nitroglycerin, and beta-blockers. These preliminary therapies can result in immediate improvement of ischemia and the ECG changes associated with ischemia.

If the first 12-lead ECG is performed upon arrival to the emergency department, the initial ischemic changes may no longer be present, which can lead to underdiagnosis of an ACS. In several European countries the prehospital ECG is routinely used to guide the administration of fibrinolytic therapy in the ambulance. The largest of the trials to examine the treatment effect of prehospital fibrinolysis was the European Myocardial Infarction Project trial in Europe. Patients who had ST-segment elevation myocardial infarction (STEMI) (N = 4767) were randomly assigned to prehospital versus in-hospital fibrinolysis. The patients randomly assigned to prehospital treatment received a fibrinolytic medication a median of 55 minutes earlier than those who received in-hospital medication. There was a trend toward a reduction in mortality, with a 30-day mortality rate of 9.7% in the prehospital group compared with 11.1% in the in-hospital group ($P = .08$) [15]. The Grampian Region Early Anistreplase Trial was a randomized, double-blind parallel-group clinical trial that enrolled 311 patients suspected of having AMI. Patients were randomly assigned to receive intravenous anistreplase (30 U) either at home or later, after arrival in the hospital. The median time saved by prehospital thrombolysis was 130 minutes. By the end of 1 year after trial entry, 17 (10.4%) of 163 patients given anistreplase at home died, compared with 32 (21.6%) of 148 patients allotted anistreplase in the hospital ($P = .007$) [16,17]. A recent meta-analysis of all prehospital fibrinolysis trials found an overall significant 20% reduction in hospital mortality favoring prehospital therapy [18]. This treatment effect is significantly greater in rural communities where transport times are prolonged and time from symptom onset to treatment can be significantly decreased by giving medication on route.

Beyond giving EMS personnel the ability to diagnose and treat AMI earlier, the prehospital ECG allows efficient triage of patients who have AMI to centers where primary angioplasty is offered. Primary angioplasty has become the preferred method of acute reperfusion therapy for many reasons. For the average patient who has STEMI, primary angioplasty confers a survival advantage over thrombolysis. A recent meta-analysis documented a 30% reduction in short-term death and nearly a 50% reduction in nonfatal reinfarction [19]. The main barrier to the universal implementation of PPCI is the availability of this technology at local hospitals. The Danish Acute Myocardial Infarction trial supported the safety

of transporting patients who had AMI to facilities with angioplasty capabilities compared with on-site thrombolysis [20]. The clear superiority of primary angioplasty has sparked a debate over prehospital triage of AMI patients. How far is too far when a patient requires reperfusion and a thrombolytic-only hospital is closer than the nearest primary angioplasty center? The issue is further clouded by political and economic factors that have complicated the formation of an organized triage system for AMI similar to the one that exists for trauma in the United States. Currently, triage of patients who have AMI by EMS personnel should be guided by the goal of prompt reperfusion, and formal protocols should exist for consideration of hospital transfer.

Emergency department

Development of logistics in the emergency department is conditioned and constrained by the goal of achieving a reperfusion time of 90 minutes. The best mode of reperfusion is dependant on the availability of primary angioplasty at that institution. Because, on average, fibrinolysis takes longer to achieve reperfusion than PCI, a door-to-needle time of only 30 minutes is the goal for fibrinolysis. Primary angioplasty is more effective than fibrinolysis provided the door-to-balloon time is less than 90 minutes. During off-hours when the angioplasty team is not on site, activating the team can take a significant amount of time. Therefore rapid upstream identification of reperfusion-eligible patients is imperative. This identification requires well-considered formal protocols to ensure that no patients who have AMI are burdened with unnecessary delay while being assessed in the emergency department. The formation of such protocols improves outcomes and is cost effective [21].

The emergency department chest pain protocol must be straightforward, robust, and user-friendly. Furthermore, with emergency department visits increasing every year, the burden logistics places on the emergency department staff must be minimized. The logistical goals in the emergency department are that every patient who has STEMI receive aspirin immediately unless contraindicated, the door-to-needle time be 30 minutes or less, and the door-to-balloon time be 90 minutes or less. The third goal translates to a door-to-catheterization laboratory time of approximately 60 minutes. Although these goals are common to every PPCI program, the way those goals are achieved—how the many details of local logistics are addressed—is unique to each institution.

It is important that an agreed-upon set of rules defining eligibility criteria for PPCI be developed and easily accessed for review for every potential candidate. Chest pain and ST-segment elevation (or new or presumed new left bundle branch block) are important inclusion criteria, but other issues also need to be addressed. Is the patient in cardiogenic shock going to be included or always transferred to a tertiary center? Do severe allergies to aspirin or contrast exclude patients? A carefully thought-out and universally agreed-upon set of criteria for considering patients for PPCI is mandatory. It is important that physician preferences not be criteria for inclusion or exclusion: having two standards of care, one for some physicians' patients and one for other physicians' patients, is a bad idea from every point of view. Emergency department physicians cannot be put in the position of having to recommend two different care standards for the same disease depending on whose patient they are seeing.

When the system required for performing PPCI fails, an agreed-upon response must be in place. For thrombolytic-ineligible patients, this response usually means transfer to a tertiary institution for PCI. For thrombolytic-eligible patients, this response may mean either administration of thrombolytic therapy or transfer to a tertiary facility. Combinations of these approaches may also be considered (so-called "drip and ship" treatment). Whatever the fallback therapy may be for these patients, it is important that they are specified, clear, reviewable by the emergency department physician as he or she is caring for the patient, and agreed upon by all concerned.

Delay in the application of PPCI is most often caused by failure to identify the patient as having a possible AMI. This failure of identification may occur at the point of triage and typically involves unusual presentations (eg, no chest pain but only fatigue or other nonspecific complaint) and a busy emergency department. These patients may be sent to the waiting room while more acutely ill patients are cared for, with acute, ST-segment elevation discovered only later on the first ECG. The patient also may not be rapidly identified because of an ECG that is unclear or equivocal.

The mechanism to determine the availability of catheterization laboratory itself and its physicians and staff is a critical piece of emergency department logistics. In the more than 40 institutions in which C-PORT has developed PPCI programs, this system almost always has been considered to be in place already. It almost never is.

It is impossible to specify how team recruitment should work in all hospitals—like so many logistical elements, its specifics depend upon the institution itself, its culture, and its resources. The goals of the system, however, are uniform. The emergency department cannot be in charge of such a system. Rather, the emergency department must be able to activate the team recruitment system with a single outgoing call to an activator. The activator then sends a call out to the team (physicians, nurses, technicians) who must then respond back to the activator. The activator, logs responses and, when the team is complete, informs the emergency department that team is assembled. If the team cannot be assembled, the activator informs the emergency department that team recruitment has failed so that fallback therapy can be instituted.

Because fallback therapy is often thrombolytic therapy, there is goal of a total elapse time of 30 minutes from arrival at the emergency department to application of thrombolytic therapy. If it takes 15 minutes to identify the patient and 5 minutes to apply thrombolytic therapy after the decision is made to do so, 10 minutes are available for team recruitment to succeed or fail. Reducing the time from arrival to patient identification to 10 minutes means 15 minutes are available. This is a very short time. Changes in the on-call schedule, pager failure, and numerous other common problems can influence the success of this system. It is critical that the system be developed and implemented in a way that identifies all potential failure points and minimizes their influence.

It is important that the emergency department and interventional physicians agree on initial care. Routine AMI laboratory tests should be obtained, but also a tube of blood should be sent to the blood bank for potential crossmatching in case of significant bleeding. All patients should receive aspirin unless otherwise contraindicated. Similarly, beta-blockers, nitrates, oxygen, and analgesics are given almost uniformly. At this time, there is a wide variety of further initial therapies that may or may not include clopidogrel, a glycoprotein IIb/IIIa receptor antagonist, unfractionated or low molecular weight heparin, and occasionally thrombolytic therapy (eg, with facilitated PCI). Within limits, agreement among interventionalists and emergency department physicians about what is done is more important than exactly what is done.

The ability to conference the interventionalist with the emergency department physician is extremely helpful in defining patient-specific treatment.

Catheter laboratory

Almost uniformly, the major issue involving the catheterization laboratory concerns staffing. Community hospitals without on-site cardiac surgery usually do not have sufficient catheterization laboratory staff to cover PPCI 24 hours a day, 7 days a week. Ideally, there are four individuals in each on-call position. Thus, if the call team is one interventionalist, two nurses, and a technician, there should be four interventionalists, eight nurses, and four technicians covering call. This staffing leads to a livable and therefore sustainable on-call schedule of approximately 1 weekday a week and 1 weekend per month (with a weekend being Friday, Saturday, and Sunday). This level of staffing can be difficult to secure, and often PPCI programs begin with fewer individuals covering call.

Coronary care unit

The CCU is the postprocedure care area for the patient who has undergone PPCI. Most hospitals without on-site cardiac surgery care for a large number of patients who have AMI, so typically the capability of the CCU staff to monitor and manage complications of AMI is already expert. There are, however, a number of issues specific to patients undergoing PPCI that need to be addressed. Chief among these is management of the procedure site, typically the femoral area. In most units, the nurse is the first line in both the detection and management of sheath complications. These individuals must, therefore, have training in identifying the signs and symptoms of postprocedure groin complications as well as training in initial management. Management of bleeding complications should include actual hands-on training of a representative group of CCU nurses who may be called on in each shift to compress a bleeding site. This training may be accomplished by compressing patients after diagnostic catheterization patients. Observational training at a high-volume tertiary center is useful for all CCU nurses who care for the patient after PCI. The details of how training is done, what kind of training is done, how many nurses are trained, and for how long is site specific. In addition to developing competency, maintenance of competency must also be defined.

Predischarge education is a critical aspect of PPCI. In addition to the usual predischarge education that includes life style, drugs, activity, rehabilitation, and so forth, discussions specific to PPCI must be added. A stent card and a closure device card should be given to the patient along with education about both devices. Particularly important is making sure that clopidogrel is available to the patient for the duration required. This requirement may mean involving social services and pharmacy early in the patient's course so that it can be confirmed that the patient can afford the drug. If not, programs by the manufacturer can be used to provide this critical medication. If the patient leaves the hospital and fails to take this drug because the patient did not recognize its importance, because of ineffective education, or because the patient cannot afford it, the entire PPCI strategy of care can be much less effective and more dangerous than thrombolytic therapy.

Summary

AMI is a life-threatening condition. Poor performance on the part of caregivers can result in the death of a patient. It is critical that a PPCI capability be developed in such a way that error is minimized. It is not enough that the system works well or very well. Aviation is often used as the example that medical systems should emulate. In developing the many interrelated systems required to function properly to ensure safe, effective, prompt, and appropriate application of PPCI, an aviation parallel should be kept in mind. If you were walking on the jetway toward a plane and were greeted by the pilot who said to you, "You know, I can land this thing 99% of the time," you would never get on that plane. It is important to develop a PPCI system that is absolutely never the cause of harm to any patient. Doing so requires exquisite attention to detail, algorithms of care when possible, redundancy, and clear orders for all drugs and procedures.

References

[1] Antman EM, Anbe DT, Armstrong PW, et al. ACC/AHA guidelines for the management of patients with ST-elevation myocardial infarction; a report of the American College of Cardiology/American Heart Association Task Force on Practice Guidelines

(Committee to Revise the 1999 Guidelines for the Management of Patients with Acute Myocardial Infarction). J Am Coll Cardiol 2004;44:E1–211.

[2] Smith SC Jr, Dove JT, Jacobs AK, et al. ACC/AHA guidelines for percutaneous coronary intervention (revision of the 1993 PTCA guidelines)—executive summary: a report of the American College of Cardiology/American Heart Association Task Force on Practice Guidelines (Committee to Revise the 1993 Guidelines for Percutaneous Transluminal Coronary Angioplasty) endorsed by the Society for Cardiac Angiography and Interventions. Circulation 2001;103:3019–41.

[3] Kainth A, Hewitt A, Sowden A, et al. Systematic review of interventions to reduce delay in patients with suspected heart attack. Emerg Med J 2004;21:506–8.

[4] Blohm M, Hartford M, Karlson BW, et al. A media campaign aiming at reducing delay times and increasing the use of ambulance in AMI. Am J Emerg Med 1994;12:315–8.

[5] Gaspoz JM, Unger PF, Urban P, et al. Impact of a public campaign on pre-hospital delay in patients reporting chest pain. Heart 1996;76:150–5.

[6] Herlitz J, Blohm M, Hartford M, et al. Follow-up of a 1-year media campaign on delay times and ambulance use in suspected acute myocardial infarction. Eur Heart J 1992;13:171–7.

[7] Luepker RV, Raczynski JM, Osganian S, et al. Effect of a community intervention on patient delay and emergency medical service use in acute coronary heart disease: The Rapid Early Action for Coronary Treatment (REACT) Trial. JAMA 2000;284:60–7.

[8] Tresch DD, Brady WJ, Aufderheide TP, et al. Comparison of elderly and younger patients with out-of-hospital chest pain. Clinical characteristics, acute myocardial infarction, therapy, and outcomes. Arch Intern Med 1996;156:1089–93.

[9] Hargarten KM, Aprahamian C, Stueven H, et al. Limitations of prehospital predictors of acute myocardial infarction and unstable angina. Ann Emerg Med 1987;16:1325–9.

[10] Brown JL Jr. An eight-month evaluation of prehospital 12-lead electrocardiogram monitoring in Baltimore County. Md Med J 1997;(Suppl):64–6.

[11] Foster DB, Dufendach JH, Barkdoll CM, et al. Prehospital recognition of AMI using independent nurse/paramedic 12-lead ECG evaluation: impact on in-hospital times to thrombolysis in a rural community hospital. Am J Emerg Med 1994;12: 25–31.

[12] Ferguson JD, Brady WJ, Perron AD, et al. The prehospital 12-lead electrocardiogram: impact on management of the out-of-hospital acute coronary syndrome patient. Am J Emerg Med 2003;21: 136–42.

[13] Kereiakes DJ, Gibler WB, Martin LH, et al. Relative importance of emergency medical system transport and the prehospital electrocardiogram on reducing hospital time delay to therapy for acute myocardial infarction: a preliminary report from the Cincinnati Heart Project. Am Heart J 1992;123:835–40.

[14] Weaver WD, Eisenberg MS, Martin JS, et al. Myocardial Infarction Triage and Intervention Project—phase I: patient characteristics and feasibility of prehospital initiation of thrombolytic therapy. J Am Coll Cardiol 1990;15:925–31.

[15] Boissel JP. The European Myocardial Infarction Project: an assessment of pre-hospital thrombolysis. Int J Cardiol 1995;49(Suppl):S29–37.

[16] GREAT Group. Feasibility, safety, and efficacy of domiciliary thrombolysis by general practitioners: Grampian region early anistreplase trial. BMJ 1992; 305:548–53.

[17] Rawles J. Halving of mortality at 1 year by domiciliary thrombolysis in the Grampian Region Early Anistreplase Trial (GREAT). J Am Coll Cardiol 1994;23:1–5.

[18] Morrison LJ, Verbeek PR, McDonald AC, et al. Mortality and prehospital thrombolysis for acute myocardial infarction: a meta-analysis. JAMA 2000;283:2686–92.

[19] Keeley EC, Boura JA, Grines CL. Primary angioplasty versus intravenous thrombolytic therapy for acute myocardial infarction: a quantitative review of 23 randomised trials. Lancet 2003;361:13–20.

[20] Andersen HR, Nielsen TT, Rasmussen K, et al. A comparison of coronary angioplasty with fibrinolytic therapy in acute myocardial infarction. N Engl J Med 2003;349:733–42.

[21] Farkouh ME, Smars PA, Reeder GS, et al. A clinical trial of a chest-pain observation unit for patients with unstable angina. Chest Pain Evaluation in the Emergency Room (CHEER) Investigators. N Engl J Med 1998;339:1882–8.

ELSEVIER
SAUNDERS

Cardiol Clin 24 (2006) 87–102

CARDIOLOGY
CLINICS

Moving from Evidence to Practice in the Care of Patients Who Have Acute Coronary Syndrome

Kelly J. Miller, MD[a], Charles V. Pollack Jr., MA, MD, FACEP[b],
Eric D. Peterson, MD, MPH[c,d],*

[a]Division of Cardiology, University of Maryland School of Medicine, 22 South Greene Street,
Baltimore, MD 21201, USA
[b]Department of Emergency Medicine, Pennsylvania Hospital, 800 Spruce Street Philadelphia, PA 19107, USA
[c]Duke University Medical Center, Box 3236, Durham, NC 27710, USA
[d]Duke Clinical Research Institute, 2400 Pratt Street, Room 7009, Durham, NC, 27705 USA

The spectrum of acute coronary syndromes (ACS), ranging from unstable angina to non–ST-segment elevation myocardial infarction (NSTEMI), to ST-segment elevation myocardial infarction (STEMI), represent major causes of morbidity and mortality for patients who have cardiovascular disease. The field of ACS management underwent a remarkable evolution during the decade of the 1990s. This change was caused primarily by a large number of randomized clinical trials studying all aspects of the diagnosis and treatment of ACS, including, but not limited to, the development of cardiac biomarker assays, early use of antithrombotic and antiplatelet drugs, beta-blockers, angiotensin-converting enzyme (ACE) inhibitors, and early invasive treatment strategies. In recognition of the importance and the breadth of these data, clinical practice guidelines (CPGs) have been developed by the American College of Cardiology (ACC) and the American Heart Association (AHA) to provide standards for the diagnosis and treatment of patients who have ACS and to construct a framework for clinical decision making [1–6]. These guidelines have also been translated into user-friendly form for emergency medicine physicians [7–9]. Despite the publication and wide distribution of these guidelines, their routine clinical application has been slow, incomplete, and often ineffective [1,2,6].

This article discusses the spectrum of ACS but focuses primarily on patients who have non–ST-segment elevation (NSTE) ACS. After reviewing the ACC/AHA guidelines for the care of NSTE ACS patients, it discusses current practice patterns as documented in several large registries including the National Registry of Myocardial Infarction (NRMI), the Global Registry of Acute Coronary Events (GRACE), and the Can Rapid risk stratification of Unstable angina patients Suppress ADverse outcomes with Early implementation of the ACC/AHA guidelines (CRUSADE). Gaps in patient management between that recommended in CPGs and actual patterns of care are discussed, and areas for improvement are suggested. A discussion on means to overcome barriers to guideline adherence through quality improvement initiatives concludes this article.

Emergency department care of the patient who has acute coronary syndromes

There are more than 5 million emergency department visits for chest pain and more than 1 million hospitalizations for acute myocardial infarction (AMI) annually in the United States alone [10,11]. Despite advances in treatment, coronary heart disease remains the leading cause of death in the United States [12]. Patients who have

---

* Corresponding author. Duke Clinical Research Institute, Box 17969, Durham, NC 27715.
 E-mail address: peter016@mc.duke.edu
(E.D. Peterson).

0733-8651/06/$ - see front matter © 2005 Elsevier Inc. All rights reserved.
doi:10.1016/j.ccl.2005.09.008

a completely occluded artery are usually identified rapidly, on their presentation to the emergency department, because they typically present with ST-segment elevation or a known-to-be-new left bundle branch block on the initial ECG. In patients who have STEMI, prompt reperfusion therapy, either with fibrinolytic therapy or primary percutaneous coronary intervention (PCI), is indicated; both approaches can reduce infarct size and improve survival [13]. Up to two thirds of patients presenting with ACS, however, do not present with ST-segment elevation on their initial ECG. These patients require further risk stratification, usually by serial evaluation, to distinguish where they fall in the spectrum of ACS, from noncoronary chest pain to unstable angina to NSTEMI. This risk stratification is a dynamic process that requires time for data collection and observation of symptoms but is critical in determining appropriate management based on patient risk.

Guidelines for evidence-based care of patients who have acute coronary syndromes

The ACC and AHA first published guidelines for the evaluation and management of unstable angina in 1994 [4]. The guidelines were revised in 2000, and after the publication of several trials pertaining to the NSTE ACS population, an update was published in 2002 [5,14]. These guidelines define classes of indications for therapy based on the strength and consistency of evidence supporting them (Box 1).

Prehospital factors leading to delays in treatment

For most patients who have ACS, the initial contact with health care providers is through the emergency department and may or may not be preceded by prehospital evaluation and transportation by ambulance. Despite public education initiatives, the time from symptom onset to the initiation of therapy in large-scale clinical trials during the last decade (Global Use of Strategies to Open Occluded Coronary Arteries I, III, and V and Assessment of the Safety and Efficacy of a New Thrombolytic II and III) has remained unchanged, with a 2.7- to 2.9-hour delay being consistently documented. Hospital-based delays in door-to-needle or door-to-drug time have improved during the last decade, but patient factors (ie, delay between onset of symptoms to activating emergency medical services) have not [15]. The Rapid Early Action for Coronary Treatment study

---

Box 1. Definitions of indications by the ACC/AHA [14]

Class I indication: Conditions for which there is evidence and/or general agreement that a given procedure or treatment is useful and eective

Class II indication: Conditions for which there is conflicting evidence and/or a divergence of opinion about the usefulness/ecacy of a procedure or treatment

IIa: Weight of evidence/opinion is in favor of usefulness/efficacy

IIb: Usefulness/efficacy is less well established by evidence/opinion

Class III indication: Conditions for which there is evidence and/or general agreement that the procedure/treatment is not useful/effective and in some cases may be harmful

The weight of the evidence was ranked highest (A) if the data were derived from multiple, randomized clinical trials that involved large numbers of patients and intermediate (B) if the data were derived from a limited number of randomized trials that involved small numbers of patients or from careful analyses of nonrandomized studies or observational registries. A lower rank (C) was given when expert consensus was the primary basis for the recommendation.

———

From Brunwald E, Antman EM, Beasley JW, et al. ACC/AHA guideline update for the management of patients with unstable angina and non-ST–segment elevation myocardial infarction–2002: a report of the American College of Cardiology/American Heart Association Task Force on Practice Guidelines (Committee on the Management of Patients with Unstable Angina). Circulation 2002;106:1893–1900.

---

examined factors that lead to a patient's delay in seeking medial attention in hopes of devising ways to improve quality [15,16]. This study, drawn from data in 20 communities across the country, demonstrates that 89.4% of community survey respondents would use emergency medical services, but only 23.2% of patients who had chest pain actually did use emergency medical services; denial of a possible cardiac cause of the chest pain played a critical role in the delay [16]. The disconnect between what people seem to understand is the right course of action in a survey and actual patient behavior points to certain modifiable situational or belief factors and supports a role for patient-focused education initiatives in improving delays in seeking medical care.

To improve these delays, the National Heart, Lung, and Blood Institute has launched several programs to educate patients about their personal risks of heart disease, symptoms of myocardial infarction, and the proper action to take if they think they are having a heart attack. The goal of these programs is to reduce the time between the onset of symptoms and treatment [15,17]. Patients too must play a role in delivering timely medical care.

Initial emergency department triage

Once a patient suspected of having ACS arrives at the emergency department, prompt and accurate triage is essential. A determination should be made in all patients who have chest discomfort as to whether the likelihood of acute ischemia caused by coronary artery disease is high, intermediate, or low. Important also is the realization that many patients, especially women and diabetics, do not always present with classic chest pain, often presenting instead with potentially confounding anginal equivalents including nausea, dyspnea, or pain in the back, neck, jaw, or epigastrium.

In the absence of ST-segment elevation on the initial ECG, differentiating NSTEMI or unstable angina from low-risk stable angina or noncardiac chest pain can be challenging. This distinction, however, is crucial in assessing risk of myocardial infarction and death and in deciding on appropriate medical therapy and management strategy. Using a composite of clinical predictors to assess risk is an important role of the emergency department physician. Besides history (tempo and severity of angina, including presence of ongoing chest pain), physical examination (detection of heart failure, other signs of vascular disease) and the ECG (ST-segment depression or transient elevation), cardiac biomarkers are an important risk-stratification tool. Elevation of cardiac troponin is a marker of high risk. In fact, the degree of troponin elevation has been correlated with in-hospital mortality in many studies. For example,

in a large community study of ACS, the mortality rate nearly doubled as serum troponin went from normal to above the upper limit of normal and then rose linearly thereafter [18,19].

Using cardiac troponin in addition to other clinical variables, multivariate models of risk assessment have been developed; the most commonly used and most validated are the Thrombolysis In Myocardial Infarction (TIMI) risk score developed by Antman and colleagues [20]. This seven-item risk scale assigns one point for the presence of each of the following: age greater than 65 years, presence of more than three coronary risk factors, prior angiographic coronary obstruction, ST-segment deviation, more than two angina events within 24 hours, use of aspirin within 7 days, and elevated cardiac markers. The risk of developing an adverse outcome—death, (re)infarction, or recurrent severe ischemia requiring revascularization—ranged from 5% to 41%, increasing with the sum of the individual variables. The score was derived from data in the TIMI 11B trial and has been validated in three additional trials— Efficacy and Safety of Subcutaneous Enoxaparin in Non-Q Wave Coronary Events, Treat Angina with Aggrastat and Determine Cost of Therapy with an Invasive or Conservative Strategy (TACTICS)-TIMI 18, and Platelet Receptor Inhibition in Ischemic Syndrome Management in Patients Limited by Unstable Signs and Symptoms [14,20–24]. Among patients who have unstable angina/NSTEMI, there is a progressively greater benefit from newer therapies such as low molecular weight heparin (LMWH), platelet glycoprotein (Gp) IIb/IIIa inhibition, and an invasive strategy, with increasing risk score [20–25]. This benefit is highlighted in the revised ACC/AHA guidelines from 2002 [14].

American College of Cardiology/American Heart Association recommendations for initial triage, ECG, and biomarker assessment

Box 2 gives the ACC/AHA recommendations for early risk stratification.

Acute medical therapies

Because of delays in or lack of bed availability in many hospitals, a large burden of caring for patients who have NSTE ACS is placed on the emergency department. Therefore, it is crucial for emergency physicians to institute evidence-based therapy as quickly, appropriately, and accurately as possible. Boxes 3 and 4

Box 2. Recommendations for early risk stratification [14]

Class I

A determination should be made in all patients who have chest discomfort of the likelihood of acute ischemia caused by coronary artery disease as high, intermediate, or low (level of evidence: C).

Patients who present with chest discomfort should undergo early risk stratification that focuses on anginal symptoms, physical findings, ECG findings, and biomarkers of cardiac injury (level of evidence: B).

A 12-lead ECG should be obtained immediately (within 10 minutes) in patients who have ongoing chest discomfort and as rapidly as possible in patients who have a history of chest discomfort consistent with ACS but whose discomfort has resolved by the time of evaluation (level of evidence: C).

Biomarkers of cardiac injury should be measured in all patients who present with chest discomfort consistent with ACS. A cardiac-specific troponin is the preferred marker, and if available it should be measured in all patients. Creatinine kinase myocardial band (CK-MB) by mass assay is also acceptable. In patients who have negative cardiac markers within 6 hours of the onset of pain, another sample should be drawn in the 6- to 12-hour time frame (eg, 9 hours after the onset of symptoms) (level of evidence: C).

Class IIa

For patients who present within 6 hours of the onset of symptoms, an early marker of cardiac injury (eg, myoglobin or CK-MB subforms) should be considered in addition to a cardiac troponin (level of evidence: C).

Class IIb

C-reactive protein and other markers of inflammation should be measured (level of evidence: B).

Class III

Total CK (without MB), aspartate aminotransferase, beta-hydroxybutyric dehydrogenase, and/or lactate dehydrogenase should be the markers for the detection of myocardial injury in patients who have chest discomfort suggestive of ACS (level of evidence: C).

From Brunwald E, Antman EM, Beasley JW, et al. ACC/AHA guideline update for the management of patients with unstable angina and non-ST–segment elevation myocardial infarction–2002: a report of the American College of Cardiology/American Heart Association Task Force on Practice Guidelines (Committee on the Management of Patients with Unstable Angina). Circulation 2002;106:1893–1900.

---

highlight the ACC/AHA-recommended approaches for anti-ischemic, antithrombotic, and antiplatelet therapies from the 2002 update. Essential also is clear and thorough communication from emergency medical services to the emergency department and from the emergency department to the coronary care unit, catheterization laboratory, or telemetry floor, to curb errors of omission.

Early invasive versus early conservative approach

Randomized clinical trial data collectively support the use of an early invasive approach with prompt cardiac catheterization, compared with an initial conservative approach that reserves cardiac catheterization for patients who develop recurrent ischemia despite medical therapy (Box 5) [23,25–27]. The TACTICS-TIMI-18 trial found that catheterization within the first 48 hours after presentation was superior to an initial strategy of medical management, particularly in patients who had elevated troponin levels or elevated TIMI risk score [23]. Similarly, The Fast Revascularization during Instability in Coronary artery disease trial demonstrated a significant reduction in long-term mortality with early invasive management for NSTE ACS [27].

Box 3. Recommendations for anti-ischemic therapy [14]

Class I

Bed rest with continuous ECG monitoring for ischemia and arrhythmia detection in patients who have ongoing rest pain (level of evidence: C)

Nitroglycerine, sublingual tablet or spray, followed by intravenous administration, for the immediate relief of ischemia and associated symptoms (level of evidence: C)

Supplemental oxygen for patients who have cyanosis or respiratory distress; finger-pulse oximetry or arterial blood gas determination to confirm adequate arterial oxygen saturation (SaO_2 > 90%) and continued need for supplemental oxygen in the presence of hypoxemia (level of evidence: C)

Morphine sulfate intravenously when symptoms are not immediately relieved with nitroglycerine or when acute pulmonary congestion and/or severe agitation is present (level of evidence: C)

A beta-blocker, with the first dose administered intravenously if there is ongoing chest pain, followed by oral administration, in the absence of contraindications (level of evidence: B)

In patients who have continuing or frequently recurring ischemia when beta-blockers are contraindicated, a nondihydropyridine calcium antagonist (eg, verapamil or diltiazem) as initial therapy in the absence of severe left ventricular dysfunction or other contraindications (level of evidence: B)

An ACE inhibitor when hypertension persists despite treatment with nitroglycerine and a beta-blocker in patients who have left ventricular systolic dysfunction or heart failure and in diabetic patients who have ACS (level of evidence: B)

Class IIa

Oral long-acting calcium antagonists for recurrent ischemia in the absence of contraindications and when beta-blockers and nitrates are fully used (level of evidence: C)

An ACE inhibitor for all post-ACS patients (level of evidence: B)

Intra-aortic balloon pump counterpulsation for severe ischemia that is continuing or recurs frequently despite intensive medical therapy or for hemodynamic instability in patients before or after coronary angiography (level of evidence: C)

Class IIb

Extended-release form of nondihydropyridine calcium antagonists instead of a beta-blocker (level of evidence: B)

Immediate-release dihydropyridine calcium antagonists in the presence of a beta-blocker (level of evidence: B)

Class III

Nitroglycerine or other nitrate within 24 hours of sildenafil use (level of evidence: C)

Immediate-release dihydropyridine calcium antagonists in the absence of a beta-blocker (level of evidence: A)

From Brunwald E, Antman EM, Beasley JW, et al. ACC/AHA guideline update for the management of patients with unstable angina and non-ST–segment elevation myocardial infarction–2002: a report of the American College of Cardiology/American Heart Association Task Force on Practice Guidelines (Committee on the Management of Patients with Unstable Angina). Circulation 2002;106:1893–1900.

National acute coronary syndromes databases—evidence meets community practice

During the last decade, several large registries have been created to examine the temporal and regional management of patients who have ACS and to provide real-world data on practice and outcomes. This wealth of data makes it possible to monitor trends in ACS care and to observe evidence-based therapy only slowly being adopted

---

Box 4. Recommendations for antiplatelet and anticoagulation therapy [14]

Class I
Antiplatelet therapy should be initiated promptly. Aspirin (ASA) should be administered as
    soon as possible after presentation and continued indefinitely (level of evidence: A).
Clopidogrel should be administered to hospitalized patients who are unable to take ASA
    because of hypersensitivity or major gastrointestinal intolerance (level of evidence: A).
In hospitalized patients in whom an early noninterventional approach is planned,
    clopidogrel should be added to ASA as soon as possible on admission and administered
    for at least 1 month (level of evidence: A) and for up to 9 months (level of evidence: B).
In patients for whom a PCI is planned, treatment with clopidogrel should be started and
    continued for at least 1 month (level of evidence: A) and up to 9 months in patients who
    are not at high risk for bleeding (level of evidence: B).
In patients taking clopidogrel in whom elective coronary artery bypass graft surgery is
    planned, the drug should be withheld for 5 to 7 days before surgery (level of evidence: B).
Anticoagulation with subcutaneous LMWH or intravenous unfractionated heparin (UFH)
    should be added to antiplatelet therapy with ASA and/or clopidogrel (level of evidence: A)
A platelet Gp IIb/IIIa antagonist should be administered, in addition to ASA and heparin,
    to patients in whom catheterization and PCI are planned. The Gp IIb/IIIa antagonist may
    also be administered just before PCI (level of evidence: A).

Class IIa
Eptifibatide or tirofiban should be administered, in addition to ASA and LMWH or UFH, to
    patients who have continuing ischemia, an elevated troponin level, or with other high-risk
    features in whom an invasive management strategy is not planned (level of evidence: A).
Enoxaparin is preferable to UFH as an anticoagulant in patients who have unstable angina/
    NSTEMI, unless coronary artery bypass graft surgery is planned within 24 hours (level
    of evidence: A).
A platelet Gp IIb/IIIa antagonist should be administered to patients already receiving
    heparin, ASA, and clopidogrel in whom catheterization and PCI are planned. The Gp IIb/IIIa
    antagonist may also be administered just prior to PCI (level of evidence: B).

Class IIb
Eptifibatide or tirofiban, in addition to ASA and LMWH or UFH, should be administered to
    patients who do not have continuing ischemia, who have no other high-risk features, and
    in whom PCI is not planned (level of evidence: A).

Class III
Intravenous fibrinolytic therapy is recommended in patients who do not have acute
    ST-segment elevation, a true posterior myocardial infarction, or a presumed new left
    bundle-branch block (level of evidence: A).
Abciximab should be administered to patients in whom PCI is not planned (level of
    evidence: A).

From Brunwald E, Antman EM, Beasley JW, et al. ACC/AHA guideline update for the management of
patients with unstable angina and non-ST–segment elevation myocardial infarction–2002: a report of the
American College of Cardiology/American Heart Association Task Force on Practice Guidelines (Committee on the Management of Patients with Unstable Angina). Circulation 2002;106:1893–1900.

---

into everyday clinical practice. During the observation period reported by these registries, there
were upward trends in the use of guideline-based
medical therapy (aspirin, beta-blockers, ACE
inhibitors, and antithrombin therapy) and

decreases in time to reperfusion. As guideline-
based therapy was adopted into practice, hospital
mortality fell (from 11.2% in 1990 to 9.4% in
1999) [28]. These registries are a reminder, however, that there are still areas for significant

---

Box 5. Recommendations for early conservative versus invasive treatment strategies [14]

Class I

An early invasive strategy is indicated in patients who have unstable angina/NSTEMI and any of the following high-risk indicators (level of evidence: A):

Recurrent angina/ischemia at rest or with low-level activities despite intensive anti-ischemic therapy

Elevated troponin T or troponin I

New or presumably new ST-segment depression

Recurrent angina/ischemia with symptoms of chronic heart failure, an S3 gallop, pulmonary edema, worsening rales, or new or worsening mitral regurgitation

High-risk findings on noninvasive stress testing

Depressed left ventricular systolic function (eg, ejection fraction < 0.40 on noninvasive study)

Hemodynamic instability

Sustained ventricular tachycardia

PCI within 6 months

Prior coronary artery bypass graft surgery

In the absence of these findings, either an early conservative or an early invasive strategy is indicated in hospitalized patients who do not have contraindications for revascularization (level of evidence: B).

Class IIa

An early invasive strategy is indicated in patients who have repeated presentations for ACS despite therapy and without evidence for ongoing ischemia or high risk (level of evidence: C).

Class III

Coronary angiography is indicated in patients who have extensive comorbidities (eg, liver or pulmonary failure, cancer), in whom the risks of revascularization are not likely to outweigh the benefits (level of evidence: C).

Coronary angiography is recommended in patients who have acute chest pain and a low likelihood of ACS (level of evidence: C).

Coronary angiography is indicated in patients who will not consent to revascularization regardless of the findings (level of evidence: C).

From Brunwald E, Antman EM, Beasley JW, et al. ACC/AHA guideline update for the management of patients with unstable angina and non-ST–segment elevation myocardial infarction–2002: a report of the American College of Cardiology/American Heart Association Task Force on Practice Guidelines (Committee on the Management of Patients with Unstable Angina). Circulation 2002;106:1893–1900.

---

improvement and many missed opportunities for intervention in the care of patients who have ACS. This difference between the recommendations and practice partially explains why real-world mortality for ACS still remains much higher than that reported in randomized clinical trials.

National Registry of Myocardial Infarction

The NRMI was initiated in July 1990 to provide participating hospitals a means of tracking the characteristics, treatment, and outcome of patients who have AMI. During the 14 years that the NRMI has been enrolling, more 2.2 million patients who have myocardial infarction have been evaluated. The NRMI thus is the largest observational registry of ACS to date [28,29].

Global Registry of Acute Coronary Events

The GRACE is an ongoing international registry enrolling patients from 94 hospitals in 14 countries in Europe, North America, South

America, Australia, and New Zealand [30]. GRACE spans a variety of care facilities, encompasses the full range of coronary syndromes, and as of 2003 has enrolled 39,000 patients. GRACE highlights the high morbidity and mortality associated with hospitalization for any ACS. Death occurred in 12% of patients who had STEMI, in 13% of those who had NSTEMI, and in 8% of those who had unstable angina. Thus, among hospitalized patients, the risk of death at 6 months was just as great among patients who had ACS presenting with NSTEMI as among those presenting with STEMI [30–32].

Get With The Guidelines

The Get With The Guidelines program is a hospital-based quality improvement initiative created by the AHA and American Stroke Association targeting secondary prevention efforts. The largest quality improvement initiative, it has targeted an initial 1800 hospitals, representing 75% of the patients in the United States who have AMI, and currently has a database of more than 80,000 patients [33,34]. A Web-based management tool is used for data collection and feedback (data are compatible with the Joint Commission on Accreditation of Health care Organizations and NRMI) and provides real-time, guideline-based, on-line reminders specifically addressing discharge management. Additionally the Web tool provides communication with primary care providers by generating a letter documenting discharge instructions and medications to enforce long-term compliance.

The Can Rapid Risk Stratification of Unstable Angina Patients Suppress Adverse Outcomes with Early Implementation of the American College of Cardiology/American Heart Association guidelines initiative

The national quality improvement initiative CRUSADE was established to promote awareness and widespread use of the ACC/AHA clinical treatment guidelines specifically directed at patients who are at high risk of NSTE ACS [19,35]. Data are being collected regarding all aspects of NSTE ACS care and will be used for reporting, feedback, and quality improvement. More than just a database, CRUSADE is also a quality improvement project and will educate hospital staff on all aspects of the ACC/AHA guidelines before participation and offer hospitals access to educational and patient care materials (eg, standardized orders sets, risk-stratification charts, discharge planning forms) with the goal of improving both acute (emergency department–based) and longer-term (postdischarge) management of this population. Moreover, CRUSADE will report back to a given institution its treatment patterns compared with national norms, coupling these reports to multispecialty educational efforts by the steering committee, including lectures and scientific publications of risk-stratification practice and success. As of mid-2005, more than 140,000 patients from more than 400 emergency departments and medical centers in 47 states across the United States had been analyzed.

Real-world patients versus selected trial populations

Registry data show that the demographics of the patients who have ACS are changing; clinicians now more frequently are faced with higher risk and more comorbidities in patients presenting with NSTE ACS. For example, during the 1990s the mean patient age in the NRMI registry increased from 65.3 to 68.0 years [28]. Furthermore, the proportion of women rose from 35.3% to 39.3%, and there is an increased incidence of associated comorbidities including heart failure, stroke, diabetes, hypertension, and previous coronary revascularization. There was also a decrease in patients presenting with STEMI (from 36.4% in 1994 to 27.1% in 1999) and an increase in the prevalence of NSTEMI (from 45% in 1994 to 63% in 1999) [28].

Although some would argue that this demographic shift makes treatment decisions more difficult by bringing to medical attention patients who would have less often been enrolled in clinical trials (if not excluded altogether), it is clear from both clinical trials and observational studies that these high-risk patients derive the most benefit from the early invasive approach. Also, this demographic shift alone does not explain the clear gaps in treatment between certain geographical areas, institution types, and among certain patient populations.

Real world management: risk stratification

Despite recommendations by the ACC/AHA for prompt evaluation and obtainment of an ECG, this guideline recommendation is met only one third of the time according to the CRUSADE quality improvement initiative [36]. Quality improvement measures focusing on the areas of timely access to care and providers may include additional nurses or ECG technicians during peak emergency department hours, synchronizing emergency department and ECG machine clocks to assess actual timing of evaluation more accurately, training additional staff in ECG acquisition, and educating triage nursing staff about atypical symptoms that could be consistent with cardiac ischemia.

Biomarkers of cardiac injury should be measured in all patients who present with chest discomfort consistent with ACS, a cardiac-specific troponin is the preferred marker. It is also recommended that biomarker results be available to the treating physician within 30 to 60 minutes after admission. Delays in biomarker turnaround are unfortunately common in clinical practice. In a study of 1340 patients at 25 CRUSADE hospitals, the overall mean "vein to brain" time (time from arrival in the emergency department as recorded in the medical chart or ambulance arrival data to notification of the treating physician of laboratory results, VTBT) was 115.7 ± 70.1 minutes. The use of point-of-care testing rather than a central laboratory was associated with a significantly shorter VTBT (68.2 ± 40.8 minutes) but was used in a minority of the emergency departments. CRUSADE also found that patients in hospitals with the shortest VTBT were more likely to receive recommended evidenced-based therapies including aspirin, beta-blockers, clopidogel, GpIIbIIIa and heparin (Peacock WF, Roe MT, Chen AY, et al. Vein-to-brain time: an emergency department quality of care marker for non–ST-segment elevation acute coronary syndromes, unpublished article).

Real world management: acute treatment for acute coronary syndromes

Despite guideline recommendations, acute medical therapies are often underused, especially in populations at highest risk. Registry data report that early in the 1990s acute therapies were grossly underused. During the latter half of the decade practices were becoming increasingly concordant with guideline recommendations but still had significant room for improvement. This trend continues into the current decade. Fig. 1 illustrates the trend in select acute therapies in the NRMI registry (in both patients who have STEMI and those who have NSTEMI) between 1994 and 2003. Table 1 illustrates usage rates of acute therapies in eligible patients who have

NSTEMI and in-hospital mortality from the GRACE and CRUSADE registries.

Beyond the global trends in care, these registries give insights into which patient populations are failing to receive evidence-based care. A disturbing trend has been noted in analysis of many registries, namely that patients who present with ACS and are at the highest risk are paradoxically treated less aggressively than those who are at the lowest risk. Additionally, there are significant disparities in treatment based on age, race, sex, and insurance status with the elderly, nonwhites, women, and the uninsured least likely to receive guideline-based therapy [37,41]. A recent study that illustrates this trend examined patterns of use of Gp IIb/IIIa inhibitors in the early management of NSTEMI patients using the NRMI 4 registry at 1189 centers across the United States [41]. The investigators noted that of 60,770 patients who had NSTEMI and who were eligible for early Gp IIb/IIIa inhibitor therapy, only 15,379 patients (25%) received such therapy. Patients receiving early Gp IIb/IIIa inhibitor treatment were significantly younger and were more likely to be white and male and to have private insurance (instead of Medicare, Medicaid, or self-pay). Treated patients were less likely to have had a prior myocardial infarction or most comorbid illnesses but were more likely to have had a coronary revascularization procedure. The overall in-hospital mortality rate was 8.0% for all patients, but patients treated early with Gp IIb/IIIa inhibitors had significantly lower unadjusted mortality than did patients not receiving such therapy (3.3% versus 9.6%; $P < .001$). Patients who had higher baseline risk were also less likely to receive early Gp IIb/IIIa inhibitor treatment. For example, whereas 45% of low-risk patients (expected risk < 2%) received early Gp IIb/IIIa inhibition, only 9% of the high-risk patients (expected mortality > 15%) received treatment. This pattern of conservative care in high-risk patients is also seen in other areas of medicine but is inconsistent with maximizing absolute benefits from therapy [41–43].

Similar patterns can be seen in the use of early invasive catheterization in patients who have ACS. Using patients enrolled in the CRUSADE registry between March 2000 and September 2002, Bhatt and colleagues [44] found that the unadjusted incidence of in-hospital mortality was 2.0% for patients who underwent early invasive management (within 48 hours) compared with 6.2% for patients who did not undergo early

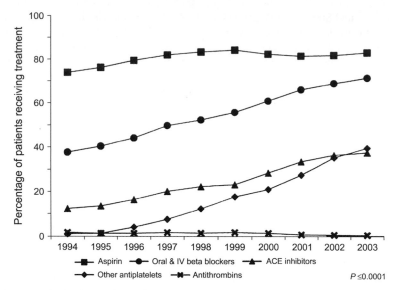

Fig. 1. Medication range in the first 24 hours from the NRMI registry (STEMI and NSTEMI patients. (*From* Gibson MC. NRMI and current treatment patterns for ST-elevation myocardial infarction. Am Heart J 2004;148:S31; with permission.)

invasive management. Patients who underwent early catheterization were younger, more often male and white, more likely to be admitted to a cardiology service, and less likely to have heart failure or renal insufficiency. Additionally, when stratified into low, medium, and high clinical risk based on the modified PURSUIT risk score (Platelet Glycoprotein IIb/IIIa in Unstable Angina: Receptor Suppression Using Integrilin Therapy [PURSUIT Trial]), patients in all three risk categories undergoing early invasive management had a significantly lower risk of unadjusted in-hospital mortality [44,45]. The patients at highest risk seemed to derive the greatest absolute benefit from early invasive management. Propensity matching of patients by early invasive management status produced groups that were similarly matched for clinical, demographic, and hospital characteristics, and in this sample of propensity-matched pairs the frequency of in-hospital mortality was lower in patients who underwent early invasive management (2.5% versus 3.7%; $P < .001$).

Concepts of quality and quality improvement

As evidenced by the data presented here and detailed in several recent prominent reports, American medicine is challenged by errors of omission or failure to ensure that evidence-based therapeutic and preventive measures reach patients as well as by errors of commission or failure to deliver treatments in a safe and appropriate manner. Failure in any of these areas can lead to poor patient outcomes and high cost [46–50]. The Institute of Medicine's report *Crossing the Quality Chasm* outlines six aims for

Table 1
Observational studies describing care and outcomes in NSTE ACS [1,31]

Care/outcome[a]	Study GRACE 1999–2000 (N = 2893)	CRUSADE 2001–2002 (N = 18937)
Aspirin (%)	91	90
Beta-blockers (%)	78	76
Heparin (%)	61	53
Low molecular weight heparin (%)	51	36
Gp IIbIIIa inhibitors (%)	20	31
Inhospital mortality (%)	6.0	4.9

[a] Treatments listed reflect usage patterns during hospitalization for eligible patients who do not have possible contraindications to the given treatments at the end of the respective evaluation periods.

Data from Roe MT, Ohman EM, Pollack CV Jr, et al. Changing the model of care for patients with acute coronary syndromes. Am Heart J 2003;146:605–12; Fox KA, Goodman SG, Klein W, et al. Management of acute coronary syndromes. Variations in practice and outcome; findings from the Global Registry of Acute Coronary Events (GRACE). Eur Heart J 2002;23:1177–89.

improvement in the United States health care system. For the treatment of ACS, these goals can be translated as follows:

Timeliness—rapid risk stratification and treatment

Effectiveness—providing the right evidence-based treatment

Safety—assuring that therapies, when given, are administered correctly with an emphasis on appropriate drug dosing and procedures done correctly

Equity—assuring all patients, regardless of race, sex, socioeconomic or insurance status, receive safe and effective care

Efficiency—avoiding overtreatment in those who do not stand to benefit

Patient centeredness—considering a treatment's risks and benefits in an individual patient and according to the patient's value system

Improving practice patterns: barriers to evidence-based care

Cabana and colleagues [51] conducted a literature review to determine the barriers to adoption of practice guidelines in clinical practice. The barriers they identified included lack of awareness, lack of familiarity, lack of agreement, lack of self-efficacy, lack of outcome expectancy, inertia of previous practice, and external barriers. Of these barriers, lack of awareness and lack of familiarity are best remedied by educational initiatives, whereas lack of self-efficacy and lack of outcome expectancy are best remedied by providing continuous feedback on guideline adherence and patient outcomes data, respectively. Unfortunately, interventions designed to enhance physician education such as continuing medical education conferences and printed materials have been shown to have little impact on improving physician performance [35,52,53].

Using the data from the NRMI, Bradley and colleagues [54] attempted to identify factors present in hospitals with higher compliance to guideline-based therapy, specifically the use of beta-blockers in the treatment of AMI. In an interesting and hypothesis-generating study using open-ended interviews of clinical staff and administrators, the investigators noted four themes that were prevalent among the hospitals with the greatest or increasing use of beta-blockers (>65%) versus those with least or declining use (<65%): (1) a high degree

of commitment among clinicians and support staff regarding the use of evidence-based therapies, (2) a substantial level of administrative support for quality improvement, (3) strong physician leadership or a physician champion, and (4) high-quality data feedback. Additional factors that have been reported in the literature to improve adherence to practice guidelines include reminder systems such as critical care pathways or computerized support programs, patient-oriented interventions, and the use of local opinion leaders in the education of physicians [55,56].

Cycle of continuous quality improvement

The process of continuous quality improvement begins with the publication of CPGs, which are generated by expert committees and based on assimilation of clinical-trial results [1]. Data must then be collected to determine rates of use of therapies and interventions recommended by CPGs, and performance indicators are developed to establish benchmarks for high-quality care. Next, multidisciplinary teams led by local opinion leaders must develop and implement plans to improve adherence to practice guidelines. Finally, patient outcomes based upon performance and adherence to practice guidelines must be measured to encourage continuous improvements in patient care (Fig. 2) [1,57]. As discussed previously, significant challenges limit the success of quality improvement initiatives designed to encourage the adoption of CPGs. Clearly an active, multidisciplinary, and multifactorial approach is needed to integrate CPGs into clinical practice, as demonstrated through the various successful AMI quality improvement initiatives outlined in Table 2.

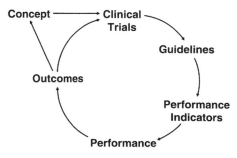

Fig. 2. The cycle of clinical therapeutics. (*Adapted from* Califf RM, Peterson ED, Gibbons RJ, et al. Integrating quality into the cycle of therapeutic development. J Am Coll Cardiol 2002;40:1896; with permission.)

Table 2
Quality improvement initiatives in patients who have myocardial infarction

Program	Population	Intervention	Initial Data Collection	Re-measurement	Improvements in guideline adherence	Mortality
Cardiac Hospitalization Arteriosclerosis Management Program (CHAMP) [3]	UCLA ~ 300 patients per collection time focusing on secondary prevention at discharge	Protocols and standing orders Retrospective data collection Quarterly feedback to clinicians	1992–1993	1994–1995	Aspirin (78% to 92%) Beta-blocker (12% to 61%) ACE inhibitors (4% to 56%) Lipid-lowering therapy (6% to 86%)	Reduction in death and recurrent myocardial infarction from 14.8% to 6.4%
Cooperative Cardiovascular Project Pilot [59]	Medicare patients in four states discharged with diagnosis of MI, focusing on both acute and discharge therapies	Feedback of performance Opinion leaders	1992–1993	1995–1996	Thrombolytics within 1 hour (57.1% to 70.8%) Thrombolytics within 30 minutes (17.6% to 30.1%) Smoking cessation counseling (28.6% to 41%) Aspirin (83.6% to 90.3%) Beta-blockers (47.5% to 68.4%) ACE inhibitors (48.5% to 62.2%)	10% relative reduction in short-term (30-day) and longer-term (1-year) mortality

Guidelines Applied in Practice (GAP) [60]	Random sample of Medicare and non-Medicare patients presenting with MI in Michigan, focusing on acute and discharge therapies	A tool kit for clinicians and patients included care maps, standing admission orders, and discharge forms. Grand rounds site visits Physician and nurse opinion leaders	1998–1999	2001	No significant difference in time to thrombolysis Aspirin (84% to 92%) Beta-blockers (89% to 93%) ACE inhibitors (80% to 86%) Smoking cessation counseling (53% to 65%) Lipid-lowering therapy (68 to 75%)	Not reported
Get With The Guidelines (GWTG) [33,34]	1800 hospitals representing 75% of the MI patients. Over 80,000 patients enrolled. Pilot data from 24 hospitals has been reported (>1700 patients)	A web-based management tool is used for data collection and feedback and provides real-time, guideline based, on-line, reminders specifically addressing discharge management.	2000	Ongoing	Significant improvements in Smoking cessation counseling (48% to 87%) Lipid lowering therapy (54% to 79%) LDL measurement (59% to 81%) BP control, Blood pressure less than 140/90 (60% to 68%) Cardiac rehabilitation referral (34% to 73%)	Not reported

Linking quality of care to outcomes

There is strong emerging evidence that improving hospital guideline compliance is associated with improved patient outcomes. Peterson and colleagues [58] used NRMI IV (2000–2002) data to review the care of more than 250,000 patients who had AMI from more than 1200 institutions. A measurement of "composite quality" was calculated by reviewing each patient's care, and scores were given for the correct application of the guideline-based therapy for which the patient was eligible. Institutions were ranked according to their composite quality scores and divided into quartiles. In the leading quartile (best care), the average inpatient mortality was 8.3%. In contrast, patients treated in the lagging quartile hospitals (worst care) had an inpatient mortality rate of 15.3%.

This association between the degree of adherence to ACC/AHA guidelines and better patient outcomes has been duplicated using data from the CRUSADE database [18]. Again, more than 400 hospitals in the United States were grouped into quartiles based on reported overall adherence to ACC/AHA guidelines. Hospitals with more than 80% adherence to these guidelines (leading quartile) were compared with hospitals that demonstrated less than 65% adherence to the guidelines (lagging quartile). As in the NRMI, the in-hospital mortality rate was 3.6% for leading-quartile hospitals, versus 5.9% for hospitals in the lagging quartile. This difference in mortality indicates that adherence to the ACC/AHA guidelines does indeed seem to result in improved outcomes for patients [18].

Summary

Both acute management and secondary prevention for patients presenting with the spectrum of ACS have evolved greatly during the last decade, as evidenced by the multitude of clinical trials and the development of CPGs. The goal of the next decade is to ensure the accurate, equal, and timely application of these therapies and management strategies in clinical practice. In the emergency department, initiation of guideline-based management is especially challenging given the dynamic process of risk stratification that must take place to ensure properly directed care. It is clear, however, that application of such therapies leads to improved outcomes. Lessons learned from previous and ongoing quality improvement initiatives will provide the tools needed to ensure that widespread adoption of guideline-based therapy is complete.

References

[1] Roe MT, Ohman EM, Pollack CV Jr, et al. Changing the model of care for patients with acute coronary syndromes. Am Heart J 2003;146:605–12.

[2] French WJ. Trends in acute myocardial infarction management: use of the National Registry of Myocardial Infarction in quality improvement. Am J Cardiol 2000;85:5B–12B.

[3] Fonarow GC, Gawlinski A, Moughrabi S, et al. Improved treatment of coronary heart disease by implementation of a cardiac hospitalization atherosclerosis management program (CHAMP). Am J Cardiol 2001;87:819–22.

[4] Braunwald E, Jones RH, Mark DB, et al. Diagnosing and managing unstable angina. Agency for Health Care Policy and Research. Circulation 1994;90:613–22.

[5] Braunwald E, Antman EM, Beasley JW, et al. ACC/AHA guidelines for the management of patients with unstable angina and non-ST-segment elevation myocardial infarction: a report of the American College of Cardiology/American Heart Association Task Force on Practice Guidelines (Committee on the Management of Patients with Unstable Angina). J Am Coll Cardiol 2000; 36:970–1062.

[6] McCarthy M. US heart-guidelines strategy makes promising start. Lancet 2001;358:1618.

[7] Pollack CV Jr, Roe MT, Peterson ED. 2002 update to the ACC/AHA guidelines for the management of patients with unstable angina and non-ST-segment elevation myocardial infarction: implications for emergency department practice. Ann Emerg Med 2003;41:355–69.

[8] Pollack CV Jr, Diercks DB, Roe MT, et al. 2004 ACC/AHA guidelines for the management of patients with ST-elevation myocardial infarction: implications for ED practice. Ann Emerg Med 2005;45:363–76.

[9] Gibler WB, Cannon CP, Blomkalns AL, et al. Practical implementation of the guidelines for unstable angina/non-ST-segment elevation myocardial infarction in the emergency department. Circulation 2005;111:2699–710.

[10] American Heart Association. 2002 Heart and stroke statistical update. Dallas (TX): American Heart Association; 2001.

[11] Nouraj P. National hospital ambulatory medical care survey: 1997 emergency department summary. Hyattsville (MD): National Center for Health Statistics; 1997.

[12] American Heart Association. Heart disease and stroke statistics—2005 update. Dallas (TX): American Heart Association; 2005.

[13] Antman EM, Anbe DT, Armstrong PW, et al. ACC/ AHA guidelines for the management of patients with ST-elevation myocardial infarction: executive summary: a report of the ACC/AHA Task Force on Practice Guidelines (Committee to Revise the 1999 Guidelines on the Management of Patients With Acute Myocardial Infarction). J Am Coll Cardiol 2004;44:671–719.

[14] Braunwald E, Antman EM, Beasley JW, et al. ACC/ AHA guideline update for the management of patients with unstable angina and non-ST-segment elevation myocardial infarction – 2002: a report of the American College of Cardiology/American Heart Association Task Force on Practice Guidelines (Committee on the Management of Patients with Unstable Angina). Circulation 2002;106: 1893–900.

[15] Gibson CM. Time is myocardium and time is outcomes. Circulation 2001;104(22):2632–4.

[16] Brown AL, Mann NC, Daya M, et al, for the Rapid Early Action for Coronary Treatment (REACT) study. Demographic, belief, and situational factors influencing the decision to utilize emergency medical services among chest pain patients. Circulation 2000; 102:173–8.

[17] Faxon D, Lenfant C. Timing is everything: motivating patients to call 9-1-1 at onset of acute myocardial infarction. Circulation 2001;104:1210–1.

[18] Peterson ED, Roe MT, Lytle BL, et al. The association between care and outcomes in patients with acute coronary syndromes: national results from CRUSADE. J Am Coll Cardiol 2004;43:406A.

[19] Ohman EM, Roe MT, Smith SC Jr, et al. Care of the non-ST-segment elevation patients: insights from the CRUSADE national quality improvement initiative. Am Heart J 2004;148:S34–9.

[20] Antman EM, Cohen M, Bernink PJ, et al. The TIMI risk score for unstable angina/non-ST elevation MI: a method for prognostication and therapeutic decision making. JAMA 2000;284:835–42.

[21] Antman EM, McCabe CH, Gurfinkel EP, et al. Enoxaparin prevents death and cardiac ischemic events in unstable angina/non-Q-wave myocardial infarction: results of the Thrombolysis In Myocardial Infarction (TIMI) 11B trial. Circulation 1999; 100:1593–601.

[22] Cohen M, Demers C, Gurfinkel EP, et al, for the Efficacy and Safety of Subcutaneous Enoxaparin in Non-Q-Wave Coronary Events Study Group. A comparison of low-molecular-weight heparin with unfractionated heparin for unstable coronary artery disease. N Engl J Med 1997;337:447–52.

[23] Cannon CP, Weintraub WS, Demopoulos LA, et al. TACTICS (Treat Angina with Aggrastat and Determine Cost of Therapy with an Invasive or Conservative Strategy)–Thrombolysis in Myocardial Infarction 18 Investigators. Comparison of early invasive and conservative strategies in patients with unstable coronary syndromes treated with the glycoprotein IIb/IIIa inhibitor tirofiban. N Engl J Med 2001;344(25):1879–87.

[24] Platelet Receptor Inhibition in Ischemic Syndrome Management in Patients Limited by Unstable Signs and Symptoms (PRISM-PLUS) Study investigators. Inhibition of the platelet glycoprotein IIb/IIIa receptor with tirofiban in unstable angina and non-Q-wave myocardial infarction. N Engl J Med 1998; 338:1488–97.

[25] The TIMI IIIB Investigators. Effects of tissue plasminogen activator and a comparison of early invasive and conservative strategies in unstable angina and non-Q-wave myocardial infarction: results of the TIMI IIIB trial. Thrombolysis In Myocardial Ischemia. Circulation 1994;89.1545–56.

[26] Fragmin and Fast Revascularisation during Instability in Coronary artery disease investigators. Invasive compared with non-invasive treatment in unstable coronary-artery disease: FRISC II prospective randomised multicentre study. Lancet 1999;354: 708–15.

[27] Wallentin L, Lagerqvist B, Husted S, et al. FRISC II investigators. Outcome at 1 year after an invasive compared with a non-invasive strategy in unstable coronary-artery disease: the FRISC II invasive randomised trial. Lancet 2000;356:9–16.

[28] Rogers WJ, Canto JG, Lambrew CT, et al. Temporal trends in the treatment of over 1.5 million patients with myocardial infarction in the US from 1990 through 1999: the National Registry of Myocardial Infarction 1, 2 and 3. J Am Coll Cardiol 2000;36(7):2056–63.

[29] Gibson MC. NRMI and current treatment patterns for ST-elevation myocardial infarction. Am Heart J 2004;148:S29–33.

[30] GRACE investigators. Rationale and design of the GRACE (Global Registry of Acute Coronary Events) project: a multinational registry of patients hospitalized with acute coronary syndromes. Am Heart J 2001;141:190–3.

[31] Fox KA, Goodman SG, Klein W, et al. Management of acute coronary syndromes. Variations in practice and outcome; findings from the Global Registry of Acute Coronary Events (GRACE). Eur Heart J 2002;23:1177–89.

[32] Eagle KA, Goodman SG, Avezum A, et al. Practice variation and missed opportunities for reperfusion in ST–segment-elevation myocardial infarction: findings from the Global Registry of Acute Coronary Events (GRACE). Lancet 2002;359:373–7.

[33] LaBresh KA, Ellrodt AG, Gliklich R, et al. Get With the Guidelines for cardiovascular secondary prevention: pilot results. Arch Intern Med 2004;164(2): 203–9.

[34] Smaha LA. The American Heart Association Get With the Guidelines Program. Am Heart J 2004; 148:S46–8.

[35] Hoekstra JW, Pollack CV Jr, Roe MT, et al. Improving the care of patients with non-ST-elevation

acute coronary syndromes in the emergency department: the CRUSADE initiative. Acad Emerg Med 2002;9(11):1146–55.

[36] Diercks DB, Roe MT, Chen AY, et al. Disparities by sex in timing of initial electrocardiogram for patients presenting with acute coronary syndromes. J Am Coll Cardiol 2005;45(3):221A.

[37] Shahi CN, Rathore SS, Wang Y, et al. Quality of care among elderly patients hospitalized with unstable angina. Am Heart J 2001;142:263–70.

[38] Scirica BM, Moliterno DJ, Every NR, et al. Differences between men and women in the management of unstable angina pectoris (the GUARANTEE registry). Am J Cardiol 1999;84:1145–50.

[39] Stone PH, Thompson B, Anderson HV, et al. Influence of race, sex, and age on management of unstable angina and non–Q-wave myocardial infarction: the TIMI III registry. JAMA 1996;275:1104–12.

[40] Giugliano RP, Camargo CA Jr, Lloyd-Jones DM, et al. Elderly patients receive less aggressive medical and invasive management of unstable angina: potential impact of practice guidelines. Arch Intern Med 1998;158:1113–20.

[41] Peterson ED, Pollack CV Jr, Roe MT, et al. National Registry of Myocardial Infarction (NRMI) 4 investigators. Early use of glycoprotein IIb/IIIa inhibitors in non-ST-elevation acute myocardial infarction: observations from the National Registry of Myocardial Infarction 4. J Am Coll Cardiol 2003;42(1):45–53.

[42] Batchelor WB, Peterson ED, Mark DB, et al. A comparison of US and Canadian cardiac catheterization practices in detecting severe coronary artery disease after myocardial infarction: efficiency, yield and long-term implications. J Am Coll Cardiol 1999;34:12–9.

[43] Pilote L, Califf RM, Sapp S, et al, for the GUSTO-I investigators. Regional variation across the United States in the management of acute myocardial infarction. N Engl J Med 1995;333:565–72.

[44] Bhatt DL, Roe MT, Peterson ED, et al, for the CRUSADE investigators. Utilization of early invasive management strategies for high-risk patients with non-ST-segment elevation acute coronary syndromes: results from the CRUSADE Quality Improvement Initiative. JAMA 2004;292(17):2096–104.

[45] Boersma E, Pieper KS, Steyerberg EW, et al, for the PURSUIT investigators. Predictors of outcome in patients with acute coronary syndromes without persistent ST-segment elevation: results from an international trial of 9461 patients. Circulation 2000;101:2557–67.

[46] Zeidel ML. Improving the quality of health care in America: what medical schools, leading medical journals and federal funding agencies can do. Am J Med 2002;112(2):165–7.

[47] Chassin MR. Improving the quality of care. N Engl J Med 1996;335:1060–3.

[48] Kohn LT, Corrigan JM, Donaldson MS. To err is human: building a safer health system. Washington (DC): National Academy Press; 2000.

[49] Allison JJ, Kiefe CI, Weissman NW, et al. Relationship of hospital teaching status with quality of care and mortality for Medicare patients with acute MI. JAMA 2000;284:1256–62.

[50] Institute of Medicine. Crossing the quality chasm: a new health system for the 21st century. Washington (DC): National Academy Press; 2001.

[51] Cabana MD, Rand CS, Powe NR, et al. Why don't physicians follow clinical practice guidelines? A framework for improvement. JAMA 1999;282:1458–65.

[52] Davis DA, Thomson MA, Oxman AD, et al. Changing physician performance: a systematic review of the effect of continuing medical education. JAMA 1995;274:700–5.

[53] Grol R. Improving the quality of medical care. Building bridges among professional pride, payer profit, and patient satisfaction. JAMA 2001;284:2578–85.

[54] Bradley EH, Holmboe ES, Mattera JA, et al. A qualitative study of increasing beta-blocker use after myocardial infarction: why do some hospitals succeed? JAMA 2001;285(20):2604–11.

[55] Soumerai SB, McLaughlin TJ, Gurwitz JH, et al. Effect of local medical opinion leaders on quality of care for acute myocardial infarction: a randomized controlled trial. JAMA 1998;279:1358–63.

[56] Cooperative Cardiovascular Project Best Practices Working Group. Improving care for acute myocardial infarction: experience from the Cooperative Cardiovascular Project. Jt Comm J Qual Improv 1998;24:480–90.

[57] Califf RM, Peterson ED, Gibbons RJ, et al. Integrating quality into the cycle of therapeutic development. J Am Coll Cardiol 2002;40:1895–901.

[58] Peterson ED, Parsons LS, Pollack CV, et al. Variation in AMI care quality across 1,085 hospitals and its association with hospital mortality rates. Circulation 2002;106:II-722.

[59] Marciniak TA, Ellerbeck EF, Radford MJ, et al. Improving the quality of care for Medicare patients with acute myocardial infarction: results from the Cooperative Cardiovascular Project. JAMA 1998;279:1351–7.

[60] Mehta RH, Montoye CK, Gallogly M, et al. Improving the quality of care for acute myocardial infarction: the Guidelines Applied in Practice (GAP) initiative. JAMA 2002;287:1269–76.

ELSEVIER
SAUNDERS

Cardiol Clin 24 (2006) 103–114

CARDIOLOGY
CLINICS

Evaluation and Management of the Patient Who Has Cocaine-associated Chest Pain

Judd E. Hollander, MD[a],*, Timothy D. Henry, MD[b]

[a]Department of Emergency Medicine, University of Pennsylvania, Ground Floor, Ravdin Building,
3400 Spruce Street Philadelphia, PA 19104-4283, USA
[b]Minneapolis Heart Institute Foundation, University of Minnesota, 920 East 28th Street,
Suite 40, Minneapolis, MN 55407, USA

Erythroxylon coca, the shrub from which cocaine is naturally derived, grows indigenously in South America. Cocaine was first identified as the active alkaloid in the coca leaf in 1857. As far back as the twelfth century, Incas used cocaine-filled saliva as local anesthesia for ritual trephinations [1]. In 1884, it was recognized medically as a local anesthetic [2]. In the early twentieth century, cocaine was used briefly as an ingredient in Coca-Cola. In 1906, the United States began to control cocaine use, and in 1914 the Harrison Narcotic Act labeled cocaine as a narcotic. It became a schedule II drug in the 1970s. During the last several decades, recreational cocaine use has increased, and reports of side effects have grown exponentially. As of 2003, 34.9 million citizens of the United States (14.7%) have used cocaine at least once, with 2.3 million citizens using cocaine within the past month [3].

Pharmacology

Cocaine is absorbed through application to the mucosa, ingestion, inhalation, and direct intravenous injection. Effects from nasal insufflation begin rapidly with peak concentrations typically reached within 30 to 60 minutes. Intravenous and inhalational routes of cocaine use produce near-immediate distribution throughout the circulation. "Crack" is the direct precipitate of free-base cocaine that results from alkalinization of aqueous cocaine hydrochloride.

The relative contributions of cocaine and its metabolites to the clinical effects remain somewhat unclear. Cocaine is hydrolyzed rapidly by liver and plasma esterases to ecgonine methylester (EME), which accounts for 30% to 50% of the parent product. Nonenzymatic hydrolysis results in the formation of the other major metabolite, benzoylecgonine (approximately 40% of the parent product). The biologic half-life of cocaine is 0.5 to 1.5 hours; Benzoylecgonine and EME, the major metabolites of cocaine, have half-lives of 5 to 8 hours and 3.5 to 6 hours, respectively [4].

Minor metabolites, norcocaine and ecgonine, account for the majority of the other degradation products. Early studies suggested that cocaine and norcocaine accounted for majority of the vascular effects of cocaine [5]. Recent studies, however, demonstrate an active role for many of the metabolites. Most studies suggest that cocaine and norcocaine are the most potent vasoconstrictors; benzoylecgonine and ecgonine have less of an effect. Some studies suggest that EME may result in mild cerebral vasodilation [6,7]. Sodium-channel antagonist effects occur with cocaine and norcocaine [8]. Sodium-channel antagonist effects do not occur with benzoylecgonine or EME [8].

Cocaethylene is a unique metabolite that results from the combined use of alcohol and cocaine [9]. In clinical studies, cocaethylene produces hemodynamic effects comparable to those of cocaine. Cocaethylene has a direct myocardial depressant effect [10] that is independent of any coronary artery vasoconstriction [11]. The permeability of

* Corresponding author.

human endothelial cells to low-density lipoproteins is increased by both cocaine and cocaethylene, potentially suggesting a mechanism for the accelerated atherosclerosis seen with cocaine [12].

Pathophysiology

Cocaine has diverse actions in humans. It directly blocks fast sodium channels, stabilizing the axonal membrane, with a resultant local anesthetic effect. Blockade of myocardial fast sodium channels causes cocaine to have type I antidysrhythmic properties [13,14]. Cocaine interferes with the uptake of neurotransmitters at the nerve terminal. Cocaine functions as a vasoconstrictive agent. These three properties account for most of the toxicity seen in the clinical setting.

The initial effect on the cardiovascular system is a transient bradycardia, secondary to stimulation of the vagal nuclei. Tachycardia typically ensues, predominantly from increased central sympathetic stimulation. Cocaine has a cardiostimulatory effect through sensitization to epinephrine and norepinephrine. It prevents neuronal reuptake of these catecholamines and increases the release of norepinephrine from adrenergic nerve terminals, leading to enhanced sympathetic effects. The vasopressor effects of cocaine are mostly mediated by norepinephrine of sympathetic neural origin, and the tachycardiac effects of cocaine are mostly mediated by epinephrine of adrenal medullary origin [15].

The pathophysiology of cocaine-associated myocardial ischemia is multifactorial. Chronic cocaine users develop left ventricular hypertrophy, premature atherosclerosis, and coronary aneurysms and ectasia [16]. Acutely, cocaine causes coronary arterial vasoconstriction, in situ thrombus formation, platelet aggregation, and increased myocardial oxygen demand. The combination of increased myocardial oxygen demand (from hypertension, tachycardia, and left ventricular hypertrophy) in the setting of decreased blood flow (from atherosclerosis, platelet aggregation, and thrombus formation) and coronary vasoconstriction results in myocardial ischemia.

Cocaine produces coronary vasoconstriction of the epicardial coronaries that can be reversed by phentolamine, an alpha-adrenergic antagonist [17] and exacerbated by propranolol, a beta-adrenergic antagonist [18]. Cocaine-induced vasoconstriction occurs in both diseased and nondiseased coronary artery segments; however, the magnitude of the effect is more pronounced in the diseased segments [19]. Tobacco smoking induces coronary artery vasoconstriction through an alpha-adrenergic mechanism similar to that of cocaine [20]. Most cocaine-using patients are also cigarette smokers, and the combination of near-simultaneous tobacco and cocaine use has a synergistic effect on epicardial coronary artery vasoconstriction [21]. Cocaine also impedes microvascular blood flow in the heart [22].

Platelet activation and thrombus formation also occur secondary to cocaine. Cocaine activates platelets directly [23] and indirectly through an alpha-adrenergic–mediated increase in platelet aggregability [24]. Adenosine diphosphate–induced platelet aggregation is enhanced [25], and tissue plasminogen activator inhibitor is increased [26] in the presence of cocaine. Thrombus formation can occur in patients who have cocaine-associated myocardial infarction (MI) whether or not underlying coronary artery disease is present [2,22].

Chronic users of cocaine may be prone to early atherosclerosis, as demonstrated by autopsy studies of young cocaine users [27–29]. Although initial reports of cocaine-associated MI emphasized a lower-than-expected prevalence of coronary artery disease, many, if not most, patients who have cocaine-associated MI have underlying coronary artery disease. Large clinical series have found that 31% to 67% of patients who have cocaine-associated MI have atherosclerotic coronary artery disease [2,16,22,27]. Coronary artery disease is less common in patients who have MI associated with cocaine than in cocaine-free patients; however, it is still more common than in controls [22]. Chronic cocaine use has also recently been associated with coronary artery ectasia and aneurysms [16]. In a consecutive series of 112 cocaine users who underwent angiography, 30% had coronary ectasia and aneurysms. MI had occurred in 65% of the patients who had coronary ectasia and aneurysms, including patients who did not have significant coronary artery stenosis [16]. Epicardial [30] and intramyocardial coronary artery disease [31] is also present in patients who have chest pain in the absence of MI.

Cocaine use has also been identified as a possible cause of aortic dissection. One study in an inner-city setting reported 38 cases of acute aortic dissection over a 20-year period, 14 of which (37%) were associated with cocaine use [32]. Although the International Registry for Aortic Dissection suggests that cocaine use is involved in less than 1% of aortic dissections, this diagnosis may be underappreciated and must be considered in patients presenting with cocaine-associated chest pain [33,34].

Initial approach to the patient in the emergency department

Patients who have potential cocaine toxicity should receive a complete evaluation including a history of cocaine use, recognition of signs and symptoms consistent with sympathetic nervous system excess, and evaluation of organ-specific complaints. It is imperative to determine whether signs and symptoms are caused by cocaine itself, underlying unrelated structural abnormalities, or cocaine-induced structural abnormalities.

The differential diagnosis of cocaine-associated chest pain is similar to the differential diagnosis of chest pain unrelated to cocaine except that the likelihood of a patient having a serious event in the absence of traditional risk factors for that particular disease is increased. Potentially serious causes of chest pain are cardiovascular, pulmonary, and vascular in origin and include myocardial ischemia and infarction, aortic dissection, pulmonary embolism, pneumothorax, pneumomediastinum, and noncardiogenic pulmonary edema [35]. Less serious causes of chest pain following cocaine use include traumatic injury and rhabdomyolysis.

The risk of MI is increased 24-fold in the hour following cocaine use [36]. Approximately 6% of patients who have cocaine-associated chest pain are actually having an acute MI [37,38], and another 15% have an acute coronary syndrome [37]. The classic patient who has cocaine-associated MI is a young, male tobacco smoker with a history of repetitive cocaine use and few other cardiac risk factors [2,37–50]; however, cocaine-associated MI has been reported in patients over 60 years old [2,37,39]. Demographic or historical factors do not reliably predict or exclude acute MI [37]. Likewise, location of chest pain, duration of chest pain, quality of chest pain, and symptoms associated with chest pain are not predictive of MI [37].

The duration of time for which a patient is at risk for MI or ischemia following cocaine use is unknown, because it has been postulated that cocaine-associated acute coronary syndromes (myocardial ischemia and infarction) can also occur secondary to cocaine withdrawal [2,37,45,47]. Spontaneous episodes of ST-elevation myocardial infarction

(STEMI) have been documented for up to 6 weeks after withdrawal of cocaine [47]. These patients often do not have classic chest pain syndromes. The chest pain can be delayed for hours to days after their most recent use of cocaine, although most cocaine-related MIs occur within 24 hours of last use [36,37,39,43,50]. Both STEMI and non-STEMI can occur [2,40,51]. Chronic cocaine use is also associated with premature atherosclerosis and coronary ectasia; these patients can present with MI that is not temporally related to cocaine use.

Electrocardiography

Interpretation of the EKG in patients who have cocaine-associated chest pain can be difficult, because patients can have nondiagnostic EKGs in the setting of ischemia as well as abnormal EKGs in the absence of ischemia. MI occurs in patients who have normal or nonspecific EKGs [37,48]. In one series, patients who had MI were as likely to present with normal or nonspecific EKGs as with ischemic EKGs, thereby, resulting in the emergency department release of 15% of patients who have MI [37]. The sensitivity of the EKG for MI is less than in other patients who have acute MI (approximately 36%) [37].

Conversely, EKGs are abnormal in 56% to 84% of patients who have cocaine-associated chest pain [37,40,50,52], and up to 43% of patients who do not have MI may meet standard EKG criteria for use of reperfusion therapy [50]. J-point and ST-segment elevation secondary to early repolarization or left ventricular hypertrophy makes the identification of ischemia more difficult in these patients [50,53].

Cardiac markers

Cardiac markers are elevated in MI, but false elevations of creatine kinase-MB fraction are common [48,54,55]. Elevations in creatine kinase and creatine kinase-MB occur in the absence of MI [54,55] because of cocaine-induced skeletal muscle injury and rhabdomyolysis. Following the use of cocaine, approximately 50% of patients have elevations in serum creatine kinase with or without myocardial injury [37]. Rising enzyme patterns are more likely to occur in patients who have MI [37,48], whereas initial elevations that rapidly decline less commonly indicate infarction [37,48]. Additionally, in the setting of an elevated absolute creatine kinase-MB, reliance should not be placed entirely on the creatine kinase-MB relative index, because the creatine kinase-MB relative index may be falsely low when concurrent MI and skeletal muscle rhabdomyolysis occur. Cardiac troponin I and T are more specific than creatine kinase-MB for myocardial injury when concomitant skeletal muscle injury exists. Use of cardiac troponin I or T may enhance the diagnostic accuracy of MI in patients who have cocaine-associated ischemia and therefore is preferred [54,55].

Urine drug testing

Patients may initially deny cocaine use. As a result, urine drug testing can be helpful. Relatively little cocaine is excreted unchanged in the urine [56]. Because of a long elimination half-life, assays for cocaine and cocaine metabolites generally will detect benzoylecgonine for up to 48 to 72 hours after use.

Other diagnostic tests

Laboratory evaluation may include a complete blood cell count, electrolytes, glucose, blood urea nitrogen, creatinine, arterial blood gas analysis, urinalysis, creatine kinase, and cardiac marker determinations. Excess sympathetic stimulation may result in hyperglycemia and hypokalemia. Patients who have acute cocaine toxicity can have severe acid-based disturbances as well as rhabdomyolysis [57]. A chest radiograph should be obtained in patients who have cardiopulmonary complaints. It may help demonstrate noncardiac causes for the chest pain.

Initial disposition decision

Patients who have acute STEMI should receive immediate reperfusion therapy. Direct percutaneous coronary intervention (PCI) is preferred in light of the frequently complex clinical presentation and risk of thrombolytics. Patients who have cocaine-associated MI who are likely to develop complications can be identified with a high degree of accuracy during the initial 12 hours of hospitalization [58]. Patients who have cocaine-associated chest pain and do not have infarction have an extremely low frequency of delayed complications [37,39,50]. Cost-effective evaluation strategies, such as 9- to 12-hour observation periods, are appropriate for many patients who have cocaine-associated chest pain, because these patients seem to have a low incidence of cardiovascular complications. Weber and colleagues [59]

demonstrated the safety of a 12-hour observation protocol in 302 patients who had cocaine-associated chest pain.

EKG evidence of ischemia, elevated cardiac markers, and cardiovascular complications occurring before or within 12 hours of arrival predict late complications [58]. These patients should be admitted to monitored beds. Other patients who have cocaine-associated chest pain can be evaluated safely in a 12-hour observation unit [59].

Initial treatment considerations

The initial treatment should focus on airway, breathing, and circulation. Specific treatments are based on the specific sign, symptom, or organ system affected. Because of the direct relationship between the neuropsychiatric and other systemic complications, management of neuropsychiatric manifestations affects the systemic manifestations of cocaine toxicity.

Patients who have suspected cocaine-induced ischemia or MI should be treated similarly to those with traditional acute coronary syndromes, with some notable exceptions. Aspirin, nitroglycerin, and heparin remain important initial therapies. Intravenous benzodiazepines should be provided as early management [2,39,44,60–62]. They will decrease the central stimulatory effects of cocaine, thereby indirectly reducing the cardiovascular toxicity of cocaine. Beta antagonists are contraindicated, because they may exacerbate cocaine-induced coronary artery vasoconstriction [39,44,61,62]. Another management difference between the management of cocaine-using patients and those who have STEMI is a preference for PCI over fibrinolysis [39,44,51,61,62]. Finally, there are anecdotal reports of the safety and efficacy of phentolamine, an alpha antagonist, for treatment of cocaine-associated acute coronary syndromes [39,44,61–62].

Studies in the cardiac catheterization laboratory have largely provided the evidence-based approach to patients who have cocaine-associated coronary vasoconstriction. In these studies, adult patients who had not previously used cocaine were given a low dose of intranasal cocaine (2 mg/kg). Patients developed an increase in heart rate, blood pressure, and coronary vascular resistance with the coronary arterial diameter narrowed by 13% [17]. With administration of phentolamine, the coronary arterial diameter returned to baseline [17]. This finding suggests that phentolamine may be useful for treatment of cocaine-induced ischemia. Based on these data, case reports, and anecdotal experience, the International Guidelines for Emergency Cardiovascular Care recommend alpha-adrenergic antagonists (phentolamine) for the treatment of cocaine-associated acute coronary syndrome [61,62].

Case series and one randomized, controlled trial show that nitroglycerin relieves cocaine-associated chest pain [60,63]. Cardiac catheterization studies demonstrate that nitroglycerin reverses cocaine-induced vasoconstriction [64]. Benzodiazepines have a salutary effect on the hyperdynamic effects of cocaine and relieve chest pain [60]. Benzodiazepines are similar to nitroglycerin with respect to effects on pain relief, cardiac dynamics, and left ventricular function in patients who have cocaine-associated chest pain [60].

The role of calcium-channel blockers for the treatment of cocaine-associated chest pain remains ill defined. Pretreatment of cocaine-intoxicated animals with calcium-channel blockers has had variable results with respect to survival, seizures, and cardiac dysrhythmias [65–71]. In cardiac catheterization studies, verapamil reverses cocaine-induced coronary artery vasoconstriction [72]. Large-scale multicenter clinical trials in patients who have acute coronary syndromes unrelated to cocaine have not demonstrated any beneficial effects of calcium-channel blockers on important outcomes such as survival. Thus, the role of calcium-channel blockers in patients who have cocaine-induced acute coronary syndrome has not yet been defined.

Cocaine induced coronary artery vasoconstriction is clearly exacerbated by the administration of propranolol [18]. An unopposed alpha-adrenergic effect may occur, which leads to vasoconstriction and an increased blood pressure [73–75]. Multiple experimental models have shown that beta-adrenergic antagonists lead to decreased coronary blood flow, increased seizure frequency, and high fatality rates [71,76–79]. The use of short-acting beta-adrenergic antagonists such as esmolol has resulted in significant increases in blood pressure in up to 25% of patients [80,81]. Therefore, the use of beta-adrenergic antagonists for the treatment of cocaine toxicity is contraindicated [39,44,61,62].

Labetalol does not seem to offer any advantages over propranolol. It has substantially more beta-adrenergic antagonism than alpha-adrenergic antagonist effects [82]. Labetalol increases the risk of seizure and death in animal models of cocaine toxicity [71] and does not reverse coronary artery vasoconstriction in humans [83]. Nitroglycerin or phentolamine is considered a better option to achieve vasodilation [39,44,61,62].

Cocaine injures the vascular endothelium, increases platelet aggregation, and impairs normal fibrinolytic pathways [84]. As a result, the use of antiplatelet and antithrombin agents makes theoretical sense [39,44,61,62,85]. Fibrinolytic administration poses problems, however. Many young patients have benign early repolarization, and only a small percentage of patients who have cocaine-associated chest pain syndromes and J-point elevation are actually in the midst of an acute MI [50,53]. Patients are frequently hypertensive, and aortic dissection must be considered. Several case reports document adverse outcomes following fibrinolytic administration in cocaine-using patients [86–88]. Patients who have cocaine-associated STEMI have a low mortality; therefore, the benefit of early fibrinolytic administration is less than in patients who have STEMI unrelated to cocaine, and the risk is higher. Therefore, fibrinolytic therapy should be reserved for patients who are definitely having STEMI and cannot receive primary PCI [36,60,61,85]. With the increasing availability of primary PCI including transfer, this situation should rarely occur. More aggressive antiplatelet therapy with glycoprotein IIb/IIIa antagonists and clopidogrel may be useful in patients who have cocaine-associated acute coronary syndromes, but they have not been well studied in this patient population [89].

Hypertension and tachycardia alone rarely require specific treatment but may need to be addressed in a patient who has definite acute coronary syndromes. In a patient with chest pain of unclear cause, hypertension and tachycardia alone should be treated conservatively. Resolution of anxiety, agitation, and ischemia often lead to resolution of the hypertension and tachycardia. When necessary, treatment directed toward the central effects of cocaine, such as the benzodiazepines, usually reduces blood pressure and heart rate. When sedation is unsuccessful, hypertension can be managed with sodium nitroprusside, nitroglycerin, or intravenous phentolamine [17,64].

Most atrial arrhythmias respond to sedative hypnotics. When they do not, verapamil or diltiazem may be indicated. The treatment of ventricular arrhythmias depends upon the time between cocaine use, arrhythmia onset, and treatment. Ventricular arrhythmias occurring immediately after cocaine use should be presumed to occur from the local anesthetic (sodium-channel) effects on the myocardium. They may respond to the administration of sodium bicarbonate, similar to arrhythmias associated with other type IA and type IC agents [14,90]. In addition, one animal model suggested that lidocaine exacerbates cocaine-induced seizures and arrhythmias as a result of similar effects on sodium channels [91]; however, this finding has not been confirmed in other animal models [14,92,93]. Bicarbonate therapy may be preferable and has been used effectively [94].

Ventricular arrhythmias that develop several hours after the last use of cocaine often occur as a result of ischemia. Standard management for ventricular arrhythmias, including lidocaine, is indicated and seems to be safe [95]. There are no data concerning the efficacy of amiodarone in clinical cocaine intoxication. Torsades de pointes is a rare complication of cocaine use [96] and should be managed with intravenous magnesium sulfate and overdrive pacing.

Other cardiovascular effects of cocaine

Cocaine also causes significant cardiovascular conditions besides those that result in chest pain. Cocaine has a direct myocardial-depressant effect [13,97]. Chronic cocaine use leads to a dilated cardiomyopathy, possibly from recurrent or diffuse ischemia with subsequent "stunned" myocardium [98]. Alternatively, it may a direct effect on myocardial contractility. Direct infusion of cocaine into human coronary arteries increases left ventricular end-diastolic pressures and end-systolic volume and decreases left ventricular ejection fraction [99]. Left ventricular function may improve when cocaine use is halted [100].

Intravenous cocaine use increases the risk of bacterial endocarditis, even more than intravenous heroin use, presumably because of the increased frequency of injection to sustain effects [101,102]. Direct effects of cocaine on endovascular tissues and the immune system may also play a role [102].

Aortic dissection is a rare but life-threatening complication of cocaine abuse and must be considered in the differential diagnosis. In a consecutive series, 37% of acute aortic dissections in an inner-city hospital were associated with cocaine use. This patient cohort was younger than expected with a high percentage of African American males with untreated hypertension [32].

Higher doses of cocaine are associated with virtually all types of tachyarrhythmias. Atrial fibrillation, atrial flutter, supraventricular tachycardias, ventricular premature contractions, accelerated idioventricular rhythms, ventricular tachycardia, torsades de pointes, and ventricular fibrillation may occur as a result of cocaine. High doses of cocaine lead to infranodal and intraventricular conduction delays and lethal ventricular arrhythmias secondary to prolonged QRS and QT intervals [103,104]. Prolonged QT intervals have been noted in patients who have recently used cocaine and who have not had arrhythmias [53]. These effects are probably mediated by the local anesthetic sodium-channel blockade. In addition to the local anesthetic effects, arrhythmias may also occur as a result of cocaine-induced acute coronary syndrome [13,95]. Low doses of cocaine can result in a transient bradycardia.

In-hospital management

There is limited specific information available regarding the in-hospital management of patients who have cocaine-related cardiovascular disease. Therefore, as a general rule, treatment guidelines follow those recommended for patients who have acute coronary syndromes not associated with cocaine Table 1 [105,106].

ST-elevation myocardial infarction

The diagnosis of STEMI can be more challenging in patients who have acute cocaine toxicity because of the atypical presentation and challenges with interpretation of the EKG, including left ventricular hypertrophy and early repolarization. Patients who have acute cocaine toxicity frequently are younger than expected and are hypertensive, and aortic dissection must be considered in the differential diagnosis. Therefore cardiac catheterization with direct PCI is the preferred method of reperfusion, and fibrinolytic therapy should be reserved for patients when cardiac catheterization is not available. With the development of transfer systems for STEMI, fibrinolytic therapy should rarely be required. The method of revascularization and subsequent management should follow guidelines for treatment of patients who do not have a history of cocaine abuse, with a few exceptions. There are no data available regarding the use of drug-eluting stents in patients who abuse cocaine, but they would be expected to decrease target lesion revascularization compared with bare metal stents.

Patients with ongoing cocaine abuse may have poor compliance with the required chronic antiplatelet regimen of aspirin and clopidogrel, which could potentially increase the risk of subacute thrombosis. Therefore each patient's potential for drug rehabilitation and compliance history needs to be considered in the stent choice. Patients who have accelerated atherosclerosis, coronary aneurysms, and ectasia require aggressive risk factor modification and antiplatelet therapy. Long-term clopidogrel should be considered in addition to aspirin. Patients who have left ventricular dysfunction should receive angiotensin-converting enzyme inhibitor therapy. Although patients who have STEMI would be expected to benefit from long-term beta blockade, caution should be used in patients expected to have continued exposure to cocaine.

High-risk unstable angina/non–ST-segment elevation myocardial infarction

Patients who have elevated cardiac enzymes or abnormal EKGs are at higher risk for subsequent events and benefit from an early invasive approach with cardiac catheterization and revascularization [107]. Although no specific data exist for cocaine-related unstable angina/non-STEMI, it is reasonable to believe these patients would benefit from a similar approach. It is important to use drug rehabilitation as well as aggressive risk factor modification in these patients, because

Table 1
Treatment summary for specific cocaine-related medical conditions

Medical Condition	Treatments
Cardiovascular complications	
Dysrhythmias	
Sinus tachycardia	observation oxygen
	diazepam 5 mg IV or lorazepam 2–4 mg IV titrated to effect
Supraventricular tachycardia	oxygen
	diazepam 5 mg IV or lorazepam 2–4 mg IV
	consider diltiazem 20 mg IV or verapamil 5 mg IV
	adenosine 6 mg or 12 mg IV
	cardioversion if hemodynamically unstable
Ventricular dysrhythmias	oxygen
	sodium bicarbonate 1–2 meq/kg
	lidocaine 1.5 mg/kg IV bolus followed by 2 mg/min infusion
	defibrillation if hemodynamically unstable
	diazepam 5 mg IV or lorazepam 2–4 mg IV
Acute coronary syndrome	oxygen
	diazepam 5–10 mg IV or lorazepam 2–4 mg IV
	soluble aspirin 325 mg
	nitroglycerin 1/150 sublingual × three every 5 minutes followed by a infusion titrated to a mean arterial pressure reduction of 10% or relief of chest pain.
	morphine sulfate 2 mg IV every 5 minutes titrated to pain relief
	phentolamine 1 mg IV; repeat in 5 minutes
	verapamil 5–10 mg IV
	heparin or enoxaparin
	percutaneous intervention (angioplasty and stent placement)
	glycoprotein IIb/IIIa inhibitors
Hypertension	observation
	diazepam 5–10 mg IV or lorazepam 2–4 mg IV titrated to effect
	phentolamine 1 mg IV; repeat in 5 minutes
	nitroglycerin or nitroprusside continuous infusion titrated to effect
Pulmonary edema	lasix 20–40 mg IV
	morphine sulfate 2 mg IV every 5 minutes titrated to pain relief or respiratory status
	nitroglycerin infusion titrated to blood pressure
	consider phentolamine or nitroprusside

Adapted from Hollander JE and Hoffman RS. Cocaine. In Godlfrank LR, Flomenbaum NE, Lewin NA, et al, editors. Goldfrank's toxicologic emergency. 6th edition. Stamford (CT): Appleton and Lange,; 1998. p. 1071–89.

there is a high likelihood of recurrence. In one review of patients who had cocaine-associated MI followed for median of 4.5 months, 12 of 24 patients had recurrent ischemic pain; 8 of whom sustained a second MI, suggesting that these patients are at high risk for subsequent events [2].

Low-risk unstable angina

Most patients who have cocaine-related chest pain have low-risk unstable angina and can be treated satisfactorily with a 12-hour observation protocol [59].

Patients who have cocaine-associated chest pain have a 1-year survival rate of 98% and an incidence of late MI of only 1% [49]. Most deaths occur because of concurrent medical problems (such as HIV disease). Because patients who have cocaine-associated chest pain are not at high risk for MI or death during the ensuing year, urgent cardiac evaluation is probably not necessary for patients in whom MI is ruled out. Evaluation for possible underlying coronary artery disease may be accomplished on a more elective basis. Continued cocaine usage, however, is associated with an increased likelihood of recurrent chest pain, and therefore aggressive drug rehabilitation may be useful [49].

The appropriate diagnostic evaluation for these patients remains unclear and therefore should follow general principles for risk stratification in patients who have coronary artery disease. In light of the underlying EKG abnormalities, most patients would benefit from imaging with stress testing, either echocardiography or nuclear. Many patients who have cocaine-related chest pain have pain related to coronary vasoconstriction or increased myocardial demand and therefore have negative stress evaluations. There have been remarkable advances in cardiac imaging in the last few years. Both cardiac MRI and CT angiography have theoretical advantages over conventional stress imaging for detection of premature atherosclerosis and coronary artery aneurysms, but there are currently no data available specific to cocaine-related chest pain.

Secondary prevention

Cessation of cocaine use is the hallmark of secondary prevention. Recurrent chest pain is less common and MI and death are rare in patients who discontinue cocaine use [49]. Aggressive risk factor modification is indicated in patients who have MI or evidence of premature atherosclerosis, coronary artery aneurysm, or ectasia. This risk factor modification includes smoking cessation, hypertension control, diabetes control, and aggressive lipid-lowering therapy with a target low-density lipoprotein level below 70. Although these strategies have not been tested specifically for patients who have cocaine-associated chest pain, they are standard of care for patients who have underlying coronary artery disease.

Patients who have evidence of MI or atherosclerosis should receive long-term antiplatelet therapy with aspirin. In addition to aspirin, clopidogrel should be given for at least 1 month with bare metal stents or for 3 to 6 months with currently available drug-eluting stents. Long-term combination antiplatelet therapy with aspirin and clopidogrel may be beneficial in patients who have extensive atherosclerosis, coronary ectasia, or aneurysm, but this possibility has not been studied. The role of nitrates and calcium-channel blockers remains speculative and should be used for symptomatic relief. The use of beta-adrenergic antagonists, although useful in patients who have had a previous MI and cardiomyopathy, needs special consideration in the setting of cocaine abuse. Because recidivism is high in patients who have cocaine-associated chest pain (60% admit to cocaine use within the next year [49]), beta-blocker therapy probably should be avoided in certain patients.

Summary

Patients who have chest pain following the use of cocaine have become more common in emergency departments throughout the United States, with approximately 6% of these patients sustaining an acute MI. The authors have described the rationale for recommending aspirin, benzodiazepines, and nitroglycerin as first-line treatments and calcium-channel blockade or phentolamine as possible second-line therapies and have summarized the controversies surrounding the use of fibrinolytic agents. Admission for observation is one reasonable approach to the management of the low-risk cohort. Evaluation for underlying coronary artery disease is reasonable, particularly in patients who have acute MI. Patients who do not have infarction can undergo evaluation for possible coronary artery disease on an outpatient basis. Routine interventions for secondary prophylaxis as well as cocaine rehabilitation should be used in this patient population, because the long-term prognosis seems somewhat dependent upon the ability of the patient to discontinue cocaine use.

References

[1] Haddad LM. 1978: Cocaine in perspective. JACEP 1979;8:374–6.

[2] Hollander JE, Hoffman RS. Cocaine induced myocardial infarction: an analysis and review of the literature. J Emerg Med 1992;10:169–77.

[3] Substance Abuse and Mental Health Services Administration. 2003 National Survey on Drug Use and Health. Available at: http://www.samhsa.gov/oas/oasftp.htm. Accessed March 5, 2005.

[4] Hollander JE, Hoffman RS. Cocaine. In: Goldfrank LR, Flomenbaum NE, Lewin NA, et al, editors. Goldfrank's toxicologic emergency. 7th edition. New York: McGraw Hill; 2002. p. 1004–19.

[5] Borne RF, Bedford JA, Buelke JL, et al. Biological effects of cocaine, derivatives I: improved synthesis and pharmacologic evaluation of norcocaine. J Pharm Sci 1977;66:119–29.

[6] Schreiber MD, Madden JA, Covert RF, et al. Effects of cocaine, benzoylecgonine and cocaine metabolites on cannulated pressurized fetal sheep cerebral arteries. J Appl Physiol 1994;77:834–9.

[7] Madden J, Powers R. Effect of cocaine and cocaine metabolites on cerebral arteries in vitro. Life Sci 1990;47:1109–14.

[8] Crumb WJ, Clarkson CW. Characterization of sodium channel blocking properties of the major metabolites of cocaine in single cardiac myocytes. J Pharmacol Exp Ther 1992;261:910–7.

[9] Brookoff D, Rotondo MF, Shaw LM, et al. Cocaethylene levels in patients who test positive for cocaine. Ann Emerg Med 1996;27:316–20.

[10] Henning RJ, Wilson LD, Glauser JM. Cocaine plus ethanol is more cardiotoxic than cocaine or ethanol alone. Crit Care Med 1994;22:1896–906.

[11] Pirwitz MJ, Willard JE, Landau C, et al. Influence of cocaine, ethanol, or their combination on epicardial coronary arterial dimensions in humans. Arch Intern Med 1995;155:1186–91.

[12] Kolodgie FD, Wilson PS, Mergner WJ, et al. Cocaine induced increase in the permeability function of human vascular endothelial cell monolayers. Exp Mol Pathol 1999;66:109–22.

[13] Bauman JL, Grawe JJ, Winecoff AP, et al. Cocaine-related sudden cardiac death: a hypothesis correlating basic science and clinical observations. J Clin Pharmacol 1994;34:902–11.

[14] Winecoff AP, Hariman RJ, Grawe JJ, et al. Reversal of the electrocardiographic effects of cocaine by lidocaine. Part 1. Comparison with sodium bicarbonate and quinidine. Pharmacotherapy 1994;14:698–703.

[15] Tella SR, Schindler CW, Goldberg SR. Cocaine: cardiovascular effects in relation to inhibition of peripheral neuronal monoamine uptake and central stimulation of the sympathoadrenal system. J Pharmacol Exp Ther 1993;267:153–62.

[16] Satran A, Bart BA, Henry CR, et al. Increased prevalence of coronary artery aneurysms among cocaine users. Circulation 2005;111:2424–9.

[17] Lange RA, Cigarroa RG, Yancy CW, et al. Cocaine-induced coronary-artery vasoconstriction. N Engl J Med 1989;321:1557–61.

[18] Lange RA, Cigarroa RG, Flores ED, et al. Potentiation of cocaine-induced coronary vasoconstriction by beta-adrenergic blockade. Ann Intern Med 1990;112:897–903.

[19] Flores ED, Lange RA, Cigarroa RC, et al. Effect of cocaine on coronary artery dimensions in atherosclerotic coronary artery disease: enhanced vasoconstriction at sites of significant stenosis. J Am Coll Cardiol 1990;16:74–9.

[20] Winniford MD, Wheelan KR, Kremers MS, et al. Smoking-induced coronary vasoconstriction in patients with atherosclerotic coronary artery disease: evidence for adrenergically mediated alterations in coronary artery tone. Circulation 1986;73:662–7.

[21] Moliterno DJ, Willard JE, Lange RA, et al. Coronary artery vasoconstriction induced by cocaine, cigarette smoking, or both. N Engl J Med 1994;330:454–9.

[22] Weber JE, Hollander JE, Murphy SA, et al. Quantitative comparison of coronary artery flow and myocardial perfusion in patients with acute myocardial infarction in the presence and absence of recent cocaine use. J Thromb Thrombolysis 2003;14(3):239–45.

[23] Togna G, Tempesta E, Togna AR, et al. Platelet responsiveness and biosynthesis of thromboxane and prostacyclin in response to in vitro cocaine treatment. Haemostasis 1985;15:100–7.

[24] Schnetzer GW III. Platelets and thrombogenesis—current concepts. Am Heart J 1972;83:552–64.

[25] Rezkalla S, Mazza JJ, Kloner RA, et al. The effect of cocaine on human platelets. Am J Cardiol 1993;72:243–6.

[26] Moliterno DJ, Lange RA, Gerard RD, et al. Influence of intranasal cocaine on plasma constituents associated with endogenous thrombosis and thrombolysis. Am J Med 1994;96:492–6.

[27] Mittleman RE, Wetli CV. Cocaine and sudden "natural" death. J Forensic Sci 1987;32:11–9.

[28] Dressler FA, Malekzadeh S, Roberts WC. Quantitative analysis of amounts of coronary arterial narrowing in cocaine addicts. Am J Cardiol 1990;65:303–8.

[29] Tardiff K, Gross E, Wu J, et al. Analysis of cocaine positive fatalities. J Forensic Sci 1989;34:53–63.

[30] Om A, Warner M, Sabri N, et al. Frequency of coronary artery disease and left ventricular dysfunction in cocaine users. Am J Cardiol 1992; 69:1549–52.

[31] Majid PA, Patel B, Kim HS, et al. An angiographic and histologic study of cocaine induced chest pain. Am J Cardiol 1990;65:812–4.

[32] Hsue PY, Salina CL, Bolger AF, et al. Acute aortic dissection related to crack cocaine. Circulation 2002;105:1592–5.

[33] Eagle KA, Isselbacher EM, DeSanctis RW. Cocaine-related aortic dissection in perspective. Circulation 2002;105:1529.

[34] Hagan PG, Nienaber CA, Isselbacher EM, et al. The International Registry of Acute Aortic Dissection (IRAD); new insights into an old disease. JAMA 2000;283:897–903.

[35] Thadani PV. NIDA conference report on cardiopulmonary complications of crack cocaine use—clinical manifestations and pathophysiology. Chest 1996;110:1072–6.

[36] Mittleman MA, Mintzewr D, Maclure M, et al. Triggering of myocardial infarction by cocaine. Circulation 1999;99:2737–41.

[37] Hollander JE, Hoffman RS, Gennis P, et al. Prospective multicenter evaluation of cocaine associated chest pain. Acad Emerg Med 1994;1:330–9.

[38] Weber JE, Chudnofsky C, Wilkerson MD, et al. Cocaine associated chest pain: how common is myocardial infarction? Acad Emerg Med 2000;7: 873–7.

[39] Hollander JE. Management of cocaine associated myocardial ischemia. N Engl J Med 1995;333: 1267–72.

[40] Amin M, Gabelman G, Karpel J, et al. Acute myocardial infarction and chest pain: syndromes after cocaine use. Am J Cardiol 1990;66:1434–7.

[41] Del Aguila C, Rosman H. Myocardial infarction during cocaine withdrawal [letter]. Ann Intern Med 1990;112:712.

[42] Hollander JE, Carter WC, Hoffman RS. Use of phentolamine for cocaine induced myocardial ischemia [letter]. N Engl J Med 1992;327:361.

[43] Hollander JE, Hoffman RS, Burstein J, et al. Cocaine associated myocardial infarction. Mortality and complications. Arch Intern Med 1995;155: 1081–6.

[44] Lange RA, Hillis RD. Cardiovascular complications of cocaine use. N Engl J Med 2001;345:351–8.

[45] Levine MAH, Nishakawa J. Acute myocardial infarction associated with cocaine withdrawal. Can Med Assoc J 1991;144:1139–40.

[46] Minor RL, Scott BD, Brown DD, et al. Cocaine induced myocardial infarction in patients with normal coronary arteries. Ann Intern Med 1991;115: 797–806.

[47] Nademanee K, Gorelick DA, Josephson MA, et al. Myocardial ischemia during cocaine withdrawal. Ann Intern Med 1989;111:876–80.

[48] Tokarski GF, Paganussi P, Urbanski R, et al. An evaluation of cocaine-induced chest pain. Ann Emerg Med 1990;19:1088–92.

[49] Hollander JE, Hoffman RS, Gennis P, et al. Cocaine associated chest pain: one year follow-up. Acad Emerg Med 1995;2:179–84.

[50] Gitter MJ, Goldsmith ER, Dunbar DN, et al. Cocaine and chest pain: clinical features and outcome of patients hospitalized to rule out myocardial infarction. Ann Intern Med 1991;115:277–82.

[51] Hollander JE, Burstein JL, Shih RD, et al. Cocaine associated myocardial infarction: clinical safety of thrombolytic therapy. Chest 1995;107:1237–41.

[52] Zimmerman JL, Dellinger RP, Majid PA. Cocaine associated chest pain. Ann Emerg Med 1991;20: 611–5.

[53] Hollander JE, Lozano M Jr, Fairweather P, et al. "Abnormal" electrocardiograms in patients with cocaine-associated chest pain are due to "normal" variants. J Emerg Med 1994;12:199–205.

[54] Hollander JE, Levitt MA, Young GP, et al. The effect of cocaine on the specificity of cardiac markers. Am Heart J 1998;135:245–52.

[55] McLaurin M, Apple FS, Henry TD, et al. Cardiac troponin I and T concentrations in patients with cocaine-associated chest pain. Ann Clin Biochem 1996;33:183–6.

[56] Jatlow PI. Drug of abuse profile: cocaine. Clin Chem 1987;33:66b–71b.

[57] Drake TR, Henry T, Marx J, et al. Severe acid-base abnormalities associated with cocaine abuse. J Emerg Med 1990;8:331–4.

[58] Hollander JE, Hoffman RS, Burstein J, et al, for the Cocaine Associated Myocardial Infarction Study Group. Cocaine associated myocardial infarction: complications and morbidity. Arch Intern Med 1995;155:1081–6.

[59] Weber JE, Shofer FS, Larkin GL, et al. Validation of a brief observation period for patients with cocaine associated chest pain. N Engl J Med 2003; 348:510–7.

[60] Baumann BM, Perrone J, Hornig SE, et al. Randomized controlled double blind placebo controlled trial of diazepam, nitroglycerin or both for treatment of patients with potential cocaine associated acute coronary syndromes. Acad Emerg Med 2000;7:878–85.

[61] The American Heart Association in collaboration with the International Liaison Committee on Resuscitation (ILCOR). Guidelines for cardiopulmonary resuscitation and emergency cardiovascular care. Circulation 2000;102:89.

[62] Albertson TE, Dawson A, de Latorre F, et al. TOX-ACLS: toxicologic-oriented advanced cardiac life support. Ann Emerg Med 2001;37:S78–90.

[63] Hollander JE, Hoffman RS, Gennis P, et al. Nitroglycerin in the treatment of cocaine associated chest pain: clinical safety and efficacy. J Toxicol Clin Toxicol 1994;32:243–56.

[64] Brogan WC, Lange RA, Kim AS, et al. Alleviation of cocaine-induced coronary vasoconstriction by nitroglycerin. J Am Coll Cardiol 1991;18:581–6.

[65] Derlet RW, Albertson TE. Diazepam in the prevention of seizures and death in cocaine-intoxicated rats. Ann Emerg Med 1989;18:542–6.

[66] Billman GE, Hoskins RS. Cocaine-induced ventricular fibrillation: protection afforded by the calcium antagonist verapamil. FASEB J 1988;2:2990–5.

[67] Nahas G, Trouve R, Demus JF, et al. A calcium channel blocker as antidote to the cardiac effects of cocaine intoxication. N Engl J Med 1985;313:519 [Letter.].

[68] Trouve R, Nahas GG, Maillet M. Nitrendipine as an antagonist to the cardiac toxicity of cocaine. J Cardiovasc Pharmacol 1987;9:S49–53.

[69] Derlet RW, Albertson TE. Potentiation of cocaine toxicity with calcium channel blockers. Am J Emerg Med 1989;7:464–8.

[70] Hale SL, Alker KJ, Rezkalla SH, et al. Nifedipine protects the heart from the acute deleterious effects of cocaine if administered before but not after cocaine. Circulation 1991;83:1437–43.

[71] Smith M, Garner D, Niemann JT. Pharmacologic interventions after an LD50 cocaine insult in a chronically instrumented rat model: are beta blockers contraindicated? Ann Emerg Med 1991;20:768–71.

[72] Negus BH, Willard JE, Hillis LD, et al. Alleviation of cocaine induced coronary vasoconstriction with intravenous verapamil. Am J Cardiol 1994;73:510–3.

[73] Ramoska E, Sacchetti AD. Propranolol-induced hypertension in treatment of cocaine intoxication. Ann Emerg Med 1985;14:112–3.

[74] Rappolt RT, Gay G, Inaba DS. Use of inderal (propranolo-Ayerst) in 1-a (early stimulative) and 1-b (advanced stimulative) classification of cocaine and other sympathomimetic reactions. Clin Toxicol 1978;13:325–32.

[75] Rappolt TR, Gay G, Inaba DS, et al. Propranolol in cocaine toxicity [letter]. Lancet 1976;2:640–1.

[76] Catravas JD, Waters IW. Acute cocaine intoxication in the conscious dog: studies on the mechanism of lethality. J Pharmacol Exp Ther 1981;217:350–6.

[77] Guinn MM, Bedford JA, Wilson MC. Antagonism of intravenous cocaine lethality in nonhuman primates. Clin Toxicol 1980;16:499–508.

[78] Spivey WH, Schoffstall JM, Kirkpatrick R, et al. Comparison of labetalol, diazepam, and haloperidol for the treatment of cocaine toxicity in a swine model. Ann Emerg Med 1990;19:467–8.

[79] Vargas R, Gillis RA, Ramwell PW. Propanolol promotes cocaine induced spasm of porcine coronary artery. J Pharmacol Exp Ther 1991;257:644–6.

[80] Pollan S, Tadjziechy M. Esmolol in the management of epinephrine and cocaine induced cardiovascular toxicity. Anesth Analg 1989;69:663–4.

[81] Sand IC, Brody SL, Wrenn KD, et al. Experience with esmolol for the treatment of cocaine associated cardiovascular complications. Am J Emerg Med 1991;9:161–3.

[82] Sybertz EJ, Sabin CS, Pula KK, et al. Alpha and beta adrenoreceptor blocking properties of labetalol and its R, R-isomer, SCH 19927. J Pharmacol Exp Ther 1981;218:435–43.

[83] Boehrer JD, Moliterno DJ, Willard JE, et al. Influence of labetalol of cocaine-induced coronary vasoconstriction in humans. Am J Med 1993;94:608–10.

[84] Rinder HM, Ault KA, Jatlow PI, et al. Platelet alpha granule release in cocaine users. Circulation 1994;90:1162–7.

[85] Hoffman RS, Hollander JE. Thrombolytic therapy in cocaine-induced myocardial infarction [editorial]. Am J Emerg Med 1996;14:693–5.

[86] Bush HS. Cocaine associated myocardial infarction: a word of caution about thrombolytic therapy. Chest 1988;94:878.

[87] Hollander JE, Wilson LD, Leo PJ, et al. Complications from the use of thrombolytic agents in patients with cocaine associated chest pain. J Emerg Med 1996;14:731–6.

[88] LoVecchio F, Nelson L. Intraventricular bleeding after the use of thrombolytics in a cocaine user. Am J Emerg Med 1996;14:663–4.

[89] Franogiannis NG, Farmer JA, Lakkis NM. Tirofiban for cocaine induced coronary artery thrombosis. A novel therapeutic approach. Circulation 1999;100:1939.

[90] Beckman KJ, Parker RB, Hariman RJ, et al. Hemodynamic and electrophysiological actions of cocaine: effects of sodium bicarbonate as an antidote in dogs. Circulation 1991;83:1799–807.

[91] Derlet RW, Albertson TE, Tharratt RS. Lidocaine potentiation of cocaine toxicity. Ann Emerg Med 1991;20:135–8.

[92] Grawe JJ, Hariman RJ, Winecoff AP, et al. Reversal of the electrocardiographic effects of cocaine by lidocaine, 2. Concentration-effect relationships. Pharmacotherapy 1994;14:704–11.

[93] Heit J, Hoffman RS, Goldfrank LR. The effects of lidocaine pretreatment on cocaine neurotoxicity and lethality in mice. Acad Emerg Med 1994;1:438–42.

[94] Kerns W, Garvey L, Owens J. Cocaine induced wide complex dysrhythmia. J Emerg Med 1997;15:321–9.

[95] Shih RD, Hollander JE, Hoffman RS, et al. Clinical safety of lidocaine in cocaine associated myocardial infarction. Ann Emerg Med 1995;26:702–6.

[96] Schrem SS, Belsky P, Schwartzman D, et al. Cocaine-induced torsades de pointes in a patient with idiopathic long QT syndrome. Am Heart J 1990;120:980–4.

[97] Hale SL, Alker KJ, Rezkalla S, et al. Adverse effects of cocaine on cardiovascular dynamics, myocardial blood flow, and coronary artery

diameter in an experimental model. Am Heart J 1989;118:927–33.

[98] Weiner RS, Lockhart JT, Schwartz RG. Dilated cardiomyopathy and cocaine abuse. Am J Med 1986;81:699–701.

[99] Pitts WR, Vongpatannasin W, Cigoarroa JE, et al. Effects of intracoronary infusion of cocaine on left ventricular systolic and diastolic function in humans. Circulation 1998;97:1270–3.

[100] Chokshi SK, Moore R, Pandian NG, et al. Reversible cardiomyopathy associated with cocaine intoxication. Ann Intern Med 1989;111:1039–40.

[101] Chambers HF, Morris DL, Tauber MG, et al. Cocaine use and the risk for endocarditis in intravenous drug users. Ann Intern Med 1987;106:833–6.

[102] Weiss SH. Links between cocaine and retroviral infection. JAMA 1989;261:607–8.

[103] Parker RB, Beckman KJ, Hariman RJI, et al. The electrophysiologic and arrhythmogenic effects of cocaine [abstract]. Pharmacotherapy 1989;9:176.

[104] Schwartz AB, Janzen D, Jones RT, et al. Electrocardiographic and hemodynamic effects of intravenous cocaine in the awake and anesthetized dogs. J Electrocardiol 1989;22:159–66.

[105] Braunwald E, Antman EM, Beasley JW, et al. ACC/AHA 2002 guideline update for the management of patients with unstable angina and non-ST-segment elevation myocardial infarction—summary article: a report of the American College of Cardiology/American Heart Association task force on practice guidelines (Committee on the Management of Patients With Unstable Angina). J Am Coll Cardiol 2002;40:1366–74.

[106] Antman EM, Anbe DT, Armstrong PW, et al. ACC/AHA guidelines for the management of patients with ST-elevation myocardial infarction—executive summary: a report of the American College of Cardiology/American Heart Association Task Force on Practice Guidelines (Writing Committee to Revise the 1999 Guidelines for the Management of Patients With Acute Myocardial Infarction). Circulation 2004;110:588–636.

[107] Cannon CP, Weintraub WS, Demopoulos LA, et al. Comparison of early invasive and conservative strategies in patients with unstable coronary syndromes treated with the glycoprotein IIb/IIIa inhibitor tirofiban. N Engl J Med 2001;344:1879–87.

CARDIOLOGY
CLINICS

Cardiol Clin 24 (2006) 115–123

Acute Congestive Heart Failure in the Emergency Department

Robert L. Rogers, MD[a], Erika D. Feller, MD[b],
Stephen S. Gottlieb, MD[b,*]

[a]Division of Emergency Medicine, Department of Medicine, University of Maryland School of Medicine,
110 South Paca Street, Sixth Floor, Suite 200, Baltimore, MD 21201, USA
[b]Division of Cardiology, Department of Medicine, University of Maryland School of Medicine,
22 South Greene Street, Baltimore, MD 21201, USA

Acute congestive heart failure (CHF) and pulmonary edema is a clinical entity commonly encountered in the emergency department. It is estimated that more than 5 million people in the United States have CHF, and it is expected that as the population ages the incidence of CHF and emergency department visits for acutely decompensated CHF and pulmonary edema will rise [1,2]. As survival rates for acute myocardial infarction continue to increase, the incidence of heart failure is expected to increase as well. The estimated prevalence of CHF in adults over the age of 75 years is 10%, with a lifetime risk of almost 20% [3]. In the Acute Decompensated Heart Failure National Registry (ADHERE), a large, national database of demographic, clinical, and outcomes data for patients hospitalized for decompensated CHF, the emergency department is the initial site of care for more than 78% of patients who have acute symptomatic heart failure [4].

The syndrome of CHF is most commonly defined as a state in which cardiac abnormalities cause cardiac dysfunction so that the heart is unable to meet the circulatory demands of the body or does so with elevated filling pressures. Clinically, this syndrome causes symptoms of reduced exercise tolerance or signs of fluid retention. Congestive heart failure commonly is

a result of systolic dysfunction but can also occur in the setting of normal systolic dysfunction.

The presentation of decompensated CHF is variable and ranges from mild dyspnea on exertion to acute, severe pulmonary edema. Critically ill patients who have acute, cardiogenic pulmonary edema pose the greatest clinical challenge. The primary role of the emergency physician is to perform a rapid assessment of the patient, develop an initial differential diagnosis for entities that could have led to the decompensation, and determine what therapies are indicated. Patients in extremis from acute pulmonary edema require the most aggressive care. In the emergency department, treatment strategies are tailored to the acuity and severity of the CHF exacerbation.

Evaluation and management in the emergency department

The emergency physician's role in the stabilization, evaluation, and treatment of the patient who has decompensated CHF is critical. Although no data exist for a "golden hour" in treating CHF, a thorough workup, triage, and treatment strategy initiated by the emergency physician is likely to have a significant impact on patient morbidity and mortality. To emphasize this point, a study by Sacchetti and colleagues [5] has shown that pharmacologic interventions started in the emergency department reduce the need for ICU admission and endotracheal intubation. Thus, emergency department treatment of

* Corresponding author.
  E-mail address: sgottlie@medicine.umaryland.edu
(S.S. Gottlieb).

0733-8651/06/$ - see front matter © 2005 Elsevier Inc. All rights reserved.
doi:10.1016/j.ccl.2005.09.004

cardiology.theclinics.com

the CHF patient has the potential to save money and lives.

A careful analysis of past medical history and chief complaint is crucial for accurately diagnosing acute CHF and its potential cause. A clear understanding of the categories and specific causes of cardiomyopathies is essential. Broad categories include dilated, hypertrophic, restrictive, and arrythmogenic right ventricle. Specific causes are ischemic, valvular, hypertensive, inflammatory, metabolic, toxic, peripartum, genetic, and idiopathic (Box 1).

The interview of a patient who has potential heart failure should include several crucial questions. The interviewer can quickly and accurately discover whether the patient has a history of CHF or risk factors for the development of heart failure: coronary artery disease, diabetes, hypertension, arrhythmias, valvular disease. It is also important to verify whether the patient has symptoms consistent with angina, which could indicate an acute coronary syndrome as an inciting event triggering CHF. In addition, a survey in search of inciting factors for acute decompensation is warranted. Common factors leading to CHF include myocardial ischemia or infarct, new-onset arrhythmias (especially atrial fibrillation),

medical noncompliance, and dietary indiscretion. Less common but certainly well-known inciting factors include infection and diuretic resistance.

Evaluation of the patient who has acute CHF (pulmonary edema) begins with a thorough assessment of the patient's airway, respiratory status, and circulation. An assessment of the patient's airway should be the first step in management, because patients who have hypoxemia or altered mental status may require immediate endotracheal intubation before further workup can proceed. Patients who are compromised but not in need of emergent intubation can be treated with noninvasive means of ventilation such as continuous positive airway pressure (CPAP) or bilevel positive airway pressure (BiPAP) as a temporizing measure. Large-bore intravenous catheters should be placed. Once it has been established that the airway is secure, an assessment of the patient's breathing and circulation can begin.

Acute medical therapy for heart failure should be considered as distinct from treatment for chronic heart failure. In the acute treatment of decompensated heart failure the goals are threefold: to stabilize the patient clinically, to normalize filling pressures, and to optimize perfusion to vital organs. Diuretics, vasodilators, and positive inotropic agents can be used to achieve these goals. In severely compromised patients mechanical support with an intra-aortic balloon pump may be warranted. In contrast, the goals for the chronic management of heart failure include improvement of morbidity and mortality.

Stabilization measures, diagnostic testing, and medical management begin in the emergency department. Vital signs should be assessed immediately, supplemental oxygen should be administered, and the patient should be placed on a cardiac monitor. All patients should have a 12-lead ECG obtained upon arrival. A complete blood cell count, renal function, and electrolytes should be obtained on all patients. Patients who have an unclear cause of their dyspnea should have a B-type natriuretic peptide (BNP) drawn, because this test may help differentiate CHF from other pulmonary disease. Patients who have the potential for ischemia should have cardiac biomarkers drawn in the emergency department to assess for myocardial infarction as the precipitant of decompensated heart failure. If available, bedside transthoracic echocardiography can be performed to assess left ventricular function and to evaluate for entities such as pericardial effusion

---

Box 1. Differential diagnosis of acute CHF/pulmonary edema

Coronary artery disease
  Acute myocardial infarction
  Myocardial ischemia
  Mechanical complications of acute
    myocardial infarction (papillary
    muscle rupture)
Valvular disease
  Aortic stenosis
  Aortic regurgitation
  Mitral regurgitation
  Mitral stenosis
Myocardial disease
  Hypertrophic cardiomyopathy
  Dilated cardiomyopathy (eg,
  idiopathic, familial)
  Myocarditis
  Hypertension
  Peripartum
  Toxic and metabolic (eg, alcohol,
    cocaine)

and valvular dysfunction. There are limited data on emergency physician–performed bedside ultrasound to estimate left ventricular function. A study by Randazzo and colleagues [6] evaluated the use of echocardiography performed by emergency physicians. It was found that after a small amount of focused training emergency physicians could assess left ventricular ejection fraction accurately in the emergency department. After stabilization of the patient, a search for the cause and precipitant of CHF/pulmonary edema should be undertaken, because detection of specific cause might have a significant impact on treatment.

Currently there are no guidelines for the management of acutely decompensated heart failure in the emergency department. DiDomenico and colleagues [7] published a set of guidelines in 2004 for the initial therapy of CHF in the emergency department. The proposed algorithm relies on a rapid assessment of the patient's overall volume status with the initial treatment approach aimed at alleviating pulmonary congestion and improving cardiac output. Patients with milder degrees of volume overload may respond to intravenous diuretics, whereas patients who have low cardiac output and moderate to severe volume overload need an approach that combines volume management, preload and afterload reduction, and inotropic support.

Noninvasive airway management

In many instances, patients do not require immediate control of their airway by endotracheal intubation but might need additional assistance to decrease their work of breathing. It has been established that noninvasive ventilation (CPAP or BiPAP) is an effective means of providing ventilatory support for critically ill patients who have acutely decompensated CHF and pulmonary edema [8]. Noninvasive ventilatory strategies using modes like CPAP work by limiting decline in functional residual capacity, improving respiratory mechanics and oxygenation, and decreasing left ventricular preload and afterload [9–11]. Two randomized studies have also found beneficial physiologic effects by showing a significant reduction in endotracheal intubation rates in patients who had acute cardiogenic pulmonary edema [12,13].

Previously, studies examining noninvasive ventilation have been performed in the ICU when respiratory failure was already present. In a study by Nava and colleagues [11], noninvasive pressure support ventilation (NPSV) was compared with conventional oxygen therapy in the treatment of acute cardiogenic pulmonary edema. In this multicenter emergency department study, 130 patients who had acute respiratory failure secondary to cardiogenic pulmonary edema were randomly assigned to traditional medical therapy including oxygen (65 patients) or NPSV (65 patients). The main outcome measured was the need for intubation. NPSV provided faster improvement in the ratio of arterial oxygen saturation to inspired oxygen concentration (Pao_2/Fio_2), respiratory rate, and dyspnea. Although the rates of intubation, hospital mortality, and duration of hospitalization were similar in the two groups, a subgroup of hypercapneic patients did benefit from the therapy and had a decreased intubation rate (2 of 33 versus 9 of 31). This study lends credence to the anecdotal evidence that noninvasive ventilation is effective in relieving the work of breathing and in some cases in preventing endotracheal intubation [11].

B-type natriuretic peptide as a diagnostic tool in the emergency department

Among the tools available to the emergency physician for the assessment of the patient who has undifferentiated dyspnea or suspected heart failure, no test has been proven as useful as BNP. This peptide is released into the circulation when ventricular stress is present and has been shown to assist in the diagnosis of CHF and to help differentiate it from other syndromes [14]. The ability to measure this peptide to aid diagnosis and to use as a prognostic indicator represents a major advance in the diagnosis and management of CHF. Some studies have shown that measurement of BNP can reduce hospitalization rates, reduce length of stay, and may help resource use and possibly even improve survival [15].

There are some limitations of using BNP as a diagnostic aid in the emergency department. Interpretation of the test should be used in conjunction with other clinical data and judgment and as an adjunct only [16]. Also, a number of other conditions have been shown to elevate BNP levels. It should never be assumed that elevated BNP levels alone indicate CHF. Box 2 reviews the reasons for a falsely elevated BNP (in the absence of heart failure) and the reasons for a falsely low BNP.

Box 2. Conditions that affect BNP levels

Conditions that can elevate BNP levels
Right-sided heart failure
Pulmonary embolism
Myocardial infarction
Advanced age
Renal failure

*Conditions that cause
lower-than-expected BNP levels*
Obesity
Acute pulmonary edema
Mitral stenosis
Acute mitral regurgitation

Several studies have investigated the use of BNP as a diagnostic test. The Breathing Not Properly (BNP) trial showed that, in patients presenting to the emergency department with acute dyspnea, the diagnostic accuracy of BNP measurement was 81% for a BNP level greater than 100 pg/mL compared with an accuracy if 74% for clinical judgment [17]. In fact, a BNP level of 100 pg/mL or greater provides a sensitivity of 90%, specificity of 76%, positive predictive value of 79%, and a negative predictive value of 89%. The overall accuracy in the study was determined to be 81%. A BNP level of 500 pg/mL or greater has been shown to indicate a 95% probability of heart failure [18]. Recent results from the Rapid Emergency Department Heart Failure Outpatient Trial (REDHOT) showed that BNP levels might also be useful in the assessment of disease severity and prognosis. This study evaluated 464 patients presenting to the emergency department with dyspnea and BNP levels greater than 100 pg/dL. BNP was found to be a predictor of events and mortality [19].

Volume management

Diuretics are the first-line therapeutic modality to consider in acute treatment of CHF. Although diuretics have no proven mortality benefit, they effectively relieve symptoms of congestion, pulmonary edema, extremity swelling, and hepatic congestion. The acute effect of diuretics in patients who have heart failure–related volume overload is to reduce left ventricular filling pressures. There is no acute increase in cardiac output.

Many patients who have chronic heart failure are taking stable doses of loop diuretics as outpatients. Therefore, it is important in the acute setting to administer a dose of intravenous diuretic to achieve the desired therapeutic effect. In general, with normal renal function, two times the oral dose is given intravenously in the acute setting. With abnormal renal function, two and half times the oral dose is generally required to achieve the desired affect.

It should be obvious within 2 hours whether a patient will respond to initial intravenous diuretic therapy. If not, and if diuretic resistance is suspected, it is likely that the patient will require hospital admission for other fluid removal therapy. These measures may include escalating doses and combination diuretic therapy, ultrafiltration, or parenteral therapy.

Vasodilator therapy

For the patient who presents to the emergency department with acutely decompensated CHF, vasodilator therapy should be initiated to achieve reduction in preload and afterload. The use of intravenous vasodilators to treat acute heart failure and pulmonary edema makes sound physiologic sense, because the underlying mechanism of dyspnea and respiratory distress relates to elevated filling pressures. Several different forms of vasodilators are currently available. Most act to reduce filling pressures and systemic vascular resistance, thereby increasing cardiac function. Therapy should be individualized [20,21].

Nitroglycerin

Nitroglycerin traditionally has been the vasodilator of choice in the treatment of acutely decompensated heart failure and pulmonary edema. Nitroglycerin acts primarily to lower preload by increasing venous capacitance. The lowered preload in turn reduces ventricular filling pressure and volume and leads to a decrease in myocardial oxygen consumption. Nitrates also cause coronary vasodilatation, which may be beneficial if ischemia is the underlying precipitant of acute heart failure. Nitroglycerin's effect on the arterial side is seen mainly when high doses are used, in excess of 30 μg per minute. In cases of acutely decompensated heart failure and pulmonary edema, nitroglycerin can be given sublingually while an intravenous drip is prepared [22]. Use of nitroglycerin should be considered for any patient who presents with acutely decompensated CHF, particularly in cases of pulmonary edema and respiratory distress. Drawbacks to its use include its contraindication in patients taking phosphodiesterase-5 inhibitors for erectile dysfunction (sildenafil, tadalafil, vardenafil) and side effects such as headache.

Angiotensin-converting enzyme inhibitors

The use of angiotensin-converting enzyme (ACE) inhibitors to treat acutely decompensated CHF and pulmonary edema has been a controversial topic among cardiologists and emergency physicians. There are anecdotal reports of rapid improvements in patients who had acute cardiogenic pulmonary edema after of sublingual or intravenous administration of ACE inhibitors. Is there, however, any evidence in the literature to support these reports?

In a study of 24 patients who had acute cardiogenic pulmonary edema, Haude and colleagues [23] showed that significant hemodynamic changes were induced by the acute administration of sublingual captopril. Captopril caused an increase in stroke volume and was also found to decrease systemic vascular resistance. Although no firm conclusions can be drawn from this study, it did indicate that ACE inhibitors could affect parameters shown to be problematic in patients who have acute pulmonary edema, namely elevated peripheral vascular resistance. Hamilton and colleagues [24] studied the effects of adding an ACE inhibitor to the usual therapy of oxygen, nitrates, morphine, and diuretics (furosemide) in the treatment of acute pulmonary edema. He found that the addition of an ACE inhibitor produced more rapid clinical improvement than the standard treatment. Again, this study was small and evaluated only 48 patients. In a placebo-controlled, randomized, double-blind trial of intravenous enalapril in patients who had acute cardiogenic pulmonary edema, Annane and colleagues [25] showed that early administration of intravenous enalapril was effective and well tolerated in patients who had acutely decompensated heart failure. Of course, vasodilation may have been the cause of the benefit seen in these small studies. Acute ACE inhibition can cause renal dysfunction in patients who are intravascularly depleted, however, and therefore should not be the vasodilator of choice in patients who have unknown renal function or intravascular volume status. To date, there has not been a large, randomized study of ACE inhibitor use in acute pulmonary edema or comparisons with other vasodilators.

Nitroprusside

Nitroprusside is a potent arterial and venous vasodilator and can be used to treat acutely decompensated heart failure in specific circumstances. Nitroprusside was one of the first vasodilators used in the management of acute heart failure. Patients who have acute mitral or aortic regurgitation may benefit from the use of nitroprusside. In addition, the drug is useful in patients who have cardiogenic pulmonary edema in the setting of severely elevated blood pressure. Caution should be exercised, however, if ischemia is a possible underlying mechanism, because nitroprusside administration has been shown to induce a "coronary steal" phenomenon and worsen cardiac ischemia. Drawbacks of nitroprusside include the need for invasive hemodynamic monitoring and the side effects of accumulation of cyanide and thiocyanate.

Nesiritide

Nesiritide is a vasodilator that has been shown to decrease pulmonary artery and pulmonary capillary wedge pressures in patients who have heart failure [26]. It has also been advocated as an acute treatment in the emergency department with the goal of decreasing hospitalization rates. The argument is that starting active therapy earlier will lead to quicker resolution of symptoms and shorter hospital stays.

Unfortunately, beneficial outcomes of nesiritide have never been documented in a randomized, blinded, controlled study. Indeed, recent studies have suggested that nesiritide may actually decrease survival [27] and increase the rate of renal dysfunction [28]. Despite a common belief that renal function and urine output improve with nesiritide, this improvement has never been documented in heart failure patients receiving currently used doses [29].

It is clear that the vasodilation caused by nesiritide can lead to clinically significant hypotension. Thus, it is contraindicated in patients who have a systolic blood pressure less than 90 mm Hg. It should be used very cautiously in patients who have ischemic heart disease, especially those suspected of having myocardial infarction, because hypotension can be particularly detrimental in these patients.

As a vasodilator, nesiritide can clearly decrease symptoms associated with increased volume and left ventricular filling pressures. Diuretics and other vasodilators have the same potential actions, however. Analyses of large databases have suggested better outcomes with nesiritide [30], but these uncontrolled studies with many potential biases should not be misused to support conclusions that can be provided only by well-designed investigations. Indeed, the findings of one analysis that patients not receiving nesiritide were more likely to be discharged to extended care facilities suggests that the patients receiving nesiritide were healthier and different from patients who received other care.

At present, nesiritide can be used in patients who have adequate blood pressure and symptomatic heart failure until the effects of more definitive therapy can take hold. It is expensive, however, and physicians should not assume that it improves outcomes or affects renal function.

Inotropes

Inotropic therapy is commonly used to treat the sickest patients. Although its potential adverse effects are now well accepted, the mainstay of treatment of patients who have worsening renal function or suggestion of other end-organ damage continues to include dobutamine or milrinone. This use arises mostly from lack of other options and has not been supported by studies; inotropic therapy which increases cAMP by receptor stimulation (dobutamine) or phosphodiesterase inhibition (milrinone) has never been shown to be beneficial. Fortunately, studies of newer interventions are being undertaken and may provide pharmacologic options for the sickest patients.

The few randomized studies of inotropic therapy have been disappointing. Chronic therapy has been shown to be detrimental [31,32], and in-hospital use has also been shown to be of no benefit. The Outcomes of a Prospective Trial of Intravenous Milrinone for Exacerbations of Chronic Heart Failure (OPTIME-CHF) study tested the hypothesis that milrinone given to patients hospitalized because of heart failure would lead to shorter hospitalizations and improved outcomes as compared with placebo [33]. The study demonstrated no improvement in patients receiving milrinone, however, and mortality, arrhythmia, and myocardial infarction rates tended to be worse. Furthermore, adverse events and the incidence of sustained hypotension were statistically worse

in patients receiving active drug. OPTIME-CHF clearly demonstrated that milrinone should not be used routinely in patients hospitalized for heart failure.

The applicability of OPTIME-CHF to sicker patients, however, is uncertain. Investigators did not randomize patients who were thought to need inotropic therapy; these patients were given active drug. Thus, the impact of milrinone in patients who have worsening renal function or refractory symptoms is unknown. Although the randomized studies of chronic inotropic use and the OPTIME-CHF study led to concern that inotropic therapy may be detrimental, the OPTIME-CHF data cannot be extrapolated to the sickest patients. There are few studies of these patients. Nevertheless, retrospective data also raise concern about the utility of conventional inotropic therapy. Of course, such data are limited by differences between groups of patients that cannot be controlled for by any statistical analysis.

Recent controlled data do support the concept that adrenergic agents and phosphodiesterase inhibitors may be harmful. Levosimendan is a novel agent that increases calcium sensitivity. In one study, the comparison of levosimendan and dobutamine showed improved survival with levosimendan [34]. Whether this improved survival reflects benefits of levosimendan or harm of dobutamine (or both) is not known. Some studies demonstrate better outcome with levosimendan than with placebo and provide hope that levosimendan will prove to increase survival and decrease symptoms [35]. The composite outcome in the ongoing Randomized, Multicenter Evaluation of Intravenous Levosimendan Efficacy Versus Placebo in the Short Term Treatment of Decompensated Chronic Heart Failure (REVIVE) study may help illuminate whether levosimendan is truly beneficial.

One problem regarding analyses of older studies of inotropic therapy is that concomitant therapies were very different. Those studies were not performed with patients taking beta-adrenergic blocking agents or even ACE inhibitors. It is certainly possible that the effects of an inotropic agent will be different in patients receiving modern therapy. For this reason studies of enoximone are in process and may lead to a better understanding of the effects of inotropic therapy.

Despite these concerns, with present knowledge and available agents, physicians appropriately still find it necessary to use dobutamine and milrinone in selected patients. When these agents are used, a few factors should be considered. First, because many patients arrive at the emergency department taking chronic β-blocking therapy, an agent that is still effective may be preferable. The effects of dobutamine are more likely to be impacted by β-blocking agents [36], and milrinone may be the preferred drug in these patients.

Tolerance to these drugs should also be considered in patients who have received them for a prolonged period. Decreased expression of receptors may lead to decreased contractility (as compared with before initiation of dobutamine) if the drug is abruptly stopped. Therefore, any patient who has been taking dobutamine for more than 1 day should be weaned off it slowly. In the sickest patients, weaning may take many days. Although changes in receptors do not affect the efficacy of milrinone, drug weaning may also be needed in patients receiving this drug.

Beta-adrenergic blockers

With the multiple studies showing marked benefit when beta-adrenergic blockers are given chronically to patients who have heart failure, these drugs are occasionally prescribed for acutely decompensated patients. These patients often have a tachycardia, which is tempting to treat. Beta-blockers are negative inotropic, however, and will decrease contractility. Although their chronic effect is to improve cardiac function, a dose of a beta-blocker will impair cardiac performance. In a decompensated patient, they are likely to lead to deterioration and should not be used.

A common question is what to do with beta-adrenergic blockers in patients who present with worsening heart failure. Although their negative inotropic properties can certainly decrease contractility in compromised patients, it is also known that abrupt withdrawal of these agents can lead to adverse consequences. Furthermore, if the drugs are not given for a prolonged period, retitration may take weeks or months. Unfortunately, there are no studies indicating how to deal with this situation.

Each case must be evaluated individually. A patient who presents with fluid overload and an anticipation of rapid improvement with diuresis probably does not need to have the beta-blocker withheld. Conversely, giving a beta-blocker to someone in cardiogenic shock will undoubtedly make the situation worse. At times, halving the dose may provide acute help while making it simple to titrate back to a therapeutic dose when the patient stabilizes.

Of course, someone who deteriorates with initiation or increasing titration of a beta-blocker (usually occurring approximately 1 week after the change) [37] may be helped by decreasing the dose. Even in some of these patients, however, all that is needed is diuresis and time to accommodate to the new dose.

Some patients present to the emergency room with primary tachycardia [38]. Atrial fibrillation with a rapid ventricular response or a supraventricular tachycardia in a patient who has poor cardiac function may be particularly difficult to treat. Although a slower rate may improve hemodynamic parameters, agents that are negative inotropic (such as calcium-channel blockers or beta-blockers) might cause deterioration. In such patients, the risk of these agents must be remembered. This situation is ideal for the use of esmolol, which can be tried but discontinued with immediate reversal of its effects. If improvement is seen in clinical status and heart rate, a longer-acting beta-blocker can be given. In contrast, deterioration can be easily reversed. If the primary problem is cardiac dysfunction, calcium-channel blockers such as diltiazem must be used cautiously, if at all.

Another agent that can be considered in these patients is amiodarone, remembering that the intravenous formulation is a vasodilator and that blood pressure must be followed carefully. Although it might be difficult to know if the tachycardia is the cause of the heart failure or its consequence, cardioversion should always be considered in a compromised patient who is presumed to have primary atrial fibrillation or supraventricular tachycardia.

Vasoconstrictors

In patients who have heart failure, low blood pressure is usually the consequence of a decreased cardiac output. Increasing the blood pressure with a vasoconstrictor results in further lowering of cardiac output and worsening of the primary problem. Thus, vasoconstrictors should be used only in a patient whose blood pressure is clearly affecting organ systems, particularly the brain. A patient who has chronic heart failure without symptoms of dizziness or lightheadedness rarely needs a vasoconstrictor. If a higher blood pressure is clearly needed, vasopressin may increase blood pressure without directly affecting the heart.

When hypotension is present, it is necessary to see if other problems might be leading to the deterioration. Sepsis should be considered, and volume must be assessed. In a patient who has heart failure, however, the routine administration of large volumes of fluid for hypotension may exacerbate the heart failure without increasing blood pressure. Volume should be given judiciously and in small boluses to ensure a positive response.

References

[1] Feinglass J, Martin GJ, Lin E, et al. Is heart failure survival improving? Evidence from 2323 elderly patients hospitalized between 1989–2000. Am Heart J 2003;146:111–4.

[2] Ansari M, Massie BM. Heart failure: how big is the problem? Who are the patients? What does the future hold? Am Heart J 2003;146:1–4.

[3] Lloyd-Jones DM, Larson MG, Leip EP, et al. Lifetime risk for developing congestive heart failure: the Framingham Heart Study. Circulation 2002; 106:3068–72.

[4] Acute Decompensated Heart Failure National Registry. 3rd quarter 2003 national benchmark report. Available at: http://www.adhereregistry.com/national_BMR/Q3_2003_ADHERE_National_BMR.pdf. Accessed January 7, 2005.

[5] Sacchetti A, Ramoska E, Moakes ME, et al. Effect of ED management on ICU use in acute pulmonary edema. Am J Emerg Med 1999;17:571–4.

[6] Randazzo MR, Snoey ER, Levitt MA, et al. Accuracy of emergency physician assessment of left ventricular ejection fraction and central venous pressure using echocardiography. Acad Emerg Med 2003;10(9): 973–7.

[7] DiDomenico RJ, Park HY, Southworth MR, et al. Guidelines for acute decompensated heart failure treatment. Ann Pharmacother 2004;38:649–60.

[8] Yan AT, Bradley D, Liu PP. The role of continuous positive airway pressure in the treatment of congestive heart failure. Chest 2001;120:1675–85.

[9] Katz JA, Marks JD. Inspiratory work with and without continuous positive airway pressure in patients with acute respiratory failure. Anesthesiology 1985;63:598–607.

[10] Katz J, Kraemer RW, Gjerde GE. Inspiratory work and airway pressure with continuous positive airway pressure delivery systems. Chest 1985;4:519–26.

[11] Nava S, Carbone G, DiBattista N, et al. Noninvasive ventilation in cardiogenic pulmonary edema: a multicenter randomized trial. Am J Respir Crit Care Med 2003;168(12):1432–7.

[12] Bernsten AD, Holt AW, Vedig AE, et al. Treatment of severe cardiogenic pulmonary edema with continuous positive airway pressure delivered by face mask. N Engl J Med 1991;325:1825–30.

[13] Lin M, Yang YF, Chiang HT, et al. Reappraisal of continuous positive airway pressure therapy in acute cardiogenic pulmonary edema. Short-term results and long-term follow-up. Chest 1995;107:1379–86.

[14] McCullough PA, Nowak RM, McCord J, et al. B-type natriuretic peptide and clinical judgment in emergency diagnosis of heart failure. Circulation 2002;106:416.

[15] Mueller C, Scholer A, Laule-Killian K, et al. Use of B-type natriuretic peptide in the evaluation and management of acute dyspnea. N Engl J Med 2004; 350:647–54.

[16] Maisel A. B-type natriuretic peptide measurements in diagnosing congestive heart failure in the dyspneic emergency department patient. Rev Cardiovasc Med 2002;3(Suppl 4):S10–7.

[17] Maisel AS, Krishnaswamy P, Nowak RM, et alfor the Breathing Not Properly Multinational Study Investigators. Rapid measurement of B-type natriuretic peptide in the emergency diagnosis of heart failure. N Engl J Med 2002;347:161–7.

[18] Silver MA, Maisel A, Yancy CW, et al. BNP Consensus Panel 2004: a clinical approach for the diagnostic, prognostic, screening, treatment monitoring, and therapeutic roles of natriuretic peptides in cardiovascular diseases. Congest Heart Fail 2004;10:1–30.

[19] Maisel A, Hollander JE, Guss D, et al. Primary results of the Rapid Emergency Department Heart Failure Outpatient Trial (REDHOT): a multicenter study of B-type natriuretic peptide levels, emergency department decision making, and outcomes in patients presenting with shortness of breath. J Am Coll Cardiol 2004;44:1328–33.

[20] Nohria A, Lewis E, Stevenson LW. Medical management of advanced heart failure. JAMA 2002; 287:628–40.

[21] Johnson W, Omland T, Collins CM, et al. Neurohormonal activation rapidly decreases after intravenous therapy with diuretics and vasodilators for class IV heart failure. J Am Coll Cardiol 2002;39: 1623–9.

[22] Abrams J. Beneficial actions of nitrates in cardiovascular disease. Am J Cardiol 1996;77:31C–7C.

[23] Haude M, Steffen W, Erbel R, et al. Sublingual administration of captopril versus nitroglycerin in patients with severe congestive heart failure. Int J Cardiol 1990;27:351–9.

[24] Hamilton RJ, Carter WA, Gallagher J. Rapid improvement of acute pulmonary edema with sublingual captopril. Acad Emerg Med 1996;3:205–12.

[25] Annane D, Bellissant E, Pussard E, et al. Placebo-controlled, randomized, double-blind study of intravenous enalaprilat efficacy and safety in acute cardiogenic pulmonary edema. Circulation 1996; 94:1316–24.

[26] Publication Committee for the VMAC Investigators (Vasodilatation in the Management of Acute CHF). Intravenous nesiritide vs nitroglycerin for treatment

of decompensated congestive heart failure: a randomized controlled trial. JAMA 2002;287:1531–40.

[27] Sackner-Bernstein JD, Kowalski M, Fox M, et al. Short-term risk of death after treatment with nesiritide for decompensated heart failure: a pooled analysis of randomized controlled trials. JAMA 2005; 293:1900–5.

[28] Sackner-Bernstein JD, Skopicki HA, et al. Risk of worsening renal function with nesiritide in patients with acutely decompensated heart failure. Circulation 2005;111:1487–91.

[29] Wang DJ, Dowling TC, Meadows D, et al. Nesiritide does not improve renal function in patients with chronic heart failure and worsening serum creatinine. Circulation 2004;110(12):1620–5.

[30] Peacock F, Emerman CL, Wynne J, for the ADHERE Scientific Advisory Committee and Investigators and the ADHERE Study Group. Early use of nesiritide in the emergency department is associated with improved outcome: An ADHERE registry analysis. Ann Emerg Med 2004;44(Suppl 4):S78.

[31] Packer M, Carver JR, Rodeheffer RJ, et al, for the PROMISE Study Research Group. Effect of oral milrinone on mortality in severe chronic heart failure: the PROMISE Study Research Group. N Engl J Med 1991;325:1468–75.

[32] Cohn JN, Goldstein SO, Greenberg BH, et al. A dose-dependent increase in mortality with vesnarinone among patients with severe heart failure. Vesnarinone Trial Investigators. N Engl J Med 1998; 339:1810–6.

[33] Cuffe MS, Califf RM, Adams KFJ, et al, for the Outcomes of a Prospective Trial of Intravenous Milrinone for Exacerbations of Chronic Heart Failure (OPTIME-CHF) investigators. Short-term intravenous milrinone for acute exacerbation of chronic heart failure: a randomized controlled trial. JAMA 2002;287:1541–7.

[34] Follath F, Cleland JG, Just H, et al. Efficacy and safety of intravenous levosimendan compared with dobutamine in severe low-output heart failure (the LIDO study): a randomized double blind trial. Lancet 2002;360:196–202.

[35] Moiseyev VS, Poder P, Andrejevs N, et al for the RUSSLAN Study Investigators. Safety and efficacy of a novel calcium sensitizer, levosimendan, in patients with left ventricular failure due to an acute myocardial infarction. A randomized, placebo-controlled, double-blind study (RUSSLAN). Eur Heart J 2002;23:1422–32.

[36] Lowes BD, Tsvetkova T, Eichhorn EJ, et al. Milrinone versus dobutamine in heart failure subjects treated chronically with carvedilol. Int J Cardiol 2001;81:141–9.

[37] Gottlieb SS, Fisher ML, Kjekshus J, et al, on behalf of the MERIT-HF Investigators. Tolerability of beta-blocker initiation and titration in MERIT-HF. Circulation 2002;105:1182–8.

[38] Shinbane JS, Wood MA, Jensen DN, et al. Tachycardia-induced cardiomyopathy: a review of animal models and clinical studies. J Am Coll Cardiol 1997; 29:709–15.

ELSEVIER
SAUNDERS

Cardiol Clin 24 (2006) 125–133

CARDIOLOGY
CLINICS

Management of Arrhythmias in the Emergency Department

R.E. Hood, MD, Stephen R. Shorofsky, MD, PhD*

*Division of Cardiology, Department of Medicine, University of Maryland School of Medicine,
22 South Greene Street, Baltimore, MD 21201, USA*

Little raises the anxiety level of a physician more than a call to the emergency department about a patient who has an arrhythmia. Despite devoting significant time in training to the mechanisms and treatment of cardiac rhythm disturbances, most physicians are uncomfortable dealing with them. This article strives to provide practical and concise advice on initial diagnosis and management of arrhythmias that present to the emergency department. There has been no attempt to be exhaustive in the descriptions. Common pitfalls and concerns are addressed. The article is divided into a discussion of tachyarrhythmias, both wide and narrow complex, bradyarrhythmias, and management of arrhythmia devices—pacemakers and defibrillators. Finally, no account of emergency department arrhythmias can be complete without some mention of syncope.

The acute treatment of cardiac rhythm disturbances is quite simple if one follows a few basic rules (Box 1). First, if the presenting arrhythmia is fast, and the patient is hemodynamically unstable, regardless of the arrhythmia mechanism, perform a direct current transthoracic cardioversion to restore normal sinus rhythm. The patient should either be unconscious or sedated before delivery of the energy. Second, if the patient presents with a bradycardia that is hemodynamically unstable, pace the heart either transvenously or transthoracically. The former is a more reliable method. For all other arrhythmias in which the patient is hemodynamically stable, obtain a 12-lead ECG; there is time to think before acting. By following these two simple rules, all acute arrhythmic emergencies can be handled appropriately.

Tachycardias

Tachycardias can be divided into two categories based on the width of the QRS complexes, narrow complex (QRS duration $\leq$ 120 milliseconds) or wide complex (QRS duration > 120 milliseconds) tachycardias. When determining the QRS width, it is important to use at least two orthogonally placed lead systems. A single-lead rhythm strip is often inadequate. In any given single-lead recording, a wide complex tachycardia may appear narrow (Fig. 1). If the arrhythmia has a narrow QRS complex, it is by definition a supraventricular tachycardia (SVT). These arrhythmias are usually benign, and often the patient can be treated and discharged from the emergency department to complete the evaluation as an outpatient. If the tachycardia has a wide QRS complex, it is either a ventricular tachycardia (VT) or, extraordinarily rarely, a SVT with aberrant conduction or pre-excitation. In contrast to the narrow complex tachycardias, these tachycardias are usually malignant and require hospitalization for further treatment.

The differential diagnosis between a SVT with aberration and VT has fascinated physicians for years. Several algorithms have been proposed to differentiate between these arrhythmias based on the 12-lead ECG pattern [1–3]. It seems as though physicians try to demonstrate their diagnostic acumen by diagnosing SVT with aberration in patients who present with wide complex tachycardias. The reality, however, is that in attempting to prove their diagnostic skills, physicians who

---

* Corresponding author.

E-mail address: sshorofsky@medicine.umaryland.edu
(S.R. Shorofsky).

diagnose a wide complex tachycardia as SVT with aberration are wrong most of the time [4]. The correct diagnosis is important, because medication given for the treatment of SVT may be harmful or fatal to a patient in VT [5–7].

In addition to characterizing the tachycardia by its QRS morphology, other important clinical and ECG information can be helpful in diagnosing the arrhythmia and treating the patient. Dissociation between the atrium and ventricle is diagnostic of VT but is recognized only about 25% of tracings [4]. The converse, however, is not true, because ventriculo-atrial association is common during VT. Other morphologic features that suggest VT include a QRS width greater than 160 milliseconds, the QRS axis in the frontal plane (far left or right), concordance of the QRS complexes across the precordium, and a time from the onset of the R wave to the nadir of the S wave in any precordial lead of more than 100 milliseconds [1,2,8,9]. Clinical data are also useful for establishing the correct diagnosis. A history of a previous myocardial infarction or structural heart disease is highly suggestive that the wide complex tachycardia is VT [8,10,11]. A careful history and physical examination often will be sufficient to establish the presence or absence of structural heart disease in the patient. If this information is insufficient, a transthoracic echocardiogram will define the patient's cardiac structure and function. Lastly, hemodynamic stability during the wide complex tachycardia is often assumed to be evidence that the tachycardia is caused by SVT with aberration or pre-excitation. This assumption is clearly incorrect. Steinman and colleagues [12] demonstrated that VT is the correct diagnosis in 85% of patients who present with a wide complex tachycardia without significant hemodynamic compromise.

Box 1. Rules for the acute management of arrhythmias

If heart rhythm is fast and the patient is hemodynamically unstable, shock the patient as quickly as possible and keep shocking until normal sinus rhythm is restored.

If the heart rhythm is slow and the patient is symptomatic, pace the heart with either a transthoracic or transvenous pacemaker.

Supraventricular tachycardias

Many articles and reviews have been written about the diagnosis and management of SVT. The reader is referred to the American College of Cardiology/American Heart Association/European Society of Cardiology guidelines for a complete review [13]. This article focuses on a simplified, practical approach to diagnosing and treating these common arrhythmias.

When approaching a patient who has SVT, it is helpful to have in mind the different arrhythmias that cause narrow complex tachycardias. An easy framework on which to base a differential diagnosis is to think anatomically, beginning where the heartbeat starts at the sinus node and ending at the atrioventricular (AV) node. SVT can be caused by sinus tachycardias (appropriate, inappropriate, or reentrant), atrial tachycardias, atrial flutter, atrial fibrillation, junctional tachycardia, AV nodal reentry, or AV reciprocating tachycardia using a bypass tract. It is important to diagnose the arrhythmia mechanism, because treatment is specific for individual arrhythmias. For example, appropriate sinus tachycardia is treated by identifying the cause for the arrhythmia, such as fever, hypovolemia, or hyperadrencrgic states rather than simply slowing the heart rhythm with beta-blockers.

Patients who have SVT usually present with palpitations. They notice a rapid heart rate and seek medical attention if it persists. They usually give a history of paroxysmal symptoms that have been present for years. Initial evaluation in the emergency department includes an ECG, history, and complete physical examination. If symptoms persist, a Valsalva maneuver or carotid sinus massage, provided there is no carotid disease, might be useful in either terminating the arrhythmia or causing the loss of ventricular capture for a single beat to allow diagnosis of the arrhythmia mechanism [14]. If the arrhythmia is not terminated by these bedside maneuvers, adenosine (6 or 12 mg intravenously) will usually cause AV nodal block, either terminating the arrhythmia or allowing the visualization of the underlying mechanism. This drug has a rapid onset and short duration of action with a half-life of less than 10 seconds. It is important to administer the adenosine rapidly and to follow the infusion with a flush of saline to affect a result. The usual side effects of flushing, dyspnea, and chest discomfort are usually short lived [15,16]. Severe complications are extraordinarily rare, but case reports of prolonged asystole,

A

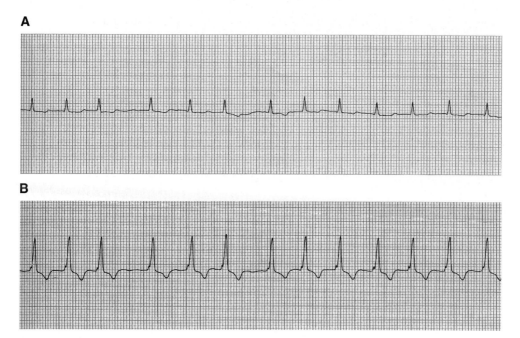

B

Fig. 1. Rhythm strips from a patient. (*A*) A rhythm strip from lead 2, which has a QRS duration of 70 milliseconds. (*B*) The simultaneous rhythm strip from lead V1. The QRS duration in this strip is 140 milliseconds.

VT and fibrillation, and bronchospasm have been published. Resuscitation capability must be immediately available. There are additional considerations to remember about adenosine. The methylxanthines, such as theophylline and caffeine, are competitive antagonists. Dipyridamole may potentiate adenosine's effects. The denervated, transplanted heart is supersensitive to adenosine [17].

Other intravenous AV nodal blocking agents such as beta-blockers or calcium-channel blockers (verapamil or diltiazem) have been used to treat SVT acutely. These drugs, however, have longer half-lives than adenosine and cause other problems such as hypotension (verapamil) or severe bradycardia (beta-blockers). Because of these potential complications, they have been largely replaced by adenosine [18].

Most SVTs are benign and can be treated in the emergency department, and the patient can be discharged home. The exception is atrial fibrillation in a patient who has Wolff-Parkinson-White syndrome who has rapid conduction in the bypass tract from the atrium to the ventricle. This arrhythmia presents as an irregularly irregular arrhythmia with QRS complexes of variable duration (Fig. 2). This arrhythmia may present with hemodynamic compromise if the ventricular rate is sufficiently fast. As mentioned earlier, any SVT with hemodynamic compromise should be treated by electrical cardioversion. This presentation is also the one case when calcium-channel blocking drugs and adenosine should be avoided. These drugs often increase conduction through the bypass tract while decreasing it through the AV node, thus increasing the ventricular response rate and causing hemodynamic compromise [5]. The ideal drug for this condition is intravenous procainamide, which slows the ventricular rate by blocking conduction through the bypass tract.

Most SVTs are caused by a reentrant circuit involving the AV node or use the AV node to conduct to the ventricle. Therefore, long-term treatment is directed at decreasing conduction through the AV node. Beta-blockers and calcium-channel blockers are particularly useful for treating these arrhythmias. Once patients have been stabilized in the emergency department, they can usually be discharged on either a long-acting beta-blocker or calcium-channel blocker to complete their evaluation in the outpatient clinic. If patients have recurrent episodes despite these medications, a referral to the electrophysiologist for consideration of an ablation is warranted. Most SVTs can be cured with an ablation [18].

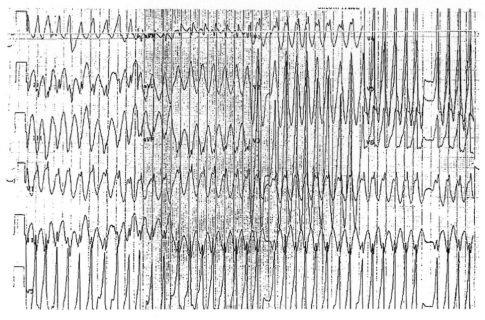

Fig. 2. Pre-excited atrial fibrillation.

Atrial flutter and atrial fibrillation

Atrial flutter and atrial fibrillation represent a special challenge to the emergency department physician. Both arrhythmias may present as incidental findings in a patient who presents to the emergency department for other complaints. These arrhythmias are common in the general population, with the incidence increasing with advancing age [19,20]. In the emergency department, the same rules apply as for other supraventricular arrhythmias. Cardioversion is the treatment of choice if the patient is hemodynamically compromised. If the patient is hemodynamically stable, control the ventricular response rate with AV nodal blocking medications such as beta-blockers and calcium-channel blockers. Digoxin is a third-line drug, which may be useful in patients who have left ventricular dysfunction. The AV nodal blocking properties of digoxin are caused by an increase in vagal tone and thus are not useful for a physically active patient. It is important to begin anticoagulation in patients who present with atrial fibrillation or atrial flutter because these arrhythmias predispose the patient to thromboembolic events [21–25]. Anticoagulation recommendations are well summarized and have been recently updated [26]. Recently, a consensus agreement has been proposed on a treatment scheme for these arrhythmias in both acute and chronic settings [27].

Of special consideration is the patient who presents with atrial fibrillation and an acute myocardial infarction. Although the diagnosis is commonly considered, few patients who present with new-onset atrial fibrillation are having an acute myocardial infarction. In fact, when atrial fibrillation occurs during an acute myocardial infarction, it is an indication of significant myocardial damage and pulmonary congestion. The treatment of choice is diuresis and hemodynamic support rather than rate control with AV nodal blocking agents [28,29].

Ibutilide, an intravenous class III anti-arrhythmic, has been used successfully for conversion of atrial fibrillation and atrial flutter, particularly when they are of short duration, and can be considered for acute cardioversion in the emergency department. Because of its potential side effects, it has been recommended that ibutilide be limited to patients who have an ejection fraction greater than 30%. There is an increased risk of torsades de pointes with lower ejection fractions, which may be minimized by pretreatment with magnesium [30–32].

Ventricular tachycardia

Again, the management of VT should not be frightening to the emergency department physician. Most patients who present with these arrhythmias have underlying heart disease. If the patient is hemodynamically unstable, perform an electrical cardioversion as quickly as possible. The rate of survival depends on the speed of cardioversion [33]. Support the patient hemodynamically following advanced cardiac life support protocols. In the acute phase of treatment, the intravenous drug of choice is amiodarone. When given to patients in the ambulance, amiodarone improves survival to admission to the hospital when compared with lidocaine [34]. Amiodarone should be administered as a 150-mg bolus, followed by an infusion at 1 mg/minute for 6 hours, decreasing to 0.5 mg/minute subsequently. One complication that is specific to intravenous amiodarone is hypotension, secondary to the detergent, polysorbate 80, used to dissolve the drug [35]. Other medications that can be used if more readily available are lidocaine and procainamide, the latter being useful when atrial fibrillation with pre-excitation is suspected. Polymorphic VT or torsades de pointes responds to intravenous magnesium (1–5 g), and VT storm often responds to intravenous beta-blockers and often with amiodarone supplementation [36–39]. Once stabilized, all patients who have VT should be admitted to the hospital for further evaluation and treatment.

Cardioversion

Cardioversion refers to the process of terminating arrhythmias either by pharmacologic agents, direct current, or a combination of both. Cardioversion is used to restore normal sinus rhythm to relieve symptoms and reduce the heart rate. Stroke risk must be assessed before every cardioversion. Hemodynamic stability provides opportunity to choose therapies, drug versus electrical. Pharmacologic cardioversion has the advantage of not requiring sedation, which may a particular concern in patients who have severe respiratory disease. Drugs commonly used for cardioversion are those already mentioned for the treatment of VT and SVT. Direct current cardioversion, however, is the most efficacious means for restoring normal rhythm. In the past, investigative efforts directed toward the optimal vector, pad/paddle size, and energy requirement have been the subject of much discussion. The one substantial improvement has been the introduction of biphasic shocks. There continues to be controversy over the ideal waveform, but from a practical perspective, the current, commercially available external defibrillators are all highly effective. Skin erythema is common. Tachyarrhythmias, bradyarrhythmias, and pulmonary edema have been rarely reported complications. If cardioversion is not successful, repeating with increased power, changing the vector, use of paddles with manual compression, or some combination often is successful.

Syncope

Syncope is the sudden, transient loss of consciousness and postural tone with spontaneous recovery, most often caused by generalized cerebral hypoperfusion [40]. Loss of consciousness must involve either both cerebral hemispheres or the reticular activating system of the brainstem. It is the result of decrease in cardiac output or loss of vascular tone or both.

The differential diagnoses of altered mental status include syncope, seizure, obtundation, delirium, dementia, coma, change in postural tone, and drop attacks. It is not regional hypoperfusion, which may present as transient ischemic attack or stroke. It may be confused with dizziness, vertigo, disequilibrium, or lightheadedness. Syncope is rarely caused by acute coronary syndrome or myocardial infarction with the possible exception of the very elderly or when an arrhythmia occurs [41,42]. Syncope is not caused by hypoglycemia.

Causes for cardiovascular syncope include (1) circulatory obstruction such as that occurring with critical aortic stenosis, hypertrophic obstructive cardiomyopathy, and pulmonary embolism; (2) arrhythmia such as VT, atrial flutter with 1:1 conduction, or occasionally bradycardia; (3) orthostatic intolerance associated with the autonomic nervous system including neurocardiogenic syncope, postural orthostatic tachycardia syndrome, and primary and secondary autonomic failure [43].

The patient's history provides the best means of elucidating the origin of a syncopal spell [44]. A description of a prodrome such as palpitations, blurred vision, nausea, warmth, diaphoresis, or lightheadedness is important, as are postevent symptoms such as nausea, warmth, diaphoresis, and fatigue. Activity, position, recurrence, family history of syncope, sudden death, unexplained accidents including drowning and motor vehicle accidents, and epilepsy are all relevant [44]. The physical examination should be directed to orthostatic vital signs, murmurs, prominent P2, gallops, and other evidence of compromised ventricular function. The 12-lead ECG should be examined for evidence of heart block, ectopy, prior myocardial infarction, and the QT interval. Very rarely, classic findings of a delta wave, epsilon wave, or Brugada syndrome will suggest a cause. The selective use of cardiac diagnostic tests should be considered. These include echocardiography, tilt table testing, ambulatory monitoring, or electrophysiologic studies. Without specific neurologic findings, extensive neurologic testing has a low yield and generally is not warranted. Another pressing question is when to hospitalize a patient who has syncope. The Task Force on Syncope from the European Society of Cardiology recommended hospitalization of those with (1) known or suspected significant heart disease, (2) ECG abnormalities suspected of arrhythmic syncope, (3) syncope during exercise, (4) syncope causing severe injury, and (5) a family history of sudden death and recommends that occasionally others be admitted to the hospital for further evaluation [45].

The outcome of patients who have syncope is largely dependent on the cause. Those with a cardiac cause fare the worst. Patients who have a noncardiac cause have an intermediate risk, and those with neurocardiogenic syncope have a mortality rate of nearly nil. Ambulatory outcome data from the Framingham study were collected on 2336 men and 2873 women whose ages were between 30 and 62 years at entry. A 26-year surveillance revealed that 3.0% of men and 3.5% of women had at least one syncopal episode In 79% of men and 88% of women who experienced isolated syncope, there was no excess risk of stroke or myocardial infarction, and there was no excess all-cause or cardiovascular mortality [46]. Quinn and colleagues [47] described 684 visits to San Francisco emergency departments for syncope. Predictors of serious outcome (defined as death, myocardial infarction, arrhythmia, pulmonary embolism, stroke, subarachnoid hemorrhage, or repeat emergency department visit with hospitalization at day 7) include abnormal ECG, dyspnea, hematocrit below 30%, systolic blood pressure below 90 mm Hg, and history of congestive heart failure.

In certain populations, syncope can also be harbinger of increased mortality. Kapoor and colleagues [48] reported on 204 patients who presented with syncope to the emergency departments, hospitals, or clinics. Causes of mortality at 1 year were 30% cardiovascular, 12% noncardiovascular, and 6.4% of unknown categories. He further reported on mortality at 24 months in a 2 × 3 matrix of elderly (60–90 years) and

young (15–59 years) persons. Mortality from cardiovascular syncope was 38.1% and 32.5%, respectively. Noncardiovascular syncope had a mortality of 21.6% and 4.7%, respectively, and unknown causes had 20.4% and 2.5%, respectively [49]. Using a risk score which assigned one point each for age above 65 years, history of cardiovascular disease, syncope without prodrome, and abnormal ECG, Colivicchi and colleagues [50] reported that the mortality of 270 patients who presented to the emergency department was 0.8%, 20%, 35%, and 57% for patients assigned 1 through 4 points, respectively [50].

Implanted cardiac devices

Besides patients who have active arrhythmias, the other large group that presents to the emergency department is those who have implanted cardiac devices. They may have unique complaints related to their hardware. Three types of devices are discussed here: pacemaker, implantable cardioverter defibrillators (ICDs), and insertable loop recorders. Devices are most commonly found in the left pectoral fossa. The right pectoral fossa and abdomen are alternate sites. Very rarely inframammary or inguinal placement is used. At the time of implantation, the device manufacturer sends the patient an identification card that provides basic information such as manufacturer, model numbers, serial numbers, and telephone numbers for contact. All patients are strongly encouraged to carry this card with them at all times.

Device-related implant problems that might appear in the acute setting include pocket hematoma, wound dehiscence, upper extremity deep venous thrombosis, pneumothorax, and lead dislodgement. Chronic device complications include battery exhaustion and catastrophic, random component failure. Time-independent problems include oversensing which results in underpacing or inappropriate shocks, undersensing producing overpacing and failure of ICD therapy, infection, and erosion.

Chief complaints that are possibly device related include syncope, near syncope, palpitations, and infections. Of course there are a plethora of chief complaints that are not device related but still impact care. For instance, patient who has an implanted cardiac device cannot undergo a MRI scan at present. CT scans are safe, but the metal may produce some scatter in chest compromising image quality. If emergent surgical procedures are contemplated, the device may require reprogramming or magnet placement to use electrocautery safely. An American Heart Association Scientific Advisory was published in 2004 on ICD management for the non-electrophysiologist [51].

Permanent pacemakers at a minimum pace at least one chamber although typically they have many more functions. Pacemakers are conventionally described by the NBG code. (The acronym NBG stands for the North American Society for Pacing and Electrophysiology [NASPE] and British Pacing and Physiology Group [BPEG] Generic.) An abbreviated description of the code identifies the chamber(s) paced (first letter), chamber(s) sensed (second letter), pacemaker response (third letter), and rate responsiveness (fourth letter). A is for atrium; V is ventricle; D is dual chamber or dual function that is both triggered and inhibited; I equals inhibited, and R is for rate responsiveness. Thus a VVIR pacemaker paces the ventricle and senses in the ventricle; its output is inhibited by a sensed event, and it is rate responsive, that is, the motion sensor is active. The most common designations seen are DDD, DDDR, VVI, and VVIR.

When a patient who has a pacemaker presents to the emergency department, the first concern is whether pacemaker malfunction could account for the presenting symptoms. If the patient has the device checked regularly, and the ECG does not demonstrate a problem, the likelihood of a pacemaker malfunction is quite small. The reliability of pacemakers is such that, if the above conditions are met, the device is almost certainly functioning as programmed. It is certainly reasonable to interrogate the pacemaker, but one must prepare for alternative causes.

All ICDs have defibrillation capability (shock therapy) as well as ventricular anti-bradycardia pacing. They often have additional features such as dual-chamber pacing, biventricular pacing, and atrial defibrillation capabilities as well a variety of diagnostic recording capabilities. If a patient presents to the emergency department with a cardiac arrest, advanced cardiac life support protocols should be followed as if the patient does not have a defibrillator. If the device has not terminated a ventricular arrhythmia, external defibrillation should be performed. The only caveat is to avoid placing the pads or paddles directly over the pulse generator. Contact with the patient as an internal shock is delivered by the ICD will not cause harm the emergency department personnel.

The most disconcerting situation for both patient and physician is that of a patient who presents with multiple ICD shocks. The physician needs to assess whether the shocks were appropriate or spurious. Repetitive, appropriate shocks indicate electrical storm. One must search for a cause such as active ischemia, electrolyte abnormalities, or deterioration of left ventricular function. This determination must be concurrent with management as described above for ventricular storm. Spurious shocks could occur as the result of rapid, non-malignant rhythms such as sinus tachycardia or rapid atrial fibrillation or a malfunctioning device (noise on the rate sensing lead). In this situation, it is important to deactivate or inhibit ICD therapy. Deactivation is done with a magnet placed over the generator or by reprogramming the device. In addition to the cardiac issues, the psychologic stress of multiple shocks should be addressed.

The insertable loop recorder is a leadless device implanted subcutaneously in the left pectoral fossa. The purpose of this device is to record spontaneous arrhythmias and triggered events. It has service life in excess of 1 year and no therapeutic capability. Except for recognizing that it is neither a pacemaker nor a defibrillator, it is not discussed here.

Magnets and devices

Each manufacturer produces a doughnut-shaped magnet for use with devices. Pacemakers and defibrillators have different responses to a magnetic field. The typical response of a pacemaker is asynchronous pacing, that is, VOO or DOO. It does not sense and does not track or inhibit; it simply paces. Defibrillators' anti-tachycardia therapies (shocks and anti-tachycardia pacing) are inhibited by a magnet. The defibrillator's anti-bradycardia pacing function is not affected by a magnet.

Making the situation more confusing, some models of pacemakers and defibrillators can have their typical magnet responses disabled, in which case the effects described above will not occur. It is uncommon to program a device with the magnet function disabled. Recently, however, one manufacturer has recommended that the magnet function on several models of defibrillator be disabled as a means for dealing with a manufacturing defect.

References

[1] Brugada P, Brugada J, Mont L, et al. A new approach to the differential diagnosis of a regular

tachycardia with a wide QRS complex. Circulation 1991;83:1649–59.

[2] Wellens HJJ, Bar FWHM, Lie KI. The value of the electrocardiogram in the differential diagnosis of a tachycardia with a widened QRS complex. Am J Med 1978;64:27–33.

[3] Marriott HJL. Differential diagnosis of subraventricular and ventricular tachycardia. Geriatrics 1970;25:91–101.

[4] Akhtar M, Shenasa M, Jazayeri M, et al. Wide QRS complex tachycardia. Reappraisal of a common clinical problem. Ann Intern Med 1988;109:905–12.

[5] Stewart RB, Bardy GH, Greene HL. Wide complex tachycardia: misdiagnosis and outcome after emergent therapy. Ann Intern Med 1986;104:766–71.

[6] Buxton AE, Marchlinski FE, Doherty JU. Hazards of intravenous verapamil for sustained ventricular tachycardia. Am J Cardiol 1987;59:1107–10.

[7] Dancy M, Camm AJ, Ward D. Misdiagnosis of chronic recurrent ventricular tachycardia. Lancet 1985;2:320–3.

[8] Wellens HJJ. Ventricular tachycardia; diagnosis of a broad QRS complex tachycardia. Heart 2001;86: 579–85.

[9] Steurer G, Gursoy S, Frey B, et al. The differential diagnosis on the electrocardiogram between ventricular tachycardia and preexcited tachycardia. Clin Cardiol 1994;17:306–8.

[10] Griffith MJ, de Belder MA, Linker NJ, et al. Multivariate analysis to simplify the differential diagnosis of broad complex tachycardia Br Heart J 1991;66: 166–74.

[11] Tchou P, Young P, Mahmud R, et al. Useful clinical criteria for the diagnosis of ventricular tachycardia. Am J Med 1988;84:53–6.

[12] Steinman RT, Herrera C, Schuger CD, et al. Wide QRS tachycardia in the conscious adult. Ventricular tachycardia is the most frequent cause. JAMA 1989; 261:1013–6.

[13] Blomstrom-Lundqvist C, Scheinman MM, Aliot EM, et alfor the European Society of Cardiology Committee, NASPE-Heart Rhythm Society. ACC/AHA/ESC guidelines for the management of patients with supraventricular arrhythmias—executive summary. A report of the American College of Cardiology/American Heart Association task force on practice guidelines and the European Society of Cardiology committee for practice guidelines (writing committee to develop guidelines for the management of patients with supraventricular arrhythmias) developed in collaboration with NASPE-Heart Rhythm Society. J Am Coll Cardiol 2003;42(8): 1493–531.

[14] Mehta D, Wafa S, Ward DE, et al. Relative efficacy of various physical manoeuvres in the termination of junctional tachycardia. Lancet 1988;1:1181–5.

[15] Lerman BB, Belardinelli L. Cardiac electrophysiology of adenosine: basic and clinical concepts. Circulation 1991;83:1499–509.

[16] Camm AJ, Garratt CJ. Adenosine and supraventricular tachycardia. N Engl J Med 1991;325:1621–9.

[17] Ellenbogen KA, Thames MD, DiMarco JP, et al. Electrophysiological effects of adenosine in the transplanted human heart. Evidence of supersensitivity. Circulation 1990;81(3):821–8.

[18] Ganz LI, Friedman PL. Supraventricular tachycardia. N Engl J Med 1995;332:162–73.

[19] Camm AJ, Obel OA. Epidemiology and mechanism of atrial fibrillation and atrial flutter. Am J Cardiol 1996;78(8A):3–11.

[20] Feinberg WM, Blackshear JL, Laupacis A, et al. Prevalence, age distribution, and gender of patients with atrial fibrillation. Analysis and implications. Arch Intern Med 1995;155:469–73.

[21] Stroke Prevention in Atrial Fibrillation Study. Final results. Circulation 1991;84:527–39.

[22] The Boston Area Anticoagulation Trial for Atrial Fibrillation Investigators. The effect of low-dose warfarin on the risk of stroke in patients with nonrheumatic atrial fibrillation. N Engl J Med 1990; 323:1505–11.

[23] Connolly SJ, Laupacis A, Gent M, et al. Canadian Atrial Fibrillation Anticoagulation (CAFA) Study. J Am Coll Cardiol 1991;18:349–55.

[24] Petersen P, Boysen G, Godtfredsen J, et al. Placebo-controlled, randomised trial of warfarin and aspirin for prevention of thromboembolic complications in chronic atrial fibrillation. The Copenhagen AFASAK study. Lancet 1989;1·175–8.

[25] Ezekowitz MD, Bridgers SL, James KE, et al. Warfarin in the prevention of stroke associated with nonrheumatic atrial fibrillation. Veterans Affairs Stroke Prevention in Nonrheumatic Atrial Fibrillation Investigators. N Engl J Med 1992;327: 1406–12.

[26] Singer DE, Albers GW, Dalen JE, et al. Antithrombic therapy in atrial fibrillation: the seventh ACCP Conference on Antithrombic and Thrombolytic Therapy. Chest 2004;126:429S–56S.

[27] Fuster V, Ryden LE, Asinger RW, et al. ACC/AHA/ESC guidelines for the management of patients with atrial fibrillation: executive summary. A report of the American College of Cardiology/ American Heart Association Task Force on Practice Guidelines and the European Society of Cardiology Committee for Practice Guidelines and Policy Conferences (Committee to Develop Guidelines for the Management of Patients With Atrial Fibrillation: developed in collaboration with the North American Society of Pacing and Electrophysiology. J Am Coll Cardiol 2001;38(4):1231–66.

[28] Asanin M, Perunicic J, Mrdovic I, et al. Prognostic significance of new atrial fibrillation and its relation to heart failure following acute myocardial infarction. Eur J Heart Fail 2005;7(4):671–6.

[29] Lehto M, Snapinn S, Dickstein K, et al. for the OPTIMAAL investigators. Prognostic risk of atrial fibrillation in acute myocardial infarction complicated by

left ventricular dysfunction: the OPTIMAAL experience. Eur Heart J 2005;26(4):350–6.

[30] Oral H, Souza JJ, Michaud GF, et al. Facilitating transthoracic cardioversion of atrial fibrillation with ibutilide pretreatment. N Engl J Med 1999; 340(24):1849–54.

[31] Kalus JS, Spencer AP, Chung J, et al. Does magnesium prophylaxis alter ibutilide's therapeutic efficacy in atrial fibrillation patients? [absract]. Circulation 2002;106(19 Suppl II):634.

[32] Kalus JS, Spencer AP, Tsikouris JP, et al. Impact of prophylactic i.v. magnesium on the efficacy of ibutilide for conversion of atrial fibrillation or flutter. Am J Health Sys Pharm 2003;60(22):2308–12.

[33] De Maio VJ, Stiell IG, Wells GA, et al, for the Ontario Prehospital Advanced Life Support Study Group. Optimal defibrillation response intervals for maximum out-of-hospital cardiac arrest survival rates. Ann Emerg Med 2003;42(2):242–50.

[34] Dorian P, Cass D, Schwartz B, et al. Amiodarone as compared with lidocaine for shock-resistant ventricular fibrillation. N Engl J Med 2002;346:884–90.

[35] Munoz A, Karila P, Gallay P, et al. A randomized hemodynamic comparison of intravenous amiodarone with and without Tween 80. Eur Heart J 1988; 9(2):142–8.

[36] Roden DM. A practical approach to torsade de pointes. Clin Cardiol 1997;20(3):285–90.

[37] Credner SC, Klingenheben T, Mauss O, et al. Electrical storm in patients with transvenous implantable cardioverter-defibrillators: incidence, management and prognostic implications. J Am Coll Cardiol 1998;32(7):1909–15.

[38] Tsagalou EP, Kanakakis J, Rokas S, et al. Suppression by propranolol and amiodarone of an electrical storm refractory to metoprolol and amiodarone. Int J Cardiol 2005;99(2):341–2.

[39] Nademanee K, Taylor R, Bailey WE, et al. Treating electrical storm: sympathetic blockade versus advanced cardiac life support–guided therapy. Circulation 2000;102:742–7.

[40] Henderson MC, Prabhu SD. Syncope: current diagnosis and treatment. Curr Probl Cardiol 1997;22(5): 242–96.

[41] Link MS, Lauer EP, Homoud MK, et al. Low yield of rule-out myocardial infarction protocol in patients presenting with syncope. Am J Cardiol 2001;88(6):706–7.

[42] Bayer AJ, Chandha JS, Farag RR, et al. Changing presentation of myocardial infarction with increasing old age. J Am Geriatr Soc 1986;34(4):263–6.

[43] Grubb BP. Neurocardiogenic syncope and related disorders of orthostatic intolerance. Circulation 2005;111(22):2997–3006.

[44] Calkins H, Shyr Y, Frumin H, et al. The value of the clinical history in the differentiation of syncope due to ventricular tachycardia, atrioventricular block, and neurocardiogenic syncope. Am J Med 1995; 98(4):365–73.

[45] Brignole M, Alboni P, Benditt D, et al. Guidelines on management (diagnosis and treatment) of syncope—update 2004. Europace 2004;6:467–537.

[46] Savage DD, Corwin L, McGee DL, et al. Epidemiologic features of isolated syncope: the Framingham Study. Stroke 1985;16(4):626–9.

[47] Quinn JV, Stiell IG, McDermott DA, et al. Derivation of the San Francisco syncope rule to predict patients with short-term serious outcomes. Ann Emerg Med 2004;43(2):224–32.

[48] Kapoor WN, Karpf M, Wieand S, et al. A prospective evaluation and follow-up of patients with syncope. N Engl J Med 1983;309(4):197–204.

[49] Kapoor W, Snustad D, Peterson J, et al. Syncope in the elderly. Am J Med 1986;80(3):419–28.

[50] Colivicchi F, Ammirati F, Melina D, et al, for the OESIL (Osservatorio Epidemiologico sull Sincope nel Lazio) Study Investigators. Development and prospective validation of a risk stratification system for patients with syncope in the emergency department: the OESIL risk score. Eur Heart J 2003; 24(9):811–9.

[51] Stevenson WG, Chaitman BR, Ellenbogen KA, et al, for the Subcommittee on Electrocardiography and Arrhythmias of the American Heart Association Council on Clinical Cardiology. Heart Rhythm Society. Clinical assessment and management of patients with implanted cardioverter-defibrillators presenting to nonelectrophysiologists. Clinical assessment and management of patients with implanted cardioverter-defibrillators presenting to nonelectrophysiologists. Circulation 2004;110(25): 3866–9.

ELSEVIER
SAUNDERS

Cardiol Clin 24 (2006) 135–146

CARDIOLOGY
CLINICS

Hypertensive Crisis: Hypertensive Emergencies and Urgencies

Monica Aggarwal, MD, Ijaz A. Khan, MD*

Division of Cardiology, University of Maryland School of Medicine, 22 South Greene Street, Baltimore, MD 21201, USA

Hypertension affects an estimated 50 million people in the United States, and it contributed to more than 250,000 deaths in the year 2000 because of end-organ damage [1]. Normal blood pressure is defined as a systolic blood pressure of less than 120 mm Hg and diastolic blood pressure of less than 80 mm Hg. Hypertension is defined as a systolic blood pressure of 140 mm Hg or higher or a diastolic blood pressure of 90 mm Hg or higher. A systolic blood pressure of 120 to 139 mm Hg or a diastolic blood pressure of 80 to 89 mm Hg is considered prehypertension, because people in this range of blood pressure have higher tendency to develop hypertension over time. There is a continuous, graded relationship between hypertension and cardiovascular risk; even a slightly elevated blood pressure increases risk for cardiovascular disease. The maximum blood pressure as well as the duration of elevated pressure determines the outcome [2,3]. Most patients who have chronically uncontrolled hypertension suffer end-organ damage over time. Patients with previously untreated or inadequately treated high blood pressures are most prone to acute rises in their blood pressures [4,5]. Patients with secondary causes of hypertension are at higher risk of acute rises of blood pressure than patients who have essential hypertension [6,7]. The terms "malignant hypertension," "hypertensive emergency," and "hypertensive urgency" were instituted to describe these acute rises in blood pressure and resulting end-organ damage.

Hypertensive crisis includes hypertensive emergencies and urgencies. Hypertensive emergency is defined as severe hypertension with acute end-organ damage, such as aortic dissection, heart failure, papilledema, or stroke. Although there is no blood pressure threshold for the diagnosis of hypertensive emergency, most end-organ damage is noted with diastolic blood pressures exceeding 120 to 130 mm Hg. In these patients, immediate but monitored reduction, often accomplished with parenteral medications, is essential in preventing long-term damage. Hypertensive urgency, on the other hand, describes significantly elevated blood pressure but without evidence of acute end-organ damage. These patients also need reductions in their blood pressures; but these reductions can be achieved over a period of days, with oral medications and usually without an intensive monitoring setting.

Historical perspective

Physicians have noticed the effects of hypertension and hypertensive crises for decades. Volhard and Fahr [8] were the first to notice the acute changes in blood pressure and the differences in pathophysiology of these changes from the chronically elevated blood pressure. They noted that patients who had severe hypertension had fundoscopic changes such as retinopathy and papilledema along with renal insufficiency and fibroid necrosis of the renal arterioles. Also, they noticed that patients who had acute elevations in blood pressure were more prone to papilledema and to acute changes in their kidneys. In 1914, they defined the term "malignant hypertension" as an elevation in blood pressure with the sign of acute end-organ damage. Subsequently, in 1921, Keith and Wagener [9] described a similar finding of

* Corresponding author.
E-mail address: ikhan@medicine.umaryland.edu (I.A. Khan).

papilledema and severe retinopathy in patients who had severe hypertension but who did not have renal insufficiency. They then realized that the end-organ eye and kidney damage were not mutually exclusive to acute hypertensive episodes and therefore broadened the definition of malignant hypertension by stating that renal insufficiency was not a necessary requirement for acute hypertensive damage. Keith and Wagener [9] also used the term "accelerated hypertension," which they defined as a syndrome with severe elevations in blood pressure in the presence of retinal hemorrhages and exudates but without papilledema. Later studies have shown that retinal hemorrhages and exudates are important in malignant hypertension and are associated with decreased survival. Notably, however, the presence or absence of papilledema is not associated with decreased survival [10,11].

In 1928, Oppenheimer and Fishberg [12] were the first to use the term "hypertensive encephalopathy" when they noted malignant hypertension associated with headaches, convulsions, and neurologic deficits in a 19-year-old student. Currently, the terms "malignant hypertension" and "accelerated hypertension" are used infrequently and have been replaced by terms such as "hypertensive crisis," "hypertensive emergency," and "hypertensive urgency" (Table 1).

Demographics

The prevalence of hypertension has increased, partially because of the stringent definition of hypertension. There are notable demographic trends in the prevalence of hypertension. Hypertension is more common in older age groups and is more common in men than in women [13]. It is 1.5 to two times more prevalent in black Americans. An analysis of data from the 1999 to 2000 National Health and Nutrition Examination Survey has shown that the combined prevalence of prehypertension and hypertension has increased to 60% of American adults (67% of men and 50% of women), and 27% of American adults have established hypertension. The combined prevalence of prehypertension and hypertension is 40% in the 18- to 39-years age group and is 88% in the greater-than-60-years age group [14]. This survey showed certain risk predictors of hypertension. Education level was a notable factor. The combined prevalence of prehypertension and hypertension increased from 54% in the high-school–educated group to 65% in the non–high-school–educated

Table 1
Definitions

Term	Definition
Prehypertension	Systolic blood pressure 120–139 mm Hg and diastolic blood pressure 80–89 mm Hg
Hypertension	Systolic blood pressure > 140/90 mm Hg
Hypertensive crisis	Hypertensive urgency or emergency
Hypertensive urgency	Acute rise in blood pressure without acute end-organ damage; diastolic blood pressure usually > 120 mm Hg
Hypertensive emergency	Acute rise in blood pressure with acute end-organ damage; diastolic blood pressure usually > 120 mm Hg

group. Obesity was also an important risk predictor in this analysis; 75% of overweight individuals were prehypertensive or hypertensive, but only 47% of the non-overweight group qualified as such.

Patients who were noted to have prehypertension were also noted to have other risk factors for stroke and cardiovascular disease, such as hypercholesterolemia, obesity, and diabetes. These risk factors were less prevalent in people who had normal blood pressures. The percentage of people who had more than one risk factor for cardiovascular disease was higher in the prehypertensive group than in patients who had normal blood pressure [14]. This cross-sectional analysis also evaluated patients who, when made aware of their hypertension, followed dietary, lifestyle, and medication changes. It was noted that 7% of patients did not adopt any lifestyle changes, and 15% of patients would not take any antihypertensive medications. The problem was more notable in younger patients and in Mexican-American patients. Of the patients taking anti-hypertensive medications, 54% had their hypertension controlled. Men and patients with higher education were more likely to have their blood pressures well controlled.

Of the estimated 50 million Americans with hypertension, less than 1% will have a hypertensive crisis [15]. In a study by Zampaglione and associates [16], hypertensive crises were found to account for more than 25% of all patient visits to a medical section of an emergency department. One third of those patients were noted to have hypertensive emergencies. In the years when treatment of hypertensive crises was difficult, because of inadequate monitoring and lack of parenteral medications, survival was only 20% at 1 year and 1% at 5 years [17]. Before antihypertensive agents became available, thoracolumbar sympathectomy prolonged survival to 40% at 6.5 years. With the advent of ganglionic blocking medications, the 5-year survival rates increased to 50% to 60% in 1960 [18]. During the past 2 decades, with the increased focus on blood pressure control and emphasis on compliance, the 10-year survival rates have approached 70% [19].

Cause

Ninety-five per cent of patients who have hypertension have no obvious underlying cause. As such, hypertension without secondary causes is defined as essential hypertension. The remaining 5% of patients have an underlying cause for their elevated blood pressures, of which certain groups have higher chances of presenting with a hypertensive crisis (Box 1). Use of recreational drugs, such as cocaine, has become a frequent cause of hypertensive crisis. Cocaine amphetamines, phencyclidine hydrochloride, and diet pills are sympathomimetic and thus may cause severe acute hypertension. Patients taking monoamine oxidase inhibitors along with tricyclic antidepressants, antihistamines, or food with tyramine are prone to hypertensive crises. Withdrawal syndromes from drugs such as clonidine or beta-blockers may also precipitate hypertensive crises [20]. Pheochromocytoma is a rare cause of hypertensive crises. Patients with spinal cord disorders, such as Guillain Barré syndrome, are also at a higher risk for hypertensive crises. These patients are prone to autonomic overactivity syndrome manifested by severe hypertension, bradycardia, headache, and diaphoresis. The syndrome is triggered by stimulation of dermatomes or muscles innervated by nerves below the spinal cord lesions.

Pathophysiology

Normal mechanisms to regulate blood pressure

Blood pressure regulation is a critical action that allows perfusion to vital organs of the body. This action is based on a balance between peripheral vascular resistance and cardiac output and is dependent on the integrated actions of the cardiovascular, renal, neural, and endocrine systems. This interdependence allows a back-up

---

Box 1. Causes of secondary hypertension

Medications
Oral contraceptive pills
Cocaine hydrochloride
Phencyclidine hydrochloride
Monoamine oxidase inhibitors
Sympathomimetic diet pills
Nonsteroidal anti-inflammatory drugs
Amphetamines
Cyclosporin
Steroids

Acute glomerulonephritis
Renal parenchymal disease
Renal artery stenosis
Hyperaldosteronism
Cushing disease
Pheochromocytoma
Pregnancy
Sleep apnea
Coarctation of aorta
Spinal cord injuries

---

system so that the body can cope with internal and external stresses such as thirst, fear, infection, and trauma. Multiple intrinsic systems are activated in the body in response to external and internal stressors [21]. The renin-angiotensin-aldosterone system is thought to be critically responsible for blood pressure changes. Renin is released from the juxtaglomerular apparatus in response to low sodium intake, underperfusion of the kidney, and increased sympathetic activity. Renin is responsible for converting angiotensinogen to angiotensin, which is not metabolically active. The angiotensin is subsequently converted to angiotensin II in the lungs by the angiotensin-converting enzyme. Angiotensin II is a potent vasoconstrictor, which leads to increases in blood pressure. Besides its intrinsic vasoconstrictive effects, angiotensin II also causes aldosterone release, which further increases blood pressure by causing salt and water retention. Studies in rats support the role of the renin-angiotensin-aldosterone system in blood pressure elevation. When rats were given the Ren-2 gene, which activates the renin-angiotensin-aldosterone system, they developed severe hypertension [22]. Further support comes from therapeutic methods, such as using angiotensin-converting enzyme inhibitors or angiotensin receptor blockers or surgical removal of an ischemic kidney, which can prevent blood pressure elevations [23].

The renin-angiotensin-aldosterone system is not considered solely responsible for changes in blood pressure. Black Americans, for instance, often have low renin, angiotensin II, and aldosterone levels and yet have a notably higher incidence of hypertension. Therefore, they are less responsive to medications blocking the renin-angiotensin-aldosterone system. Theoretically, patients who have low renin states might have noncirculatory local renin-angiotensin paracrine or epicrine systems. These systems have been found in the kidney, arterial tree, and the heart; and are probably responsible for local control of blood pressure [24].

The sympathetic nervous system also affects blood pressure, especially in times of stress and exercise. The sympathetic nervous system can cause arterial vasoconstriction and can raise cardiac output. It is thought that initially the sympathetic nervous system increases the cardiac output without affecting peripheral vascular resistance. The raised cardiac output increases flow to the vascular bed, and as the cardiac output increases, the autoregulatory response of the vascular bed is activated. This autoregulatory response results in constriction of the arterioles to prevent the pressure from reaching the capillaries and affecting cell hemostasis [21].

In addition, endothelial function plays a central role in blood pressure maintenance. The endothelium secretes nitric oxide, prostacylin, and endothelin, which modulate vascular tone. Nitric oxide is released by endothelial agonists such as acetylcholine and norepinephrine and in response to shear stress [21]. Endothelin-1 has great vasoconstrictive activities and may cause a salt-sensitive rise in blood pressure and a rise in blood pressure by triggering the renin-angiotensin-aldosterone system [24]. Other vasoactive substances involved in blood pressure maintenance include bradykinin and natriuretic peptides. Bradykinin is a potent vasodilator that is inactivated by angiotensin-converting enzyme. Natriuretic peptides are secreted from the heart in response to increase in blood volume and cause an increase in sodium and water excretion.

Altered mechanisms in hypertension and hypertensive crises

The pathophysiology of hypertensive crisis is not well understood. It is thought that an abrupt rise in blood pressure, possibly secondary to a known or unknown stimulus, may trigger the event. During this abrupt initial rise in blood pressure, the endothelium tries to compensate for the change in vasoreactivity by releasing nitric oxide. When the larger arteries and arterioles sense elevated blood pressures, they respond with vasoconstriction and subsequently with hypertrophy to limit pressure reaching the cellular level and affecting cellular activity. Prolonged smooth muscle contraction leads to endothelial dysfunction, loss of nitric oxide production, and irreversible rise in peripheral arterial resistance. Without the continuous release of nitric oxide, the hypertensive response becomes more severe, promoting further endothelial damage, and a vicious cycle continues. The endothelial dysfunction is further triggered by inflammation induced by mechanical stretch. The expression of inflammatory markers such as cytokines, endothelial adhesion molecules, and endothelin-1 is increased [25,26]. These molecular events probably increase the endothelial permeability, inhibit fibrinolysis, and, as a result, activate coagulation. Coagulation along with platelet adhesion and aggregation results in deposition of fibrinoid material, increased inflammation, and the vasoconstriction of the arteries, resulting in further endothelial dysfunction. The role of the renin-angiotensin-aldosterone system also seems to be important in hypertensive emergency. There seems to be an amplification of this system that contributes to vascular injury and tissue ischemia [27].

The blood pressure at which the acute end-organ damage starts occurring is different in each individual. Patients who are more chronically hypertensive have had more smooth muscle contraction and subsequent arterial hypertrophy, which lessens the effect of acute rise in blood pressure on the capillary circulation. Although malignant hypertension is defined as a diastolic blood pressure greater than 130 mm Hg, normotensive patients who have not had time to establish compensatory autoregulatory mechanisms are more sensitive to elevations in blood pressure and may suffer end-organ damage when diastolic blood pressure becomes greater than 100 mm Hg.

Clinical manifestations

Hypertensive crisis shares all of the pathologic mechanisms and end-organ complications of the milder forms of hypertension [27]. In one study of the prevalence of end-organ complications in hypertensive crisis, central nervous system abnormalities were the most frequent. Cerebral infarctions were noted in 24%, encephalopathy in 16%, and intracerebral or subarachnoid hemorrhage in 4% of patients. Central nervous system abnormalities were followed in incidence by cardiovascular complications such as acute heart failure or pulmonary edema, which were seen in 36% of patients, and acute myocardial infarction or unstable angina in 12% of patients. Aortic dissection was noted in 2%, and eclampsia was noted in 4.5% of patients [16]. The end-organ damage is outlined in Box 2.

Acute neurologic syndromes

The cerebral vasculature must maintain a constant cerebral perfusion despite changes in blood pressure. Cerebral autoregulation is the inherent ability of the cerebral vasculature to maintain this constant cerebral blood flow [28,29]. Normotensive people maintain a constant cerebral blood flow between mean arterial pressures of 60 mm Hg and 120 mm Hg. As the mean arterial pressure increases, there is disruption of the cerebral endothelium and interruption of the blood–brain barrier. Fibrinoid material deposits in the cerebral vasculature and causes narrowing of the vascular lumen. The cerebral vasculature, in turn, attempts to vasodilate around the narrowed lumen, which leads to cerebral edema and microhemorrhages [30]. The changes in cerebral vasculature and cerebral perfusion seem to affect primarily the white matter in the parieto-occipital areas of the brain [31]. The predilection toward the parieto-occipital

---

Box 2. End-organ damage in hypertension

Acute neurologic syndromes
Hypertensive encephalopathy
Cerebral infarction
Subarachnoid hemorrhage
Intracranial hemorrhage

Myocardial ischemia and infarction
Acute left ventricular dysfunction
Acute pulmonary edema
Aortic dissection
Retinopathy
Renal insufficiency
Eclampsia

---

regions possibly results from decreased sympathetic innervation of the vessels in this region [32]. There are also reports of brainstem involvement, however [33].

Normotensive patients may develop endothelial dysfunction at lower mean arterial pressures, whereas chronically hypertensive patients can tolerate higher mean arterial pressures before they develop such a dysfunction. Chronically hypertensive patients have the capacity to autoregulate and have cerebral blood flow and oxygen consumption similar to those in normotensive persons [34]. Changes in the structure of the arterial wall cause increased stiffness and higher cerebrovascular resistance, however [35]. Although a higher threshold must be reached before they have disruption of their autoregulation system, hypertensive patients, because of the increased cerebrovascular resistance, are more prone to cerebral ischemia when flow decreases [30].

Hypertensive encephalopathy is one of the clinical manifestations of cerebral edema and microhemorrhages seen with dysfunction of cerebral autoregulation. It is defined as an acute organic brain syndrome or delirium in the setting of severe hypertension. Symptoms include severe headache, nausea, vomiting, visual disturbances, confusion, and focal or generalized weakness. Signs include disorientation, focal neurologic defects, focal or generalized seizures, and nystagmus. If not adequately treated, hypertensive encephalopathy can lead to cerebral hemorrhage, coma, and death, but with proper treatment it is completely reversible [36]. The diagnosis of hypertensive encephalopathy is a clinical diagnosis. Stroke, subarachnoid hemorrhage, mass lesions, seizure disorder, and vasculitides need to be ruled out.

Cerebral infarction, caused by an imbalance between supply and demand, is another neurologic sequela of severe acute rises in blood pressure [37]. Intracranial and subarachnoid hemorrhages are other possible neurologic complications of hypertensive crisis. The risk is increased in patients who have intracranial aneurysms and in those taking anticoagulant medications.

Myocardial ischemia

Hypertension affects the structure and function of the coronary vasculature and left ventricle. Activation of the renin-angiotensin-aldosterone system in hypertension constricts systemic vasculature and, thereby, increases myocardial oxygen demand by increasing left ventricular wall tension.

Increasing wall tension leads to hypertrophy of the left ventricular myocytes and to deposition of protein and collagen in the extracellular matrix of the ventricular wall. These actions increase ventricular mass, which further increases oxygen demand on the heart. A second effect of the hypertrophy is that the newly thickened ventricle can cause coronary compression and decreased luminal blood flow. Thirdly, hypertension can increase the epicardial coronary wall thickness, which increases the wall-to-lumen ratio and decreases coronary blood flow reserve. Concomitant atherosclerosis worsens the wall-to-lumen ratio, further decreases coronary flow reserve, and leads to coronary ischemia [38]. Acute rise in blood pressure also results in endothelial injury at the level of the coronary capillaries.

Left ventricular failure

Another effect of hypertensive crisis on the heart is left ventricular failure and acute pulmonary edema. In certain cases, despite increasing wall tension, the left ventricle cannot hypertrophy enough to overcome the acute rise in systemic vascular resistance. This inability to compensate leads to left ventricular failure and a backup of flow causing pulmonary edema. Secondly, neurohormonal activation of the renin-angiotensin-aldosterone system leads to increased sodium content and increased total body water. In addition, left ventricular hypertrophy leads to focal ischemia and subsequent inadequate diastolic filling, which can result in imbalance between left ventricular contraction and relaxation, leading to pulmonary edema [5]. Clinically, patients show signs of volume overload or signs of reduced tissue perfusion such as cool limbs.

Aortic dissection

Aortic dissection is the most rapidly fatal complication of hypertensive crises. Risk factors for dissection include untreated hypertension, advanced age, and diseases of the aortic wall. Dilation of the aorta caused by atherosclerosis and high blood pressures tear the intima of the vessel, allowing a surge of blood into the aortic wall. The blood driven by pulsatile pressure separates the arterial wall into two layers [39]. Clinically, patients complain of retrosternal or interscapular chest pain that migrates to the back. If dissection extends proximally, it can lead to aortic insufficiency or a pericardial effusion. Dissection can lead to compression or occlusion of a branch

of the aorta and subsequently lead to organ ischemia. Clinical signs that are notable with dissection include discrepancies between pulses, murmur of aortic insufficiency, and neurologic deficits [40]. Diagnosis of aortic dissection can be confirmed with transesophageal echocardiography, CT, or MRI [41].

Hypertensive retinopathy

Retinopathy was one of the first signs of hypertension, noted in 1914. In the early years fundoscopy was considered a definitive tool in diagnosing hypertensive encephalopathy. Papilledema was noted in patients who had hypertensive encephalopathy but was not necessary for diagnosis [42]. Retinal hemorrhages and exudates were considered indicative of malignant hypertension. Since 1914, multiple studies have looked at retinopathy in the setting of hypertension. In mild to moderate hypertension, the degree of focal narrowing of arterioles has been associated with the level of blood pressure rise. No relationship has been found between retinal changes and the end-organ damages such as ventricular hypertrophy or microalbuminuria, however [43]. Ophthalmoscopy may be useful in recognizing acute hypertensive target-organ damage such as hypertensive encephalopathy, but the absence of retinal exudates, hemorrhages, or papilledema does not exclude the diagnosis [11].

Acute renal insufficiency

Acute renal insufficiency may be a cause or result of rapidly progressive hypertension. Important causes of hypertension are parenchymal disease, such as acute glomerulonephritis or renal artery stenosis, or cyclosporine use in kidney transplant patients. Renal insufficiency could also be a result of hypertension and hypertensive crisis, however. Normal renal autoregulation enables the kidney to maintain a constant renal blood flow and glomerular filtration rate for mean arterial pressures between 80 and 160 mm Hg. Under normal conditions, autoregulatory vasodilation is maximal at a mean arterial pressure of about 80 mm Hg. In chronic hypertension, the small arteries of the kidney, including the afferent arteriole, undergo pathologic changes that alter renal autoregulation, showing signs of endothelial dysfunction and impaired vasodilation. Structural changes initially are probably protective of the kidney, but over time progressive narrowing of the preglomerular vessels results in ischemic injury, tubular atrophy, and fibrosis. With the impairment of the renal autoregulatory system, the intraglomerular pressure begins to vary directly with systemic arterial pressure [44]. As such, the afferent vasculature becomes a passive conduit and cannot prevent the kidney from being affected by fluctuations in pressure and flow, leading to acute renal ischemia in cases of hypertensive crisis.

Pregnancy-induced hypertension

Pre-eclampsia is characterized as a syndrome of pregnancy-induced hypertension, edema, and proteinuria in a pregnant woman after the twentieth week of gestation [27]. Eclampsia is the end result of this spectrum and is associated with acute hypertension, edema, proteinuria, and concomitant seizures. Although the pathophysiologic mechanisms of pre-eclampsia and eclampsia are not well understood, blood pressure elevation is characterized by an increased responsiveness to vasoconstrictors, especially angiotensin II. There is also decreased sensitivity to endothelium-derived vasodilators [27]. Pregnancy-induced hypertension usually resolves spontaneously after delivery of baby.

Postoperative hypertension

The postoperative hypertensive crisis is classically an acute rise in blood pressure within the first 2 hours after surgery and is typically short in duration, with most patients requiring treatment for 6 hours or less [45]. Although postoperative hypertensive crises can occur with any surgery, they are more common with cardiothoracic, vascular, head, neck, and neurosurgical procedures [45]. In one study of patients undergoing radical neck dissection, the frequency of hypertensive crisis ranged from 9% to 25% [46]. A feared complication of postoperative hypertensive crisis is bleeding from operation site [47]. The pathophysiology of postoperative hypertensive crisis is probably related to stimulation of the sympathetic nervous system and catecholamine surge [48].

Clinical evaluation

History and detailed physical examination are important in all patients who present with severe hypertension. A thorough history is important to determine the time since diagnosis of hypertension, the severity, and the baseline blood pressures at home. Determining the presence of end-organ damage and other comorbidities is important, because both are crucial factors influencing the

choice of antihypertensive drugs. Knowledge of the patient's medications and compliance with these medications, including over-the-counter medications and recreational drugs, is essential, because both could contribute to an acute rise in blood pressure. Blood pressure should be checked in both arms and should be done in supine and standing positions, if possible, to determine volume status. Neurologic examination is important to determine the focal signs of an ischemic or hemorrhagic stroke. The presence of delirium, nausea, vomiting, and seizures suggests hypertensive encephalopathy. Fundoscopic examination could be of help, because the presence of exudates, hemorrhage, or papilledema supports the diagnosis of hypertensive encephalopathy. Cardiovascular examination includes listening for new murmurs of aortic insufficiency associated with dissection or of ischemic mitral regurgitation. A gallop or left ventricular heave could suggest heart failure. Crackles in the lung fields suggest pulmonary edema. Laboratory studies should include serum electrolytes, blood urea nitrogen, serum creatinine level, blood cell count, and peripheral smear. An ECG should be taken for myocardial ischemia and left ventricular hypertrophy, and a chest radiograph should be obtained for cardiac enlargement and widened mediastinum. Urine analysis is indicated for assessment of proteinuria and tubular casts. Plasma renin and aldosterone levels could be obtained if patient is not taking diuretics or other medications that could have affected these levels [22].

Treatment

Hypertensive urgency can be treated in a non-ICU setting with oral medications over 24 to 48 hours. Medications such as beta-blockers, diuretics, angiotensin-converting enzyme inhibitors, and calcium-channel blockers can be titrated initially as an inpatient; then the patient can be discharged with close follow-up. If there is acute end-organ damage, however, the patient should be admitted to the ICU and treated with intravenous medications. The goal of therapy is prompt but gradual reduction in blood pressure. The most reasonable goal is to lower the mean arterial pressure by about 25% or to reduce the diastolic blood pressure to 100 to 110 mm Hg.

Medication options for treatment

There have been no large clinical trials to determine the optimal pharmacologic therapy in hypertensive emergency patients, primarily because of the heterogeneity among the patients and their end-organ damage. As such, management of hypertensive crisis should be dictated by individual presentation and should be specific to the end organ at risk (Tables 2, 3).

Sodium nitroprusside is the drug of choice for most hypertensive emergencies because it has an immediate onset of action and can be titrated quickly and accurately. The duration of effect is 1 to 2 minutes. The mechanism of action of this agent is probably similar to that of endogenous nitric oxide. Sodium nitroprusside is an endogenous arteriolar and venous dilator and has no effects on the autonomic or central nervous system [49]. The venous dilation decreases preload to the heart and subsequently decreases cardiac output, whereas the arterial dilation inhibits the reflex rise in blood pressure from the drop in cardiac output. Because sodium nitroprusside is a direct vasodilator, one might think that it increases cerebral blood flow and intracranial pressure. The fall in systemic pressure, however, seems to inhibit the rise in cerebral blood flow, and patients who have neurologic damage respond well to this agent [18]. Sodium nitroprusside must be administered as an infusion and thus requires continuous surveillance with intra-arterial monitoring. An end product of nitroprusside is thiocyanate, a precursor to cyanide that can causes nausea, vomiting, lactic acidosis, and altered mental status. Cyanide toxicity can be rapidly fatal. Sodium nitroprusside is broken down by the liver and cleared through the kidney, and thus thiocyanate levels must be followed in patients who have hepatic or renal insufficiency to ensure prevention of a toxic buildup [21].

Labetalol is another first-line agent for hypertensive emergency. It is a combined alpha- and beta-blocking agent; the beta-blocking activity of labetalol is five- to tenfold that of the alpha component [50]. The beta effects of labetalol are only about one fifth the activity of propranolol, however [18]. Its onset of action is within 5 to 10 minutes, and the duration of action is about 3 to 6 hours. Labetalol can be used safely in most patients, but caution should be exercised in patients who have severe bradycardia, congestive heart failure, or bronchospasm.

Fenoldopam is the first selective dopamine-1 receptor agonist approved for in-hospital shorterterm management of severe hypertension up to the first 48 hours of treatment [51–54]. The mechanism of action involves activating dopamine at the level of the kidney. Dopamine is a well-known vasoconstrictor and is sympathomimetic at intermediate to high doses. At low doses, however, dopamine lowers diastolic blood pressure and, importantly, increases renal perfusion and promotes diuresis. Fenoldopam is administered by parenteral continuous infusion and has 50% of its maximal effect within 15 minutes. Its duration of action is about 10 to 15 minutes; thus, it can be discontinued swiftly if the decrease in blood pressure is too rapid. The efficacy of fenoldopam in renal perfusion is equal to or possibly better than that of sodium nitroprusside. There are no toxic metabolites of fenoldopam; however, the onset of action is slower, and the duration of effect is longer than that of sodium nitroprusside. Patients develop tachyphylaxis to fenoldopam after 48 hours, and headache can be a side effect.

Table 2
Medications used in hypertensive emergencies

Name	Dosing	Onset of Action	Duration of Action	Preload	Afterload	Cardiac Output	Renal perfusion
Sodium nitroprusside	IV 0.25–10 µg/kg/min	within seconds	1–2 min	decreased	decreased	no effect	decreased
Labetolol	IV (20- to 80-mg bolus/10 min)	5–10 min	2–6 hr	no effect	decreased	decreased	no effect
Fenoldopam	IV 0.1–0.6 µg/kg/min	10–15 min	10–15 min	no effect	decreased	increased	increased
Nicardipine	IV 2–10 mg/hr	5–10 min	2–4 hr	no effect	decreased	increased	no effect
Esmolol	IV 80-mg bolus over 30 seconds, followed by 150 µg/kg/min infusion	6–10 min	20 min	no effect	no effect	decreased	no effect
Methyldopa	IV (250-to 1000-mg bolus every 6 hr)	3–6 hr	up to 24 hr	no effect	decreased	decreased	no effect
Hydralazine	IV bolus (10–20 mg)	10 min	2–6 hr	no effect	decreased	increased	no effect

Abbreviation: IV, intravenous.

Table 3
Major side effects of medications

Name	Comments	Major Side Effects
Sodium nitroprusside	Need to measure thiocyanate levels, caution in renal insufficiency	Cyanide toxicity: nausea, vomiting, altered mental status, lactic acidosis,death
Labetolol	Alpha and beta blocker, contraindicated in acute heart failure	Bradycardia, bronchospasm, nausea
Nicardipine	Safe in coronary bypass patients	Reflex tachycardia, flushing
Esmolol	Short-acting beta blocker, contraindicated in acute heart failure	Bradycardia, bronchospasm
Methyldopa	Safe in pregnancy, needs renal dosing	Drowsiness, fever, jaundice
Hydralazine	Safe in pregnancy	Reflex tachycardia, lupus-like syndrome

Nicardipine is a calcium-channel blocker administered parenterally by continuous infusion for hypertensive crises. The onset of action of this drug is 5 to 10 minutes, and the duration of action is 1 to 4 hours. Adverse reactions are reflex tachycardia and headache [55]. Nicardipine is contraindicated in patients who have heart failure.

Esmolol is a cardioselective beta-blocker with a short duration of action. It reduces the systolic blood pressure and mean arterial pressure as well as heart rate, cardiac output, and stroke volume. There is a notable decrease in myocardial oxygen consumption. Peak effects are generally seen within 6 to 10 minutes after a bolus dose. The effects resolve 20 minutes after discontinuation of infusion. The elimination half-life of esmolol is about 8 minutes.

Choice of agent

The choice of pharmacologic agent to treat hypertensive crisis should be tailored to each individual based on risks, comorbidities, and the end-organ damage. The lower limit of cerebral blood flow autoregulation is reached when blood pressure is reduced by 25%, and the cerebral ischemia can be precipitated with rapid reductions of blood pressure of greater than 50% [35]. Hence,

the goal of therapy in hypertensive encephalopathy is to reduce the mean arterial pressure gradually by no more than 25% or to a diastolic blood pressure of 100 mm Hg, whichever is higher, during the first hour. If neurologic function worsens, the therapy should be suspended, and blood pressure should be allowed to increase [20]. In intracerebral or subarachnoid hemorrhage, blood pressure reduction is necessary to stop the bleeding and can be facilitated by decreasing pressures by 25%. It is important to reduce blood pressure slowly to prevent cerebral hypoperfusion to the already ischemic areas [36]. Often after a stroke there is a loss of cerebral autoregulation in the infarct/ischemic region. This loss of cerebral autoregulation makes blood pressure reduction cautionary, because the ischemic region is more prone to hypoperfusion during blood pressure reduction. As such, blood pressure reduction is not recommended after stroke, except in cases of extreme blood pressure elevation (diastolic blood pressure > 130 mm Hg). If neurologic function deteriorates with reduction of blood pressure, therapy should be suspended, and blood pressure should be allowed to rise. Blood pressure usually declines spontaneously to prestroke levels within 4 days of an acute ischemic stroke without any antihypertensive treatments [37]. Sodium nitroprusside is the drug of choice for treatment of acute neurologic syndromes in hypertensive crisis. Labetolol is a good alternative unless there is evidence of severe bradycardia associated with the cerebral edema. Clonidine and methyldopa should not be used, because they can cause central nervous system depression and complicate the clinical picture.

Severe acute hypertension often results in myocardial ischemia even with patent coronary arteries. In this situation, intravenous nitroglycerin is effective in reducing systemic vascular resistance and improving coronary perfusion. Nitrates should be given until symptoms subside or until diastolic blood pressure is 100 mm Hg. Beta-blockers and calcium-channel blockers are also potential options; both can decrease blood pressure while improving myocardial oxygenation. Calcium-channel blockers should be used with caution in patients who have possible heart failure. Acute pulmonary edema that is precipitated by hypertension is best treated with sodium nitroprusside. The concomitant venous and arterial dilation improve forward flow and cardiac output. This agent should be used in conjunction with morphine, oxygen, and a loop diuretic [49].

Treatment of an aortic dissection depends on location of the injury [41]. Type A or proximal aortic dissections need immediate institution of antihypertensive medications and immediate surgery, but type B or distal aorta dissections can be controlled medically. The medical therapy of aortic dissection is aimed at reducing the shear stress on aortic wall. This reduction is achieved by lowering diastolic blood pressure to less than 100 to 110 mm Hg and by decreasing heart rate. This reduction is best achieved with a combination of an intravenous beta-blocker and sodium nitroprusside to decrease both the blood pressure and the heart rate. Another option is the use of labetolol, which has both alpha- and beta-blocking effects.

Renal insufficiency is a cause and a consequence of severe hypertension. These patients need reduction of systemic vascular resistance without compromising renal blood flow or glomerular filtration rate. Fenoldopam is a good choice in these patients because of the improvement in renal perfusion, diuresis, and lack of production of toxic metabolites. Tolerance does develop to fenoldopam after 48 hours [53]. Sodium nitroprusside can also be used, but there is a risk of thiocyanate toxicity, and the thiocyanate level needs to be closely monitored. Calcium-channel blockers are effective and well tolerated in renal transplant patients. Beta-blockers are also useful agents in hypertension in kidney disease. Calcium-channel blockers and beta-blockers have no clinically important effects on glomerular filtration or renal hemodynamics [44]. Patients who have renal insufficiency should not be treated with angiotensin-converting enzyme inhibitors or angiotensin receptor blockers.

In pre-eclampsia and eclampsia, blood pressure control is essential. Many of the traditional antihypertensive medications are contraindicated in pregnancy because of their detrimental effects on the fetus. Angiotensin-converting enzyme inhibitors and angiotensin receptor blockers can adversely affect fetal development and increase fetal morbidity. Calcium-channel blockers reduce blood pressure but decrease uterine blood flow and can inhibit labor. Methyldopa is the mainstay of treatment of blood pressure in pregnant patients. It works centrally in reducing blood pressure and heart rate. Methyldopa can be administered orally or intravenously. With renal dysfunction the doses need to be adjusted. The side effects are drowsiness, fever, and jaundice. The medication does cross into the placenta but is considered class B in pregnancy [2]. Hydralazine is another agent that is safe in pregnancy and can be administered safely parenterally. Hydralazine may cause reflex tachycardia and fluid retention because it activates the renin-angiotensin-aldosterone system [27]. Data show that labetolol is probably effective in reducing blood pressure in treatment of eclampsia without inducing fetal distress [56].

Pheochromocytoma is a rare cause of paroxysmal or sustained blood pressure and can induce hypertensive crisis. The treatment of choice in these patients is labetolol or phentolamine (an alpha-blocking agent). It is important not to use beta-blockers alone, because then there is an unopposed alpha activity that will worsen the vasoconstriction, resulting in a further increase in blood pressure. A reflex hypertensive crisis can develop in patients who have abruptly stopped taking antihypertensives, particularly clonidine or beta-blockers. The treatment in these cases is to restart previous medications after the initial reduction of blood pressure with labetolol or sodium nitroprusside. Postoperative hypertension is typically related to catecholamine surge from activation of the sympathetic nervous system. Therefore, the treatment of choice for postoperative hypertensive crisis is with a beta-blocker or labetolol.

Summary

Hypertensive crisis is a serious condition that is associated with end-organ damage or may result in end-organ damage if left untreated. Causes of acute rises in blood pressure include medications, noncompliance, and poorly controlled chronic hypertension. Treatment of a hypertensive crisis should be tailored to each individual based on the extent of end-organ injury and comorbid conditions. Prompt and rapid reduction of blood pressure under continuous surveillance is essential in patients who have acute end-organ damage.

References

[1] Heart disease and stroke statistics—2004 update. Dallas (TX): American Heart Association; 2003.

[2] Chobanian AV, Bakris GL, Black HR, et al. Seventh report of the Joint National Committee on Prevention, Detection, Evaluation, and Treatment of High Blood Pressure. Hypertension 2003;42: 1206–52.

[3] Stamler J. Blood pressure and high blood pressure: aspects of risk. Hypertension 1991;18:I95–I107.

[4] Bennett NM, Shea S. Hypertensive emergency: case criteria, sociodemographic profile, and previous care of 100 cases. Am J Public Health 1988;78:636–40.

[5] Varon J, Marik PE. The diagnosis and management of hypertensive crises. Chest 2000;118:214–27.

[6] Kincaid-Smith P. Malignant hypertension. J Hypertens 1991;9:893–9.

[7] Calhoun DA, Oparil S. Hypertensive crises since FDR: a partial victory. N Engl J Med 1995;332:1029–30.

[8] Volhard F, Fahr TH. Die Brightsche Neirenkrankheit: KlinikPathlogie und Atlas, vol. 2. Berlin: Springer Verlag; 1914. p. 247–65.

[9] Keith NM, Wagener HP, Keronohan JW. The syndrome of malignancy hypertension. Arch Intern Med 1928;4:264–78.

[10] Ahmed ME, Walker JM, Beevers DG, et al. Lack of difference between malignant and accelerated hypertension. BMJ 1986;292:235–7.

[11] Bakker RC, Verburgh CA, van Buchem MA, et al. Hypertension, cerebral edema and fundoscopy. Nephrol Dial Transplant 2003;18:2424–7.

[12] Oppenheimer B, Fishberg AM. Hypertensive encephalopathy. Arch Intern Med 1928;41:264–78.

[13] He J, Whelton PK. Epidemiology and prevention of hypertension. Med Clin North Am 1997;81:1077–97.

[14] Wang Y, Wang QJ. The prevalence of prehypertension and hypertension among US adults according to the new Joint National Committee guidelines. Arch Intern Med 2004;164:2126–34.

[15] Gudbrandsson T. Malignant hypertension: a clinical follow-up study with special reference to renal and cardiovascular function and immunogenic factors. Acta Med Scand Suppl 1981;650:1–62.

[16] Zampaglione B, Pascale C, Marchisio M, et al. Hypertensive urgencies and emergencies: prevalence and clinical presentation. Hypertension 1996;27:144–7.

[17] Keith NM, Wagener HP, Barker NW. Some different types of essential hypertension: their course and prognosis. Am J Sci Med 1939;197:332–43.

[18] Kaplan N. Management of hypertensive emergencies. Lancet 1994;344:1335–8.

[19] Webster J, Petrie JC, Jeffers TA, et al. Accelerated hypertension patterns of mortality and clinical factors affecting outcome in treated patients. Q J Med 1993;96:485–93.

[20] Calhoun DA, Oparil S. Treatment of hypertensive crisis. N Engl J Med 1990;323:1177–83.

[21] Vaughn CJ, Delanty N. Hypertensive emergencies. Lancet 2000;356:411–7.

[22] Mullins JJ, Peters J, Ganten D. Fulminant hypertension in transgenic rats harbouring the mouse Ren-2 gene. Nature 1990;344:541–4.

[23] Laragh JH. Vasoconstriction-volume analysis for understanding and treating hypertension: the use of renin and aldosterone profiles. Am J Med 1973;55:261–74.

[24] Beevers G, Lip GY, O'Brien E. The pathophysiology of hypertension. BMJ 2001;322:912–6.

[25] Okada M, Matsumori A, Ono K, et al. Cyclic stretch upregulates production of interleukin-8 and monocyte chemotactic and activating factor/monocyte chemoattractant protein-1 in human endothelial cells. Arterioscler Thromb Vasc Biol 1998;18:894–901.

[26] Verhaar MC, Beutler JJ, Gaillard CA, et al. Progressive vascular damage in hypertension is associated with increased levels of circulating P-selectin. J Hypertens 1998;16:45–50.

[27] Blumenfeld JD, Laragh JH. Management of hypertensive crises: the scientific basis for treatment decisions. Am Heart J 2001;14:1154–67.

[28] Lassen NA. Cerebral blood flow and oxygen consumption in man. Physiol Rev 1959;39:183–238.

[29] Van Lieshout JJ, Wieling W, Karemaker JM, et al. Syncope, cerebral perfusion, and oxygenation. J Appl Physiol 2003;94:833–48.

[30] Traon AP, Costes-Salon MC, Galinier M, et al. Dynamics of cerebral blood flow autoregulation in hypertensive patients. J Neurol Sci 2002;195:139–44.

[31] Garg RK. Posterior leukoencephalopathy. Postgrad Med 2001;77:24–8.

[32] Beausang-Linder M, Bill A. Cerebral circulation in acute arterial hypertension: protective effects of sympathetic nervous activity. Acta Physiol Scand 1981;111:193–9.

[33] Grond M, Reul J. Brainstem edema during a hypertensive crisis with vasogenic and cytotoxic concerns. Deutsch Med Wochenschr 2003;128:2487–9.

[34] Immink RV, van den Born BJ, van Montfrans GA, et al. Impaired cerebral autoregulation in patients with malignant hypertension. Circulation 2004;110:2241–5.

[35] Strandgaard S, Paulson OB. Cerebral autoregulation. Stroke 1984;15:413–6.

[36] Lavin P. Management of hypertension in patients with acute stroke. Arch Intern Med 1986;146:66–8.

[37] Wallace J, Levy LL. Blood pressure after stroke. JAMA 1981;246:2177–80.

[38] Frohlich ED. Target organ involvement in hypertension: a realistic promise of prevention and reversal. Med Clin North Am 2004;88:1–9.

[39] Robicsek F, Thubrikar MJ. Hemodynamic considerations regarding mechanism and prevention of aortic dissection. Ann Thorac Surg 1994;58:1247–53.

[40] Khan IA. Clinical manifestations of aortic dissection. J Clin Basic Cardiol 2001;4:265–7.

[41] Khan IA, Nair CK. Clinical, diagnostic and management perspectives of aortic dissection. Chest 2002;122:311–28.

[42] McGregor E, Isles CG, Jay JL, et al. Retinal changes in malignant hypertension. BMJ 1986;292:233–4.

[43] Dimmitt SB, West JN, Eames SM, et al. Usefulness of ophthalmoscopy in mild to moderate hypertension. Lancet 1989;20:1103–6.

[44] Palmer BF. Renal dysfunction complicating the treatment of hypertension. N Engl J Med 2002; 347:1256–61.

[45] Haas CE, LeBlanc JM. Acute postoperative hypertension: a review of therapeutic options. Am J Health Syst Pharm 2004;61:1661–80.

[46] McGuirt WF, May JS. Postoperative hypertension associated with radical neck dissection. Arch Otolaryngol Head Neck Surg 1987;113:1098–100.

[47] Gal TJ, Cooperman LH. Hypertension in the immediate postoperative period. Br J Anaesth 1975;47:70–4.

[48] Roberts AJ, Niarchos AP, Subramanian VA, et al. Systemic hypertension associated with coronary artery bypass surgery. J Thorac Cardiovasc Surg 1977;74:856–9.

[49] Shepherd AM, Irvine NA. Differential hemodynamic and sympathoadrenal affects of sodium nitroprusside and hydralazine in hypertensive subjects. J Cardiovasc Pharmacol 1986;8:527–33.

[50] Kirsten R, Nelson K, Kirsten D, et al. Clinical pharmacokinetics of vasodilators. Clin Pharmacokinet 1998;35:9–36.

[51] Murphy MB, Murray C, Shorten GD. Fenoldopam: a selective peripheral dopamine-receptor agonist for the treatment of hypertension. N Engl J Med 2001; 345:1548–57.

[52] Panacek EA, Bednarczyk EM, Dunbar LM, et al. Randomized, prospective trial of fenoldopam vs sodium nitroprusside in the treatment of acute severe hypertension. Acad Emerg Med 1995;2:959–65.

[53] Tumlin JA, Dunbar LM, Oparil S, et al. Fenoldopam, a dopamine agonist, for hypertensive emergency: a multicenter randomized trial. Acad Emerg Med 2000;7:653–62.

[54] Goldberg ME, Cantillo J, Nemiroff MS, et al. Fenoldopam infusion for the treatment of postoperative hypertension. J Clin Anesth 1993;5:386–91.

[55] Squara P, Denjean D, Godard P, et al. Enoximome vs nicardipine during the early postoperative course of patients undergoing cardiac surgery: a prospective study of two therapeutic strategies. Chest 1994;106: 52–8.

[56] Lunell NO, Nylund L, Lewander R, et al. Acute effect of an antihypertensive drug labetolol, on uteroplacental blood flow. Br J Obstet Gynaecol 1982;89:640–4.

ELSEVIER
SAUNDERS

Cardiol Clin 24 (2006) 147–152

CARDIOLOGY
CLINICS

Index

Note: Page numbers of article titles are in **boldface** type.

0733-8651/06/$ - see front matter © 2005 Elsevier Inc. All rights reserved.
doi:10.1016/S0733-8651(05)00108-6

cardiology.theclinics.com

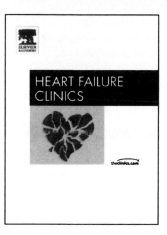

Changing Your Address?

Make sure your subscription changes too! When you notify us of your new address, you can help make our job easier by including an exact copy of your Clinics label number with your old address (see illustration below.) This number identifies you to our computer system and will speed the processing of your address change. Please be sure this label number accompanies your old address and your corrected address—you can send an old Clinics label with your number on it or just copy it exactly and send it to the address listed below.

We appreciate your help in our attempt to give you continuous coverage. Thank you.

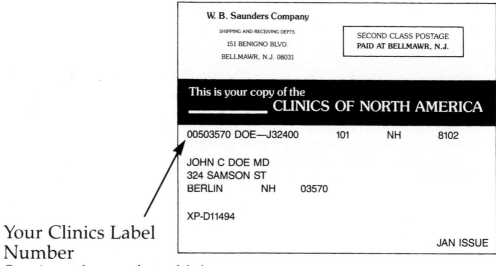

Your Clinics Label Number

Copy it exactly or send your label
along with your address to:
W.B. Saunders Company, Customer Service
Orlando, FL 32887-4800
Call Toll Free 1-800-654-2452

Please allow four to six weeks for delivery of new subscriptions and for processing address changes.